TEN GREEK PLAYS

IN CONTEMPORARY TRANSLATIONS

RIVERSIDE EDITIONS

RIVERSIDE EDITIONS

UNDER THE GENERAL EDITORSHIP OF

Gordon N. Ray

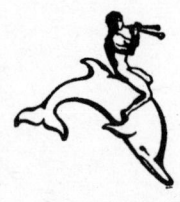

HOUGHTON MIFFLIN COMPANY · BOSTON

TEN GREEK PLAYS

IN CONTEMPORARY TRANSLATIONS

EDITED AND IN PART TRANSLATED

WITH AN INTRODUCTION BY

L. R. Lind

UNIVERSITY OF KANSAS

HOUGHTON MIFFLIN COMPANY · BOSTON

To My Students

in Humanities 51 and 52,

Past and Present

ACKNOWLEDGMENTS

GRATEFUL ACKNOWLEDGMENTS for permission to print or reprint these plays are made to:

Faber and Faber, Ltd., London, and to Louis MacNeice for his *Agamemnon* (1936).

John Lane The Bodley Head, Ltd., London, and to Rex Warner for his *Prometheus Bound* (1947).

Longmans, Green and Company, Inc., New York, and to Charles T. Murphy for his *Lysistrata*, from *Greek Literature in Translation*, edited by W. J. Oates and C. T. Murphy (1944).

Frederick Muller, Ltd., London, and to Kathleen Freeman for her *Philoctetes* (1948). Application for permission to perform the play should be made to The Walter H. Baker Co., 569 Boylston Street, Boston, Mass.

Chatto and Windus, London, and to Richard Aldington for his *Alcestis* (1930), of which he sent me an autographed copy.

Shaemas O'Sheel for his privately printed *Antigone* (1931), also an autographed copy.

Henry Birkhead for his hitherto unpublished *Bacchae*.

Albert Cook for his hitherto unpublished *Oedipus Rex*, first staged in 1948 by The Tributary Theater in Boston.

L. R. LIND

CONTENTS

ARISTOPHANES

INTRODUCTION

An Approach to Greek Drama

BY L. R. LIND

I

To the modern reader and spectator the ancient Greek drama must sometimes seem an odd mixture of a Christmas pageant and that old fashioned amusement known to our grandparents as "living statues." This impression is easy to form because these plays, contrary to modern custom, emphasize neither action on stage nor scenery, while the chorus contributes to the effect of statuesque immobility. In contrast to the often prodigious physical activity of the modern play, the Greek drama makes its strongest impact through a generally subtle representation of emotional stress. It is through a gradually loosened repression, a slowly revealed psychological transformation, an outward expression of an inner conflict that we see Antigone, Orestes, Heracles, Oedipus, Alcestis, and Medea rise to that level of human suffering which is the essence of Greek tragedy.

In spite of this impression of external simplicity there is a highly sophisticated and intricate technique in Greek drama. It overcame the apparent and actual disadvantages of a relatively static chorus, few actors who performed several rôles each, and insufficient stage machinery or scenery, to create dramatic situations of an intellectual and emotional intensity out of proportion to its limited physical resources. In relying upon the imagination of the audience and the ingenuity of the dramatist the Greeks attained heights in drama which moderns, with far more facilities for staging, may well envy. One might almost say that the technique of Greek drama in the management of exits and entrances, shifts of actors and scenes, and in the development of a plot was forced to become highly skillful precisely because of external limitations of story-material, the religious concepts which formed the basis of drama, and an elaborate tradition of play-structure which not even Euripides, with his radical innovations, could completely alter.

But it is in the world-view of Greek tragedy that we find its real complexity and its enduring claim to our attention. Rising above most of the social ideas familiar to modern drama, Greek drama exploits the possibilities for spiritual self-knowledge which human beings can reach by long and intense thought about the contest of man against man, man against nature, and man against the gods. Greek drama is very largely concerned with ethical problems of a high order which the characters must solve or surrender their individual responsibility for the maintenance of an aristocratic society. What must a high-born girl do when her own impulsive and determined nature clashes with that of an equally determined ruler over the burial of her brother? How can a noble son murder his mother (who had murdered his father) and still live conscience-free? Where can a man with more than normal curiosity and intelligence, deeply concerned over his obscure antecedents, find refuge from his unwitting sins and the horrible truth to which his stubborn inquiries have driven him? Why must a benefactor of mankind suffer torture for his kindness — and from a god? What part do fate, free will, or sheer luck play in the lives of men and women?

These simplifications do not, of course, give more than a slight indication of the great variety of interpretation which exists for each of the plays to which they refer. Nor does Greek drama always move on such a high plane. Occasionally, as in the plays of Euripides, sheer sensational thrills seem to be more important than the morality of the action. The well-known progression of moral concepts — olbos (prosperity), koros (satiety), hybris (insolent assault, arrogant pride), and ate (retribution) is not applicable to every Greek drama. But the moral questions arise from the action of the play and from the choices made by the actors within their separate situations.

The world-view of Greek drama includes the supernatural much more than does that of modern drama. God Himself as well as the gods has disappeared from the contemporary play, but the Greek plays are fundamentally religious and not only because they were presented to honor Dionysus. Actually Dionysus plays only a small part in extant Greek drama; the *Bacchae* of Euripides, that strange, solitary exhibition of the defeat of conservative reaction by religious fanaticism, is the single exception: its chief actor is Dionysus. While he presided over the fertile generative forces of drama during its entire history he remains in the background; it is the other gods who hold the stage in the plays themselves.

It is another distinction between ancient Greek drama and modern Western drama that the latter can present the supernatural only as fantasy, that it is limited to human, not divine forces, in conceiving its themes or building its plots. With their extraordinary ability for viewing things separately without invidious or inappropriate connotations, the Greeks could at one and the same time regard the gods as able to move about like spirits and to work wonders as well as to display in themselves all the faults and weaknesses of men. When two anthologists of Greek drama write of dramatic action as the result of the struggle between the dignity of man, a sense of free will, and a belief in divine power on one hand, and the problem of evil on the other, they are merely setting up a neat but inadequate formula which does not conform to the facts. Since there is no ethical purpose in the earliest Greek views of the world's creation, Greek religion and drama, as distinct from philosophy, does not know a problem of evil as stated in our terms. The Greeks did not speak of the contradiction involved in the idea of a good God who permitted evil to flourish; they do not seem to have puzzled over the inconsistencies in an unmoral universe. The most they ventured to express on the subject were some vague ideas about fate, which both gods and man obeyed.

Nor is Greek drama to be explained entirely in terms of fate, or fatalism. Moira, the Greek word for fate, means many things but chiefly "that which is one's due, lot, or portion of good fortune or ill," "that which is meet, proper, and right," or, in plural personification, the Fates. The Greek fate is not exclusively what *must* happen to one because it is foreordained but that which actually happens to one as his lot, partly due to his own actions, partly due to heredity and circumstances. So narrow a conception as mere fatalism in the modern sense would make puppets of the dramatic heroes. Such a theory corresponds to nothing in modern thought more faithfully than to that desolate sense of frustration so common in our society and the psychological isolation which it produces.

The Greek heroes act on their own responsibility, take all the consequences of their actions, and suffer like brave men; they are not cogs in a machine. The Greek drama was the democratic art of a free people. It arose in an historical environment of foreign wars and in the shadow of totalitarianism. Its atmosphere was one of public festivals, of a religion of many separate cults which regarded the gods almost as superior human beings, and it was the product of minds which saw human life as a series of struggles with forces, within and without the human soul, which had to be faced without flinching. The *Persians* of Aeschylus, the single historical drama we have, is a tribute to the national bravery of the Greeks. The symbols of Greek tragedy were drawn from the great mythological sagas, but as in all the finest art, these symbols did not become substitutes for reality; they became the powerful vehicle for expressing a deep sense of the realities of life. Some of these realities were recognized by the Greeks in the idea of moderation, or its lack, in all forms of conduct; in obedience, or disobedience, to established customs, laws, or taboos; in respect for one's elders, family, friends, superiors, or people (expressed by the Greek word aidos), or the disastrous transgression of this respect. These were realities which the gods themselves observed and upheld. One might say that Greek drama is the representation of the tragic consequences which result from a violation of basic human rights, institutions, or social beliefs.

II

The *Poetics* of Aristotle is perhaps the one indispensable document in the history of all literary criticism. It presents us with practically all we know of the ancient history and theory of drama together with a number of puzzles in interpretation. We do not have the discussion of comedy which Aristotle promised in a passage of the *Poetics:* "we shall speak later about comedy" (Chap. 6). He combines in this small treatise a discussion of both epic and dramatic poetry, although he regards Homer too as something of a *dramatic* poet. The following much debated and still obscure statements give us the essence of his understanding of the origins of Athenian drama; it must be remembered that he wrote at a long remove in time from those origins. Tragedy arose from the leaders of the dithyramb (in its earliest form an improvised drinking song, in its later a sort of simple oratorio sung by a chorus with a leader; see the example from Bacchylides, *The Coming of Theseus*, translated by Richmond Lattimore, in his *Greek Lyrics*, 1955). Tragedy then passed through a satyric stage, when it was apparently performed by a chorus dressed as satyrs (half-goats, half-men, a creation of mythological fancy like the Centaur), and came from the Peloponnesus (southern Greece) to Athens, where the language of the chorus still preserved the broad vowels of its Dorian speech. Aeschylus introduced a second actor to accompany the original protagonist of the drama; Sophocles added a third actor. Three actors thereafter continued to distribute all the rôles among themselves; the nine, ten, or even eleven roles of Euripides must have strained the actors' versatility. Yet even this limitation was made into a virtue. There were two chief parts in a tragedy: choric songs and dialogue. The time limit for a play was approximately one revolution of the sun or, more exactly, the time needed to bring about happiness from an unhappy situation or vice versa. The general ethos (tone or character) of tragedy was noble and serious; it imitated real actions and thus exploited in an artistic form the educative talent for imitation possessed by human beings, the most imitative of animals. Dramatic action grew out of a binding, then a loosing process as its motivation; this was the plot, an element much admired by Aristotle. Probability and necessity were required in the sequence of episodes of a plot. Thus far Aristotle, to whom we shall return.

The sociological origins of both Greek tragedy and comedy arose undoubtedly from primitive fertility rites and worships of a sort still to be found among living primitive people. The dying god who appears in some religions, and who has been studied by J. G. Fraser in *The Golden Bough,* represented the recurrence of the seasons and the growth of crops; he was part of the original pattern of these religions, and the structure of the plays which developed from such worships included a Contest, a Death, transformations, lamentations, and recognition-scenes. Atonement for sin, self-knowledge through suffering, reconciliation and renewal of faith were elements in the early form of Greek drama (whose nature we can merely conjecture) as well as in the latest form to be seen in the works of Aeschylus, Sophocles, and Euripides. The writings of Gilbert Murray, Jane Harrison, Frances Cornford, and George Thomson throw light upon these particular aspects of our subject.

No expense was spared in staging the plays by the rich men who defrayed the costs as a public service or liturgy, a "work for the folk." As much as 3,000 drachmas is recorded for such expenses. This sum was worth about $480 at pre-World War I values, perhaps three times that amount at current values; about half the expense recorded for tragedy is listed for comedy. A chorus teacher or director trained the chorus under the supervision of the archon, or public commissioner, in charge of drama at Athens. First, second, and third prizes in money were awarded to the poets for the trilogies they presented, or the groups of three plays with a connected theme plus a satyr-play, usually a coarse burlesque or farce. The single surviving example of a satyr-play is the *Cyclops* of Euripides.

Public applause must have greatly influenced the decision of the five judges: the Greeks even had a word for this situation — theatrocracy. A flute player accompanied the marching or standing chorus songs; a mutilated piece of the music which accompanied lines 338–344 of Euripides' *Orestes* is all that remains from the music of the fifth-century dramas, probably composed by Euripides himself since music was a fundamental part of all Greek education. The plays were presented on the round flag-stoned dance floor of the theater that lies on the southwest slope of the Acropolis at Athens; similar theaters were built in other parts of Greece, the islands, Asia, and Sicily, for example, at Epidaurus (the best-preserved of them all), at Delphi, Delos, Eretria, Megalopolis (the largest of all the theaters), Priene, and at Segesta in Sicily, where the theater stands high on a hill overlooking a beautiful valley toward Agrigento. An altar, perhaps a survival from early cult practices and certainly indicating the religious associations of drama, stood in the middle of the orchestra, or dancing-place. Scene changes were avoided, and most of the action took place before a temple or palace-front except for scenes from nature like those in the *Prometheus Bound* or *Philoctetes*. No curtain or lighting effects were used; a few plays, Aeschylus' *Eumenides*, Sophocles' *Antigone*, began at dawn, the time when the play-presentation itself regularly began. The plays were given on Elaphebolion 11–13 (in March-April) for 7 to 8 hours each day.

The chorus was maintained through tradition by the later playwrights, although it could be very useful in a structural sense also, as modern playwrights have discovered by adapting it to some of their plays. The action began with the entrance of the chorus except where a prologue (either monologue as with Euripides or a dialogue as with Sophocles) was spoken; the chorus rarely left the stage except at Aeschylus, *Eumenides* 230, Sophocles, *Ajax* 814, Euripides, *Helen* 330, and *Alcestis* 747. The chorus served to represent the broad foundation of timeless and popular views of life and to provide a background for motivation and commentary or advice on individual actions. The chorus was in a sense the "average man" who sat in the audience and nodded approval at its sage expressions of opinion. At times the chorus behaves ridiculously, as it does in the *Agamemnon* of Aeschylus, but it is always in character and true to its origins and environment. The actors had to speak within the range of understanding which the chorus, often made up of humble people, old men, women, girls, foreign slaves, or sailors among them, possessed. To put it another way, the audience sat or stood both in front of and behind the actors: in front, the people of Athens, behind, the chorus. It is a tribute, however, to the intelligence of the Athenian play-going public to say that there was little talking-down to them by way of the chorus. The first chorus-entrance (parodos; some plays have two entrances: the second is called epiparodos) was generally done with briskness, their song set to meters which reflected a march tempo: anapaestic measures, or reversed dactyls, feet of two short syllables followed by a long syllable. The chorus-leader (coryphaeus) often stepped forward and held a dialogue with an actor. He received reports, asked questions, gave advice, praise, or blame, and expressed many pious wishes or prayers. After Sophocles, he announced the entrance of a new actor.

According to Aristotle, the basic general elements of tragedy are plot, character, diction, thought, scenery, and song; plot and character (ethe, a word he uses in the plural, meaning apparently the moral impressions made by the play or the players in the large sense; he speaks of the parallel with painting and the impressions made by certain painters, perhaps what we might call their "style") are for him the most important of these elements. The technical parts or quantitative forms of a play are the prologue, episode or dialogue passages, parodos, stasima or chorus songs, kommoi or laments, and the exodus or finale. The entire drama usually included a reversal of fortune (peripeteia), a recognition-scene (anagnorisis), and a form of individual suffering (pathos) which might be defined as action of a destructive or painful nature (murders, tortures, wounding). A chorus and several actors who shared more than one part or rôle among them, a simple setting of palace-façade or temple, and a crowd of spectators in a semi-circular theater were the remaining features of the tragic presentation. The play was as long as it needed to be in order to bring about a satisfactory reversal of fortune and the proper purging of the spectator's soul through the emotions of fear and pity. The paradoxical fascination and delight of tragedy were said to consist in self-complacent gloating, if we are to believe a certain comic poet named Timocles, whose words I translate here without placing too much weight upon them:

> Look at the tragic poets, if you will, and notice how they help us all: for the poor man when he sees Telephus on the stage and discovers that the latter is poorer than himself already begins to bear his own poverty more easily; he who suffers from some mental disease obtains comfort from Alcmaeon (who became mad); should anyone suffer from eye-trouble, there are the daughters of Phineus, blinder than he; if some one has lost a child, Niobe will cheer him up; Philoctetes makes the lame man

feel better, and Oineus relieves the aged; in fact, all of us can bemoan our misfortunes the less as we see on the stage people who suffer from even greater misfortunes.

This cannot, of course, be the true view of Aristotle's catharsis, or purging of the emotions by means of the spectacle of tragedy, but it may reflect the interpretation of the purpose of tragedy which the average Greek spectator had formed. Certainly common sense can go no further in analyzing its salutary effects.

People equipped by birth and fortune to dare and suffer great and dreadful deeds populated the dramas. They were endowed with unusual energy, force of will, and sense of honor and duty. Some acted in full knowledge of the situation, others like Oedipus in ignorance of the facts, and still others in an ignorance which is dispelled in time to avoid grievous deeds. The events in the plays are greater, however, than the actors themselves and emphasize the universality of the moral predicament involved. Larger issues than the heroes themselves are often implied as in the plays about Orestes or the Seven Against Thebes, where whole families are the target of a blood curse which works its way through several generations. Certain types appear from the aristocracy, common people, seers or prophets, tyrants, constitutional kings. Pairs of characters serve as foils for each other. Some fight the gods themselves only to fail, as Hippolytus and Pentheus. Their motives are revenge, honor, duty, the protection or rescue of a loved one, the passion of love itself, or a battle for justice. Fame is a secondary theme; Achilles is not a hero in our dramas. The decision not to live under humiliation moves some of the heroes; they commit suicide or blind themselves, although a higher power sometimes intervenes to save them from themselves. The heroines especially show at times a warm human quality which takes shape in fear and sorrow contrasting strongly with their noble and decisive actions. They open their hearts to the chorus or to their closest relatives in outbursts of weakness and despair.

The more than human proportions of the heroes were exaggerated by heavy, ornamented costumes, high boots, a bushy topknot on the hair, breast and stomach pads, long trailing robes, and masks. The chorus was made up of lesser folk native to the spot in which the action was supposed to take place except in such a play as the *Suppliants* of Euripides. Choruses from other regions appear in at least nine plays; Euripides first developed the traveling "saviors" as a chorus. Of the dramatist's saga material, the Trojan, Tantalid, and

Theban cycles of legend were most commonly used, that is, the stories about the Trojan war, the descendants of Tantalus at Argos, and the family of Oedipus. The sagas of Aetolian heroes, Hercules, the Argonauts, Perseus, and Dionysus himself were less frequently employed. We know the titles of 525 plays, of which 34 are preserved intact, or almost intact; 24 per cent of the titles (hence subjects) are used again and again. At least 500 actors are known from the second century B.C. alone, and the names of 141 playwrights, including those of the great age of drama, the fifth century B.C. at Athens.

Not all of the plays end tragically, as we think of the term tragedy, that is, in sorrow. Six of those we have end happily: Aeschylus, *Eumenides*; Sophocles, *Electra, Philoctetes*, and *Oedipus at Colonus*; Euripides, *Alcestis* and *Iphigenia in Tauris*. To these might be added the *Suppliants* and *Andromache*, which end with the successful attainment of definite goals: the burial of those who attacked Thebes and the release of Andromache from imminent death. The subjects of the dramas involved the actions and sufferings of heroes and heroines, but single personalities did not always receive sole focus; events and circumstances, even the chorus itself, could provide the necessary tragic unity. The so-called tragic "unities" of time, place, and action are a much later invention and are not set down as such by Aristotle; they are not universally preserved even by the seventeenth-century Neo-Classical French playwrights for whom these unities were so important at least in theory. For example, Orestes has little individuality apart from the startling events of the trilogy by Aeschylus which bears his name, the *Oresteia*; and the personalities in the *Suppliants* and the *Persians* of Aeschylus are secondary. Tragic actions comprised episodes (in the modern sense, not as a technical division of Greek drama) from the lives of the heroes as they overstepped proper bounds against the gods, or engaged in family feuds, vengeance, incest, adultery, fratricide, matricide, patricide, or plain homicide. There was little space for character-development in our sense, even in the trilogies; the longest single play, Sophocles' *Oedipus at Colonus*, has only 1,779 lines. This fact has led to some questionable German writing on the lack of unity in the dramas, but there is surely a progression at least in the figure of Zeus in the lost plays of the *Prometheia* of Aeschylus; even Oedipus becomes more resigned and patient, if not reconciled to his sons and to Creon.

The very term "character," meaning a part or rôle in a play, is not applicable to Greek drama: their word for that was "prosopon," meaning "face, countenance," then a "mask." Of character in the more general modern sense there is no hint in the word. Even those brief descriptions of individual human behavior, the "Characters" of Theophrastus, the student of Aristotle and the first of familiar essayists, are really "types." Neither type nor character is the proper term for the great personalities of drama; they are unlike each other and exist as individuals in their own right. Neither their antecedents nor their environment wholly explain or determine the actions of these personalities. It is usually one tremendous urge — "excess" in the Greek view of the matter — toward justice, truth, vengeance, self-sacrifice or love, an excess of pride, egotism, constancy, stubbornness, or anger which drives them toward their doom. We do not see them behaving, as we see modern characters behaving in plays, under more than one aspect of their nature; it is their disposition toward excess arising from their nature (*physis*, whence comes physical) which makes their tragedy. The "tragic flaw" so much discussed is nothing more than Aristotle's *hamartia*, a missing of the mark of moderate behavior, hence excess. "Flaw" gives a quite erroneous idea of the Aristotelian word, substituting an image from pottery or glass-making for the original image drawn from archery or spear-throwing, whence comes also the New Testament Greek word for "sin." *Hamartia* means error in general; significantly, it occurs three times in Sophocles' *Trachiniae* 1123–1136, in the form of the verb, signifying harm done through self-will. Aristotle rightly says, "All human happiness or misery takes the form of action; the end for which we live is a certain kind of activity, not a quality. Character [his word is *ethe*] gives us qualities, but it is in our actions — what we do — that we are happy or the reverse." This is the lesson of Greek tragedy.

III

It is impossible in a brief introduction to give an adequate idea of the inner structure of Greek drama, its character-portrayal, motivation of action, management of exits, entrances, cues, irony, both verbal and dramatic, of surprise, suspense, and ingenious dénouement. The literature on drama is very large; the short bibliography printed in this book gives only the essential books, and there is no single one which handles thoroughly all the subjects mentioned above. It is perhaps in this area of play-technique that much of the most fruitful research remains to be done. Only one analysis from the modern point of view as it is revealed in the new criticism has yet appeared; of course many sound articles on these matters have appeared in the learned journals of the classical scholar. Francis Fergusson's *The Idea of a Theater* (1949) draws upon the results of Gilbert Murray's examination of myth and ritual in Euripides, upon the general method of the Cambridge University school of anthropological classicists, and upon Kenneth Burke's summation of "Purpose, Passion, Perception" in drama. Fergusson says, "I propose to use *Oedipus* as a landmark and to relate subsequent forms of drama to it. For it presents . . . a way of life and action which is still at the root of our culture." The steadily mounting contemporary interest in the literary uses of myth, symbol, and legend makes it only a matter of time before the modern critics give the Greek dramas the same careful examination they are now giving to the works of Henry James, Conrad, Joyce, or Kafka. The academic classicists have already provided modern criticism with a wealth of material and information upon which to advance toward a more thorough understanding of drama. R. F. Goheen's excellent study, *The Imagery of Sophocles' Antigone* (1951) is another step in that direction.

In the critical examination of the Greek plays it is essential to recognize the individual differences in treatment, point of view, and in temperament revealed by each of the three great playwrights, Aeschylus, Sophocles, and Euripides. It must also be borne in mind that their work is all that has survived out of a much larger mass written by many other dramatists and that thus their production may give us a distorted impression of the total panorama consisting of hundreds of plays by hundreds of playwrights, many of them no doubt quite as prolific as the big three and some of them perhaps equally profound thinkers. The vast amount of Greek drama which has perished points up its tremendous popularity among the Athenians.

Aeschylus (525–456 B.C.) has left us seven plays [1] out of a total of ninety; we have the titles of seventy-nine. He won fifty-two first prizes with thirteen tetralogies during his lifetime and fifteen after his death. Bound by a somewhat uncompromising conception of human responsibility to society, Aeschylus emphasizes the blood-guilt motive and its attendant vengeance, the inexorable dictates of situation and circumstance. For him justice is God, and learning is always through suffer-

[1] *Suppliants*, produced between 488 and 465 B.C.; *Persians*, 472; *Seven Against Thebes*, 467; *Prometheus Bound*, not yet dated with accuracy but probably presented between 467 and 458; the trilogy *Agamemnon*, *Choephoroi* (*Libation Bearers*), and *Eumenides*, 458.

ing. He is also interested in the political implications of guilty actions and is the most open of the three dramatists to the anthropological and ethnological approach used by George Thomson in his edition of the *Oresteia* and his book *Aeschylus and Athens.*

Sophocles (497–406 B.C.) wrote more than 123 plays; we have the titles of 114.[2] He won at least seventy-two first prizes during his lifetime. His plays show a struggle against mighty forces, even if that struggle is hopeless; no particular emphasis on a generic family bloodguilt or curse; a disinclination on the part of his characters for compromise with circumstances; and a heart-breaking loneliness of decision and action which sets in relief the importance Sophocles placed upon free will. Unhampered moral choice is the characteristic of all his major personalities. Kitto aptly says, "Sophocles sees not the simplicities but the complexities of life." Matthew Arnold may have had such a thought in mind when he wrote of Sophocles as one "who saw life steadily and saw it whole." Hoelderlin's elegiac distich on Sophocles is less well known; he is writing of the dramatist's work:

> Many have tried in vain to speak joyously of greatest joy:
> Here at last it speaks to me, here out of Sorrow itself.

Euripides (481–406 B.C.) wrote at least eighty-eight plays [3] but won only five victories during his lifetime. Euripides is less moderate in a number of respects than Aeschylus or Sophocles. He handles traditional material more freely while sometimes casting into stronger relief the ritualistic element in Greek drama. He brings to the stage psychological as well as social problems and a disturbing rationalism which is akin to the thinking of the fifth-century sophists criticized in Plato's dialogues. Like Ibsen, he questions accepted ideas and conventions of social organization, religion, and the relations between the classes and

[2] His seven extant plays are: *Ajax*, before 442; B.C.; *Antigone*, 442; *The Women of Trachis*, possibly 413; *Oedipus Rex*, 439–412; *Electra*, around 410; *Philoctetes*, 409; and *Oedipus at Colonus*, 401.

[3] The nineteen we have are: *Alcestis*, 438 B.C.; *Medea*, 431; *Hippolytus*, 428; *Heraclidae*, or *The Children of Hercules*, 427; *Andromache*, 426 (?); *Hecuba*, 425; *Cyclops*, 423; *Suppliants*, 421; *Hercules*, 421 or later; *Ion*, 417; *Troades*, or *The Trojan Women*, 415; *Iphigenia in Tauris*, 414–412; *Electra*, 413; *Helen*, 412; *Phoenissae*, or *The Phoenician Women*, 409; *Orestes*, 408; *Iphigenia in Aulis*, 405; *Bacchae*, 405; and *Rhesus* (?); the latter is considered spurious, that is, written by someone else and attributed to Euripides by mistake. Gilbert Norwood has recently made a strong case for assigning part at least of the *Suppliants* to a later poet, but all the other plays in the list are genuine.

the sexes. He brings the epic saga to its ultimate conclusions and thoroughly explores its possibilities as the vehicle of drama with a spirit of scepticism and sophistication. In technique he emphasizes single plays and allows the tetralogy — the original group of three tragedies plus a satyr-play — to go by the boards. He uses the prologue and the "god from the machine," who appeared toward the end of the play from the scene-building behind the orchestra or stage, more often and more mechanically than other playwrights. He subordinates the chorus to a lesser rôle as a mouthpiece for his own judgments. In his plays the view of inherited guilt fades rapidly in the light of what resembles modern sociological analysis. The idea of luck, on the other hand, grows in importance in his work. Some of his plays are sheer thrillers; others are studies in morbid psychology, in jealousy, revenge, love, and madness. Realism and naturalism in his personalities grow often into melodrama. He may be compared to Racine among the classical French dramatists, as Sophocles or Aeschylus may be compared to Corneille, in his special interests and in the contrast his work shows to that of the earlier dramatists of his time. Of all of them, Euripides has perhaps more to say to the modern mind because his own so closely resembles it.

IV

Greek comedy is represented in this anthology by the *Lysistrata* of Aristophanes. His dates are from about 450 to 385 B.C., and we have eleven of the forty plays attributed to him. Each of these takes the form of a problem to be solved or a plan to be carried out by the characters. The pattern followed most generally is, first, to present the idea of the play in the prologue, then to bring on the chorus and proceed to a debate between proponents and opponents of the play's idea. When the opposition has been silenced, the chorus once more appears to sing the parabasis, a song in which Aristophanes speaks to the audience, through the chorus, on a matter of current and pressing interest: this need not be closely related to the essential idea of the play. The actors then return to demonstrate how the idea works out in actual practice in a series of short episodes. Then the exodus is sung, and both actors and chorus indulge in a short burst of revelry called the comos.

Lysistrata (411 B.C.) shows the analysis of such a problem: an attempt by the women of Athens to stop the war with Sparta by applying their own peculiar form of passive resistance to it. It is one of Aristophanes' anti-war plays: others are the *Acharnians* (425), the *Peace* (421), and to some extent the *Birds* (414), considered by many as his masterpiece. The other seven extant plays are the *Knights* (424), an attack on the demagogue Cleon; the *Clouds* (423), in which Socrates is ridiculed; the *Frogs* (405), which charges Euripides with contributing to the decay of Athenian morals; the *Thesmophoriazusae*, or *Women at the Festival of Demeter* (410), where Euripides is tried for slandering the female sex; the *Wasps* (422), which satirizes the Athenian obsession for serving on juries and listening to law suits; the *Ecclesiazusae*, or *Women in the Assembly* (392), ridiculing such Utopian schemes of social reform as are found in Plato's *Republic*; and the *Plutus* (388), in which the blind god of Wealth is made to see and at last in proper justice imparts his gifts to the good man and not to the bad.

Aristophanes discusses Athenian politics, the Peloponnesian War, women's rights, education, literature (that is, the drama), and certain habits of his fellow-citizens, all with numerous contemporary allusions and more or less veiled jokes and jibes at prominent people. His satire is frank and hearty, spiced with obscenity, and full of the joy of life. His plays form part of that stage in the art which has been called Old Comedy to distinguish it from the more subtle and restricted comedy of manners represented by Middle and New Comedy; Menander (342–292 B.C.) is the most famous writer of the latter type: Diphilus and Philemon were also prominent playwrights in this kind of drama, and all three were used as sources and models by the Roman playwrights, Plautus (254–184 B.C.) and Terence (195–159 B.C.). Old Comedy arose out of a fertility cult connected with the worship of Dionysus. In the hands of Aristophanes Old Comedy, while not losing its obvious connection with an earthy kind of religious practice, became a powerful weapon of social and personal criticism. During the time of Aristophanes six comedies were given annually in the theater of Dionysus at Athens, three on separate afternoons at the festival of the Lenaea in January and three more at the festival of the City Dionysia in March. Three actors and twenty-four members of the chorus were employed.

A startlingly ingenious and fantastic imagination characterizes the work of Aristophanes. His protagonists conceive of the most amazing enterprises: to bring back Euripides to earth from Hades; to establish an empire in the land of the birds, the upper air; to fly to heaven upon the back of a huge beetle; to bring a dog and his puppies into court to plead for him while he is being tried for stealing a cheese; and to throw the cities of Greece into a huge mortar and to grind them up. Heinrich Heine, in his *Travel Pictures*, spoke of "the profound idea for overturning the world itself which lies at the base of each Aristophanic comedy, and which therein, like some fanciful ironic magic tree, shoots up with its blooming decoration of thoughts, the nests of singing nightingales, and climbing monkeys." This description sums up cleverly, in the words of another famous humorist, the vigorous wit, prolific imagination, and huge appetite for wild ridicule which we find in the plays of Aristophanes. The beauty of his lyrics, some of which have been cleverly reproduced in Gilbert and Sullivan meters by Benjamin Bickley Rogers, is often in striking contrast to his subject-matter; horse-play and common sense are mingled with the most delicate poetic nuances and shades of meaning, subordinated to a supreme command of both Greek language and meters. Aristophanes is one of the world's greatest comic poets; very few others can be set beside him.

v

Greek tragedy and comedy were the result of an artistic combination of language, meters, song, and dance, in a kind of opera mingled with elements of the oratorio and with the ceremonious group movement of a simple ballet. Their language was the old Ionic dialect in the dialogue mixed with broad-voweled Doric in the chorus-parts; a few Homeric (or Aeolic) words were scattered through the plays. Whether the Doric words (roughly analogous to Highland Scots in comparison with standard English) were a survival from the Peloponnesian origins of drama or the remnants of the early choric-dialogue of the dithyramb is hard to say. The popular speech may have had some mixture of both Doric and Attic (sprung from Ionic). Local color, picturesque characterization, and many heightened special effects were attained by the use of dialects, especially in comedy. A brogue would at once reveal a foreigner, as the Egyptian herald in Aeschylus' *Suppliants*. Each tragedy had its own special vocabulary, the several hundred words most adapted to its needs and which were not peculiar to any other tragedy. The number of such words ranges from 329 to 782 in Aeschylus' plays, from 285 to 432 in the plays of Sophocles.

Language was, of course, the common bond between the audience and the stage, since much of the audience was made up of Greeks from other parts of the Mediterranean world. The drama had a strongly educative force upon its spectators, nourished on a common fund of myth, meter, and song. The earliest vase-paintings, for instance, show how important mythology was among these people since it is used by the painters even before it was used by the dramatists. The knowledge of mythology seems to have declined by the time of Euripides, who is obliged to tell the audience the outlines of myths in his prologues. The introduction of free tickets (theorica) no doubt brought some less well educated elements of the population into the theater. What the audience could not understand intellectually among the ideas of drama, like Shakespeare's groundlings they could comprehend by way of the emotions. Many emotions — love, wonder, pity, fear, anger, loathing, excitement, pleasure, and sorrow — were stirred by the plays, which also appealed to the Greek fondness for solving puzzles and riddles.

The versification of the Greek dramas is intricate and highly artistic, designed to achieve many effects of rhythm and sound no longer perceptible to our ears. The six-foot iambic meter of the dialogue predominates, since it is the meter of all the interchange between character and character. It is also used in comedy, with more frequent substitutions or use of equivalent sound-values. The meters of the choruses (stasima) are made up, first, of dactylic (– ∪∪), anapaestic (∪∪ –), iambic (∪ –), and trochaic (– ∪) meters, which recur in recitative; these were also used in various kinds of non-dramatic poetry. Exclusively lyrical were other meters: the cretic (– ∪ –), with its resolved or substituted forms, the paeon (– ∪∪∪, ∪∪∪ –), and the bacchiac (∪ – –). The dochmiac meter was the only foot original with drama; in its commonest form (∪ – – ∪ –) it has a relationship with the cretic and iambic. The Ionic (∪∪ – –) and Aeolic measure or foot, divided into two forms (a) choriambic (– ∪∪ –) and (b) prosodiac-enoplian (– ∪∪ – ∪∪ – ∪ – –), (∪̲ – ∪∪ – ∪∪ – ∪ – –), are further choric meters. The final meters to be mentioned are the dactylo-epitrite, a large group formed in combinations called cola. They are made up of dactyls (– ∪∪) or spondees (– –) and the epitrite, the equivalent of seven short syllables occurring in these combinations: ∪ – – –, – ∪ – –, – – ∪ –, – – – ∪.

These meters were used to express various kinds of emotions and situations, in slow rhythms to indicate sadness, rapid rhythms to show excitement, in that variety of simultaneous music, dance, and recitative which constituted the dramatic chorus. They were constructed in intricate patterns of strophe, antistrophe, and epode (groups of lines bearing a relation of responsion to each other) uttered to the accompaniment of a flute obbligato and a dance. The dance was called emmeleia in tragedy, cordax in comedy, and siccinis in the satyr-play. We can imagine their nature only from vase-paintings where they are depicted and from the numerous excellent scholarly articles on the ancient dance written by Professor Lillian B. Lawler. A similarity exists between the tragic choruses and the odes of Pindar which is useful for the study of both.

Since poetry in English and other European modern languages is accentual in nature, that is, dependent upon alternating stresses of pronunciation for the creation of pleasurable rhythms, it is impossible to apply to it any such elaborate system of quantitative measurement as the Greek or ancient Latin meters. Our only analogy here is music, whose essence is quantitative and whose eighth and quarter notes may be taken as equivalents of the short and long Greek syllables. It might interest the student to listen to the readings from Greek drama, Homer, and prose authors made by the late W. H. D. Rouse on Linguaphone records. Useful though by no means elementary writings on Greek metrics are G. Norwood, *Greek Comedy*, Chap. 8, Meter and Rhythm in Greek Comedy (1931) and A. M. Dale, *The Lyric Meters of Greek Drama* (1948).

These translations vary considerably in their handling. Only one or two employ prose; all choruses are done into verse of one kind or another, as they should be in any translation from Greek drama. Rex Warner, Henry Birkhead, and I attempt to approximate the meter of the original in the iambic trimeter (or senarius) of the dialogue, where the basic iambic pattern in groups of two feet each, called dipodies, may be varied with "irrational" iambi, or apparent spondees, in the first, third, and fifth feet. The English approximation usually consists of six iambic feet with a stress on the second syllable of each foot. The choruses are much more complex and cannot be approximated in English except by the obvious and clumsy stratagem of using lines of more or less similar length to those of the original, which may contain rhythms vaguely resembling in their stresses the meters of the original. Some translators use rhyme effectively for the choruses, but it must be remembered that the original Greek never uses rhyme in either chorus or dialogue. All stage directions in these translations are added by the translators as their imaginations have suggested them; no stage directions appear in the originals except for a few remarks by the scholiasts and the writers of the arguments, or "hypotheses," prefixed to the texts of the Greek plays.

VI

Translations of the Greek dramas into the idiom of our day began to appear with W. B. Yeats' *Oedipus Rex* (1928) and Richard Aldington's *Alcestis* (1930). Of these, Yeats' translation has had a vogue unjustified by its merits, for it suffers from serious faults, as I have pointed out in my review of Dudley Fitts's anthology (for the reference see the bibliography, page 417). Yeats took outrageous liberties with the text, omitting at least fifteen per cent of the original and heavily condensing the rest. His choruses, often reduced to a mere quatrain, are turned into ridiculously inappropriate thirteen- and fourteen-syllable verses. He supplies entire lines which have no basis in the Greek; his prose dialogue is colorless although free from the inversions, archaic language, and inflated rhetoric which make earlier translations so unsatisfactory.

His translation, however, paved the way for others in the language of the present day and demonstrated the obvious truth that versions from the Greek dramas did not need to be written in a language that was not spoken in any age, even the Victorian. Richard Aldington's *Alcestis* was the first adequate translation to follow; today, probably a third of the dramas have been turned into the idiom of our time. They can be read without boredom and spoken aloud without embarrassment. The revival of translation they represent is probably no more than the fruit of that normal demand each generation makes for translations contemporary to itself, but this revival takes place at a time when criticism, Greek scholarship, and the art of poetry are at their peak of accomplishment.

Louis MacNeice's *Agamemnon* is a vigorous example of the new group of translations and at the same time indispensable to an anthology which seeks, as this one does, to give a representative view of the best works of the three great Greek dramatists. The *Agamemnon* is the most moving of all Aeschylus' plays. It has a brooding, sinister quality maintained consistently from the watchman's foreboding speech at the beginning through the profound depths of the magnificent choruses to Cassandra's wild desperate wails toward the end. Clytemnestra, whose name the play would bear were it a modern creation, is one of literature's three or four most powerful villainesses. The play has a surging force rare even in Greek drama and is a perfect vehicle for Aeschylus' convictions about sin, fate, and retribution.

The *Prometheus Bound* belongs here as the first and best account in poetry of one of the few truly seminal myths that apply to the destiny of modern man. A. J. Toynbee has made the myth fundamental to the third volume of his A *Study of History*. Comparing Prometheus with Job and Faust, Toynbee typifies Prometheus as the human urge for change, for reason, and for revolt against static tyranny. Prometheus is the world's first culture-hero and still a powerful symbol of man's struggling spirit. He was not a romantic figure, however, to Zeus; he was a transgressor against divine law and order, harsh as these were.

The story of Prometheus deserves more details here. Zeus wished to destroy mankind for their sinful neglect of the gods. Prometheus tricked a willing Zeus at Sicyon, where the gods and men were disputing their respective prerogatives, with a sacrifice of bull-bones covered in fat. Zeus in anger deprived men of fire, but Prometheus stole it from heaven again in a hollow reed of fennel. For this he was punished as the play relates; but the secret he withheld from Zeus — that in the thirteenth generation Hercules, another great culture-hero of the Greeks, was to be born and to release Prometheus — was even more a source of vexation to the father of gods and of men. The myth is the Greek way of symbolizing the universal conflict at the heart of things: liberalism against reaction, human liberty against oppression, the endurance of the human spirit struggling toward a free civilization. In the remaining plays of the Prometheus-trilogy it appears that Zeus relented and a reconciliation took place, as it does in the *Oresteia*.

The *Oedipus Rex*, Aristotle's favorite play and the one which most readily gives rise to the mistaken notion that Greek tragedy deals with puppets helpless in the toils of fate, is presented here in the most literal verse translation yet made. Mr. Cook's version does not, however, sacrifice poetic quality and readability to accuracy. Fortunately the choruses in this play are not particularly outstanding so that they do not suffer beyond what may be expected in any faithful translation. The plot is the supreme attraction in the play, and this is why Aristotle liked it.

Mr. O'Sheel's American redaction of Sophocles' *Antigone* is the earliest example known to me of modern translation of the dramas in this country, with the exception of Witter Bynner's version of Euripides' *Iphigenia in Tauris* (1915), unfortunately not complete. The *Antigone* is a play which arouses perennial questions and is a favorite with students. It gives another variety of Greek drama among the changing patterns of idea, attitude, and development which characterize these plays.

The *Philoctetes* of Sophocles has not been translated before as much in the modern manner as by Kathleen Freeman, nor in as exemplary an acting version. In this play a Greek castaway escapes at last from his island home through the devotion to fair play shown by the son of Achilles. It contains some of Greek drama's most haunting evocations of beauty in nature. The struggle between Neoptolemus and the cunning Odysseus is carried on against the romantic background of glens and coves which the lame Philoctetes, left behind on Lemnos by the Greek army with the talismanic bow and arrows by which Troy may be taken, has loved so long and which he is at the end so loth to leave.

The *Bacchae*, here presented in a new and distinctive version by Henry Birkhead, is one of the most fascinating of all Greek plays and still largely a riddle. The last of Euripides' plays, we can regard it as his final utterance on the relation of what Nietzsche called the Dionysian and Apollonian elements in the Greek nature. The god of orgiastic release, rejected in his pride and conservatism by Pentheus, the Theban king, wreaks fearful revenge, in a play notable for its primitive nature-worship and human sacrifice. Pentheus, the victim in a double sense, is mistaken by Agave in her madness for the animal whose body was torn to pieces in the ritual of one of those obscure ceremonies which must bear a close prehistoric relation to the origins of drama. In the last great Greek play we return to the source of drama itself and, by a unique coincidence, close the cycle that began before Thespis, the traditional father of Western theater, in the midst of those grotesque and weird religious rites out of which the Greeks created their drama.

Each play is preceded by a short introduction written either by the translator or by myself in which the essential facts about the play are set down. Dramatic criticism is not the function of these introductions; they convey simple basic information which may assist readers in understanding the plays. I have introduced in the margin the line numbers corresponding to the original Greek lines for facility of reference.

I am grateful to all the translators who have allowed me to reprint their work. My thanks are also due to my friend and colleague, Professor C. K. Hyder, for some valuable criticisms he has made of the book.

AESCHYLUS

PROMETHEUS BOUND

Translated by Rex Warner

INTRODUCTION

The Story

THE STORY of the *Prometheus Bound* of Aeschylus is, on the face of it, a simple one. Prometheus, the Titan, is one of those rather shadowy divine powers who were in existence before Zeus conquered his father Kronos and established himself as dictator of the gods. Unlike the rest of the older gods, Prometheus went over to the side of Zeus and it was partly owing to his advice that Zeus was successful in gaining absolute power. Prometheus (the name means "forethought") differed from his brothers in having grasped the fact that intelligence, not brute force, was to be the governing power of the universe. Also he was the champion of mankind. Zeus had wished to destroy men utterly and make another race instead. Prometheus saved them from this fate and went further still. He initiated men into all the arts and sciences which make civilisation possible and, to secure his object of raising mankind from the beasts, he stole from heaven the gods' prerogative of fire, and gave this final gift to men.

For this he was seized by Zeus and bound in fetters on a rocky mountain. It is at this point that the play starts. Hephaistos, the god of fire, unwillingly executes the order of his master, Zeus. Prometheus complains of the ingratitude and the injustice shown by "the new dictator of the gods." He is comforted in his misfortunes by the daughters of Ocean, representatives, like himself, of the old order, before Zeus established his power.

There is little obvious "action" in the play. Ocean himself comes and attempts to persuade Prometheus that it is a wise thing to submit to the powers that be, and his advice is proudly rejected. Prometheus is strong in the possession of a secret. Zeus, he knows, will, unless warned of it, make a marriage from which will come a son mightier than the father, and Prometheus is determined not to divulge the secret. Then, arriving as it were by accident, there appears another victim of Zeus's injustice, Io, a girl who has been selected as Zeus's paramour, driven out of her home, given the shape of a heifer, and is now pursued from country to country by a gad-fly. All this is the direct result of the jealousy of Hera, Zeus's wife, yet, indirectly, Io's sufferings are plainly caused by Zeus himself. Io continues on her wanderings after Prometheus has given her an account of both her future and his own.

Then Hermes, the messenger of Zeus, arrives and demands to know the secret of which Prometheus has been boasting. If Prometheus remains obdurate, sufferings far worse than his present ones will be let loose upon him. He will be plunged beneath the earth in an earthquake and at length brought back to the light, when, day after day, an eagle will come and gnaw his continually restored liver. Prometheus is wholly unmoved by threats. He will resist to the end, and the play closes in thunder and lightning and convulsions of the earth.

Problems of the Story

On the face of it the play appears as a glorification of the revolutionary who, strong in his own mind and convinced of the justice of his cause, will never bow to oppression. This version of its meaning has always appealed to romantic revolutionaries, and is best shown in Shelley's *Prometheus Unbound*. It is not, however, the whole story according to Aeschylus. The *Prometheus Bound* is only one play in a trilogy, and neither of the other two plays survives. We do know, however, that in Aeschylus' *Prometheus Unbound* there has been a reconciliation between the apparently irreconcilable forces represented by Prometheus and Zeus. Precisely how this reconciliation took place we do not know, but, from our knowledge of Aeschylus' way of thought, it seems fair to assume that the reconciliation was the result of some compromise or development by which Zeus, growing wiser, became less tyrannical and Prometheus came to recognise that an attitude of mere defiance, however splendid, is ineffective.

To Aeschylus, therefore, Prometheus is not, as he was to Shelley, the perfect hero. He is certainly a grand and sympathetic figure, — as grand as and more sympathetic than Milton's Satan, that other cosmic revolutionary. Right — ordinary human right — seems to be on his side. By all human standards Zeus is behaving monstrously. Yet it is a fact that nature, and what the Greeks called "necessity" do not proceed in accordance with human standards of justice and morality and, so Aeschylus seems to suggest, a failure to recognise this is a dangerous and unjustifiable form of pride. Not that this suggestion is any solution to the main problem. A solution to the problem of the evident inhumanity of the processes of the universe must lie somewhere beyond reason in a faith that somehow and somewhere injustice will be found to have been justified in the end. So Io's misfortunes will not last for ever. Finally she will give birth immaculately to the child of Zeus, and Prometheus himself will be restored to his old honours.

But there is more than this in Aeschylus' thought. Though he makes it clear that rebellions against God can never be finally justified, he, no less than Shelley, shows the grandeur of such a rebellion as that of Prometheus. Though Prometheus is proud, he is certainly heroic. Moreover the effect of his splendid sin is, after years of suffering, to produce a change in the nature of God himself. The very idea of such a change in "eternal changelessness" seems impossible to us, but it must be remembered that in the confused Greek mythology there were a succession of supreme beings, and the possibilities of even omnipotence changing its form or omniscience yielding to persuasion might be considered and debated.

Enough, however, has been said to show that this play, in spite of its great romantic appeal, is not merely the glorification of a romantic idea. It is an investigation into the problem of the injustice of life and, since the rest of the trilogy is lost, it is a partial investigation. It is a play where the "action" is supplied by symbols of philosophical ideas, where the interest is allegorical and the meaning somewhere rather beyond the words, prophetic, as is the style and thought of this great dramatist.

Rex Warner

PROMETHEUS BOUND

◨

SCENE. *A savage scene in mountains. Enter* HEPHAISTOS, *with* POWER
and VIOLENCE, *who are leading* PROMETHEUS.

POWER: Now we have come to the plain at the end of the earth,
the Scythian tract, and an untrodden wilderness.
And you, Hephaistos, must turn your mind to the orders
the father gave you, — to discipline and pin down
this outlaw here upon the lofty ragged rocks
in unbreakable bonds of adamantine chains.
It was your flower, the gleam of civilising fire,
he stole and handed it over to mortals. Therefore
he must pay the price of such a sin to the gods,
that he may be taught to bend to the dictatorship
of Zeus, and give up his ideas of helping men. 10

HEPHAISTOS: Power and Violence, for you the command of Zeus
    has reached fulfilment. There is nothing left to do.
    But I have not the heart to bind a brother god
    violently to this stormy cleft in the mountains.
    Yet every way I am forced to find the heart for it,
    since it is hard to leave undone the father's word.

    (*He turns to* PROMETHEUS.)

O you deep-scheming son of rightminded Themis,
    against your will and mine with ineluctable brass
    I am nailing you down to this rock away from men,   20
    where you will never hear the voice or see the sight
    of any mortal, and, scorched by the sun's bright fire,
    the flower of your flesh will shrivel, and you will be glad
    when rich-clothed night shall hide away the day, and when
    once more the sun scatters the frost at dawn. Always
    the load of what you suffer at the moment will
    oppress you, since your saviour has not yet been born.
    This is your reward for your idea of helping men.
    Yourself a god, you did not shrink from wrath of gods,
    and gave to man promotion beyond what is right.   30
    And therefore you will now be sentry of this joyless rock,
    standing upright, not sleeping, not bending the knee.
    There will be many sighs and many useless groans
    that you will utter. Zeus's mind is hard to turn
    by prayer, and all whose power is new are hard hearted.
POWER: Enough of this. Why the delay? Why the empty pity?
    Why do you not hate the god most hated by the gods,
    the one who betrayed to men your own prerogative?
HEPHAISTOS: There's a strange force in kinship and fellow-feeling.
POWER: I agree. But to leave unheard the father's command,   40
    how is that possible? Do you not fear that more?
HEPHAISTOS: Oh, you are pitiless always and empty of feeling.
POWER: Yes, since there is no cure in singing dirges for him.
    Waste not your own trouble on what will do no good.
HEPHAISTOS: O my master skill of the hand, how much I hate you!
POWER: And why hate that? Your skill, if I may put it plainly,
    has nothing whatever to do with your present trouble.
HEPHAISTOS: Still I wish it had fallen to another, not me.
POWER: All things are burdensome, except power over gods,
    since there is no one except Zeus who has freedom.   50
HEPHAISTO: I know it by these chains, and have no more to say.
POWER: Then be quick to throw the bonds around this man here,
    lest the father look upon you and find you idling.

HEPHAISTOS: Here, ready to our hands are the chains for checking him.

POWER: Throw them about his arms! In your powerful strength
strike, strike with the hammer! Nail him to the rocks!

HEPHAISTOS: This work is nearly done, and is not done in vain.

POWER: Strike harder! Press the bonds tight, and leave nothing loose.
He is one to find ways out even from hopelessness.

HEPHAISTOS: This arm at least is fixed and hard to be released.   60

POWER: And now pin down the other fast, that he may know
his brilliant mind moves slower than the mind of Zeus.

HEPHAISTOS: No one but he can have the right to reproach me.

POWER: Now the unfeeling tooth of a spike of adamant!
Use all your strength and nail it right through his breast!

HEPHAISTOS: Alas, Prometheus! I am sorry for your pain.

POWER: Will you shrink back and be sorry for Zeus's enemies?
Take care. You may have to moan for yourself one day.

HEPHAISTOS: You see a sight most hard for eyes to look upon.

POWER: I see one here who is getting what he deserves.   70
Come, fasten about his body the restraining bonds.

HEPHAISTOS: I am forced to do this. Do not urge me on too far.

POWER: Be sure I'll urge you and shout encouragement besides.
Go down, put rings of violence about his legs!

HEPHAISTOS: See now, the task is done, and did not take too long.

POWER: Now use your strength and strike the bolts in the fetters.
Hard, as you know, is the overseer of this work.

HEPHAISTOS: All of a piece the words of your tongue and your shape.

POWER: Be soft yourself, but as for my unyieldingness
and my toughness of temper, do not blame them on me.   80

HEPHAISTOS: Let us go. Now he has the chains about his limbs.

POWER: (*speaking to Prometheus*): Now, where you are, behave
outrageously and steal
and give to things of a day prerogatives of gods!
Can mortals help you out from any of these pains?
The gods who called you 'Forethought' gave you a false name.
You need forethought yourself if you would find a way
to break out into freedom from this work of art.

> (HEPHAISTOS, POWER *and* VIOLENCE *go, leaving* PROMETHEUS
> *alone.*)

PROMETHEUS: O heavenly air, and breezes swift upon the wing,
fountains of rivers and innumerable laughter
of the waves of the sea, and earth, mother of all,   90
and you, all-seeing circle of the sun, I call,
see what I suffer, a god at the hand of gods.
O see in what bitter shame,

worn out through the countless years,
my race is set.
This is the bondage of shame for me
found out by the new lord of the blessed gods.
Alas, alas, I cry for the woe that is here,
for the woe that is coming, and where will they ever,
my torments, be destined to come to an end? 100
Yet what is this I say? I know what is coming,
all of it exactly, and not a single evil
can reach me unforeseen, and I must bear the fate
allotted to me as best I may, because I know
one cannot fight with the power of necessity.
Yet neither silence nor full speech is possible
for me in these misfortunes. For giving to men
God's gift I am tied down wretched in compulsion.
For I am he who sought the stolen fount of fire,
stored in a stalk, which proved to be the teacher of 110
all kind of craft to mortals and their great resource.
This was the sin for which I pay the punishment
nailed hard and fast in chains beneath the open sky.

(A *sound of wings is heard. It is the* CHORUS *of the daughters
of* OKEANOS, *who have come to comfort him.*)

Ah, what is the sound and what is the fragrance
that floats to me viewless?
Is it of gods or of mortals or both?
Has one come to this rock at the end of the world
to survey my disaster, or why has he come?
You see me a captive, a god ill-fated,
Zeus's enemy, one grown hateful 120
to everyone of the gods who enters
Zeus's palace, because of my
excessive kindness to men.
O what can it be that I hear close by me?
The rustle of bird-wings? With light beat of feathers
all the air trembles, and all that comes near me
is matter for fear.
CHORUS: Fear no danger. It is a troop of friends
which in quick rivalry
of wing has reached this rock, and hardly won 130
by prayer the father's mind to let us come.
Swift-speeding breezes have borne me.
Through cavern depths there pierced the sound of a blow

of iron and summoned forth my shame grave-eyed.
With feet unsandalled in my wingéd car I came.
PROMETHEUS: Alas!
  You children of Tethys, mother of many,
  daughters of old father Okeanos,   140
  he who with sleepless stream engirdles
  all of the world,
  look at me, see in what cruel bondage,
  nailed to the topmost crags of this mountain,
  I shall watch here unenvied.
CHORUS: I see, Prometheus, and a mist of fear
  has leapt upon my eyes,
  a mist that's full of tears, when I look
  upon your body wasting on the rocks
  in infamous bondage of adamant.
  New rulers now hold power in Olympus,
  and in new-fangled law Zeus blindly lords it.   150
  Titanic powers of old can now be seen no more.
PROMETHEUS: I wish he had hurled me under the earth,
  lower than Hades, keeper of corpses,
  into the limitless gulf of Tartaros,
  In cruel bondage of chains unbreakable,
  so neither god nor any creature
  had joyed in my sorrow.
  Now in my misery made air's plaything,
  I suffer what pleases my foes.
CHORUS: No god is so hard hearted   160
  as to be pleased with this.
  All are indignant at your wrongs,
  all except Zeus, and he,
  ever angry with a mind set,
  never bending, crushes down the sons
  of Ouranos, nor will he cease before he sates his heart,
  or by some force another steals his empire hard to win.
PROMETHEUS: Still I can swear to you that the president
  of the immortals will find out his need for me,
  for all the maltreatment of these strong chains.
  He will need me to tell the new plan by whose working   170
  he will be stripped of his sceptre and honour.
  And then by no honey-tongued charms of persuasion
  will he win my mind over.
  Nor shall I ever shrink from his terrible
  threats and reveal it,
  till he has loosed me from these cruel chains,

and is willing to pay
recompense for my shame.
CHORUS: O you are bold, unyielding
   in all your bitter pain;
   Your speech's freedom goes too far.   180
   A piercing fear is stirring
   up my heart, and for your fortune
   terror fills me, and I know not where
   fate will have you end your voyage and see the end of pain.
   Mood immovable and heart of stone has Kronos' son.
PROMETHEUS: I know of his harshness, I know that Zeus measures
   what is just by his interest. And yet
   soft-minded he will be
   in time, broken down as I say.
   He will settle his obstinate anger.   190
   As eager as I in time he will come
   claiming peace and alliance.
CHORUS: Uncover everything and tell us all the story.
   What was the accusation on which Zeus took you,
   and now so bitterly and shamefully wrongs you?
   Tell us, if nothing prevents you from the telling.
PROMETHEUS: It causes pain to me even to tell the story,
   and there is pain in silence. Each way is misery.
   Now, first, when the gods entered upon their anger,
   when they split into parties, and strife rose among them,   200
   some wishing to cast Kronos out of his empire,
   so that this Zeus of ours might reign, and the others
   as eager to prevent Zeus ever ruling gods, —
   at this time, though I planned to give the best counsel
   to my Titan brothers, children of Heaven and Earth,
   my effort was unavailing. In their proud minds
   they saw no place for the trickery of intelligence:
   by right of might they assumed they would rule unchallenged.
   But to me my mother Themis, and not once only,
   and Gaia, one person beneath the varied names,   210
   had foretold what was the future dispensation —
   that the way of fate was not by strength or force of might:
   victory and power proceeded from intelligence.
   But when I had set out this before them in words,
   they thought it all not worth a moment's attention.
   So, with all this before me then, what seemed the best
   was to take my mother with me and show that good will
   which Zeus showed too, and take my stand together with him.
   By my device it was the deep dark hiding place

of Hell now covers up, with all who fought with him,
Old Kronos. And now the dictator of the gods,   220
after receiving all this benefit from me,
has paid me back with bitter wrong that you behold.
This is a sickness, it seems, that goes along with
dictatorship — inability to trust one's friends.
Now for your question, which was — on what accusation
he now maltreats me. This I shall make plain to you.
When first he took his seat upon his father's throne,
he divided out at once the various privileges   230
to the gods in turn and brought his empire into shape.
As for long suffering men, he took no care at all;
indeed his plan was to make the whole of their race
extinct and then to form another race instead.
Except for me no one opposed his purpose here.
I dared to stand against him and I saved mankind
from being broken to pieces and sent down to Hell.
For this, I tell you, I am bowed in sufferings
painful to feel and pitiful to look upon.
When I felt pity first for mortals I thought not
that I would be the sufferer, yet, as you see,   240
I am forced to harmony, a sight of shame for Zeus.

CHORUS: Of iron heart, Prometheus, fashioned out of rock
   must be the man who shares not your indignation
   at your hard toil. I would not have chosen to see
   a sight like this, and, seeing it, my heart is sore.
PROMETHEUS: For friends to see, yes, I am one to be pitied.
CHORUS: But did you not perhaps go further than all this?
PROMETHEUS: Yes. I stopped mortals from seeing their fate in advance.
CHORUS: What cure did you find to charm away that sickness?
PROMETHEUS: I settled unseeing hopes to dwell among them.   250
CHORUS: Here was great kindness in the gift you gave to men.
PROMETHEUS: And after that I gave to them the gift of fire.
CHORUS: Do creatures of a day now own the flame-faced fire?
PROMETHEUS: They do, and they will learn from it all kinds of arts.
CHORUS: Is this, then, all the accusation for which Zeus —
PROMETHEUS: Maltreats me, and in no way grants a pause from
   suffering.
CHORUS: Is there laid down no ending-place for your ordeal?
PROMETHEUS: No end at all, except when it seems good to Zeus.
CHORUS: How can that ever be? What hope is there? Do you not see
   you were wrong? In what way wrong it hurts me to say,   260
   and gives you no pleasure either. Let us leave
   that subject. Try to find release from your ordeal.

PROMETHEUS: It is a light thing for those who take their stand outside
the place where evil is to give advice to one
who feels the evil. I knew of all this before.
I did the wrong, and meant it, and I admit it.
In helping mortals I found trouble for myself,
though I never thought that in such punishment as this,
upon these airy cliffs, that I should waste away,
my portion being the unneighboured desolate rock.   270
So do not weep for the pain I feel at present.
Come down to earth, listen as I tell of the moving
forward of fate, and hear the story to the end.
Come, listen to me, as I ask. Show fellow-feeling
for one who is now unhappy. Suffering roves
from one to another, and settles on all alike.
CHORUS: We are willing, Prometheus,
to do as you tell us,
and now on a light foot, leaving my rushing
chariot and holy
bird-path of air, I   280
come to this rough rock, and long
to hear all the tale of your sorrow.

      (*Enter* OKEANOS *on a winged monster.*)

OKEANOS: At the end of the long road,
Prometheus, I come to you,
and steer by my will, without any bridle,
this wing-swift flyer.
Be sure that I grieve with you in your misfortunes.
Kinship, I know, must
force me to do so;   290
but, apart from all blood-ties, I know of no one
for whom I would wish to do more than for you.
You will realise the truth of my words, since I cannot
speak fair and not mean fair.
Now tell me how you wish me to help you.
You will never be able to say that you have
a friend truer than I am.
PROMETHEUS: Now what is this I see? It is you who have come
to look upon my pain? How did you find the heart
to leave the stream you name, the self-made vaulted caves   300
of rock, and come to the earth, the mother of iron?
Was it to be spectator of these my sufferings,
and to join me in indignation that you came?
Here is the sight to see — it is I, the friend of Zeus,

the one who helped him establish his dictatorship,
in suffering he sent upon me now bowed down.
OKEANOS: I see it, Prometheus, and, though I know your subtle mind,
I wish to give to you the best advice I can.
Recognise your own weakness, learn to adapt your ways
to new ways. In heaven we have a new dictator.   310
For, if you hurl abroad these bitter razor-edged words,
Zeus, though his throne is far above you, may hear you,
and then all this crowd of trouble which you have now
will come to seem to you nothing more than child's play.
No, my poor friend, put aside the anger you feel,
and try to find a way of release from your pain.
You may think the words I speak to you old-fashioned,
and yet, Prometheus, such sufferings as these ones
are the usual wages of tongues that speak too proudly.
You are not yet humble, you do not yet give way   320
to your affliction. Instead you seek more still of it.
So, if you listen to the advice I give to you,
you will not kick against the pricks, in the knowledge
that a stern monarch rules with power uncontrolled.
Now I shall go my way and shall, if I am able,
attempt to win for you release from your pain.
You must lie low and check the pride of your language.
I am sure that you, so wise, know this for a fact —
the reward of empty language is always punishment.
PROMETHEUS: I envy you your luck in being free from blame,   330
though you dared all and took your share in all with me.
Now leave things as they are, do not concern yourself.
You will never persuade him. He is not to be won over.
Look close to yourself, lest you suffer by your errand.
OKEANOS: You are far better at giving advice to others
than to yourself, and here I judge by facts not words.
Yet now I have started, do not pull me back again,
since I am sure and confident that Zeus will give
this gift to me, to free you from your sufferings.
PROMETHEUS: For this I am grateful to you, and always will be   340
You show no lack of any willingness to help.
Yet do not trouble. Wasteful and profitless will be
the trouble you take for me, if you must take it.
Lie low, I say, and keep yourself out of harm's way.
I am not one who, just because of my ill-luck,
would wish unhappy as many others as might be.
Far from it. The sorrows too of my brother Atlas
afflict me, Atlas who in regions of the West

stands still and bears upon his shoulders the pillar
of heaven and earth, no easy burden on the arms. 350
Yes, and I pitied when I saw him the earth-born
dweller in the Cilician caves, the terrible
monster, the hundred-headed one, laid low by force,
furious Typhon, who took his stand against the whole
of heaven, and hissed out horror from his grisly jaws,
and from his eyes he flashed grim-visaged gleam of fire,
bent to destroy by force the tyranny of Zeus.
But the unsleeping bolt of Zeus came down on him,
the precipitous thunder-stone, breathing out fire,
and knocked the proud words out of him and the boasting. 360
Struck through to the very heart he became mere dust
and ashes, and his strength was blasted out of him.
Now useless to him, stretched out at length, his body
lies by the narrow Mediterranean waters
weighed down beneath the weight of the roots of Etna.
And, sitting on the peaks, Hephaistos forges masses
of molten metal, and from these one day will burst
rivers of fire, devouring with their savage jaws
the smooth Sicilian meadows in that land of fruit.
So Typhon, in hot heavings of insatiable 370
fire-breathing spray will force his anger boiling up,
though burnt to ashes by the thunderbolt of Zeus.
You are not ignorant. You have no need of me
to be your teacher. Save yourself, as you know how to.
And I shall fulfil to the end my present fortune,
until the mind of Zeus shall rest from its anger.

OKEANOS: This point, Prometheus, you must recognise, — that words
can act like medicine for a spirit in distress.

PROMETHEUS: Yes, if one soothes the heart when the heart is ripe for it,
not if one represses by force a bursting anger. 380

OKEANOS: Tell me, what is the punishment you see involved
in being willing to help, and in showing daring?

PROMETHEUS: Excessive trouble and empty-headed simplicity.

OKEANOS: Let me then suffer from this sickness, since I know
the safest thing is to be wise and not thought wise.

PROMETHEUS: That is an error for which I shall have the blame.

OKEANOS: Your words are plainly sending me back home again.

PROMETHEUS: Yes, in case your pity for me should bring you hatred.

OKEANOS: From him who newly sits upon the almighty throne?

PROMETHEUS: Yes, watch him, in case one day his heart grows
angry. 390

OKEANOS: Your own fortune, Prometheus, is my instructor.

PROMETHEUS: Now go, set off, keep to the purpose you have now.
OKEANOS: You urge me on now that I am about to go.
My four-foot flyer with his wings brushes the smooth
paths of the air, and he will, I know, be happy
to bend his knee again in the familiar stable.

(OKEANOS *goes away on his winged monster*.)

CHORUS: Weeping for you, your deadly fate, Prometheus,
Welling with tears, down from my delicate eyes
shedding the stream, I wet   400
my cheek with dewy fountains.
Here Zeus unhappily
rules by the laws he made himself,
to the gods of old revealing
arrogant tyranny.

Now the whole earth has raised a cry of mourning.
All men lament the dying out of the splendid
time-honoured noble fame
of yours and of your brothers.   410
All mortals dwelling in
houses and homes of holy Asia
in your hard grievous suffering
weep and lament with you,

and the maidens who are fearless in the fight,
they who dwell in Kolchis' land,
and the hordes who are in Scythia, and there
at the furthest point of earth
live around Maeotis' lake;

and the battle-honoured flower of Aria,*   420
men who hold by Caucasus
their precipitous and rocky citadel,
savage armies roaring out
in the biting of the blade.

I saw before one other Titan god,
and one alone so broken down in pain.
It was tremendous Atlas, ever strong,

---

* Aria, Hartung's emendation, is accepted here. The scholiast to the
Libation Bearers and the lexicographer Hesychius explain this word as referring to Persia. "Arabia" of the manuscripts is impossible both metrically and
geographically.

who groaning, bears upon his back
earth and the heavenly pole.   430
The ocean wave breaks in a roar of woe,
the deep sea groans, and the black hole of hell
mutters beneath the earth, and all the fountains
of lucid-flowing rivers mourn
in pity for your pain.

PROMETHEUS: Think not that I am silent because of arrogance
or stubbornness. No, it is thought consumes my mind
when I look upon myself insulted as I am.
Yet who was it but I who, from the first to the last,   440
handed out to these new gods of ours their honours?
Enough of that. I should be telling that story
to you who know it. Listen though to the sufferings
in mortals — how I found them all helpless at first,
and made them able to reflect and use their wits.
I shall tell the story, not from any grudge to men,
but simply to declare the kindness of my gifts.
They, then, at first had eyes, but all their sight was vain;
they had ears, but did not hear. Instead they were like
the shapes we see in dreams, and all through their long life
they mingled all things aimlessly, and never knew of   450
houses, brick-built and warm, or the art of wood-work.
They lived in burrows, like the light and nimble ants
down in the deep sunless recesses of their caves.
Nor had they any certain sign by which to know
the times of winter, spring with its flowers, or fruitful
summer. Instead they acted in every matter
without intelligence, till I revealed to them
the risings of the stars and settings hard to judge.
And then I found for them the art of using numbers,
that master science, and arrangement of letters,   460
and a discursive memory, a skill to be
mother of muses. I was first to bring the beasts
to serve under the yoke and saddle, that they might
take on themselves the greatest burdens of mortals.
And it was I who brought, and made them love the rein,
horses to chariots, the pride of lordly wealth.
And no one else but I discovered for sailors
the sea-wandering vessels with their canvas wings.
These were the arts I, foolish I, devised for men,
and for myself I have no device of science   470
by which to escape from the suffering I feel now.

CHORUS: You have suffered shamefully, and now you are astray,
  driven out of your wits, and, like some bad physician,
  fallen ill, you lose your courage and know not yourself
  and how to find the drugs by which you can be cured.
PROMETHEUS: When you have heard my tale out, you will wonder more
  at all the arts I discovered and the sciences.
  This was the greatest. In the past, when men fell ill,
  there was nothing to help them, no food they might take,
  no ointment for the skin, or medicine to drink.   480
  Through lack of drugs they withered away, until I
  showed them the ingredients of soothing medicines
  by means of which they keep all illnesses at bay.
  Then I laid down the lines of many ways of prophecy.
  I first discerned from dreams the elements destined
  to be true in waking life, and of sounds hard to judge,
  I taught the interpreting, and I clearly defined
  omens met in the way, the flight of crook-clawed birds,
  which ones were of the lucky sort, and the others
  unlucky, and the way of living each kind had,   490
  what enmities there were between the different kinds,
  what bonds of friendship and what associations.
  I taught men too about the smoothness of entrails
  and of what colour they should be to please the gods,
  the auspicious shape of the gall-bladder and liver.
  And then, by burning fat-enveloped limbs and loins
  of sacrifices, I set mortals on the path
  of a science hard to judge, and to the signs in flames
  I made their eyes bright that before were dim and dark.
  So much for these things. Then what was beneath the earth 500
  stored up and hidden for the benefit of men,
  bronze, iron, silver, gold, — who is there who could claim
  to have found all these out before me? No one could,
  no one, unless he wished to make an empty boast.
  In this short word learn all the story together:
  Prometheus gave all arts and sciences to men.
CHORUS: In doing good to mortals now unseasonably
  do not forget yourself and your misfortunes. I
  am full of hope that a day will come when you,
  freed from these chains, will hold a power no less than Zeus. 510
PROMETHEUS: No, not yet is fulfilling Fate fixed to accomplish
  things in this way. Instead bowed down by innumerable
  sufferings and pains, thus only shall I win freedom.
  Science is weaker a long way than necessity.
CHORUS: Whose hand is it that holds the tiller of necessity?

PROMETHEUS: The threefold Fates, and the remembering Erinyes.
CHORUS: Is Zeus, then, weaker than the Fates and Erinyes?
PROMETHEUS: He will not run away from what Fate has in store.
CHORUS: But what is Zeus's fate except to rule always?
PROMETHEUS: You must not learn this yet, so do not seek to know.
CHORUS: This is some holy secret which you fold away.   521
PROMETHEUS: Think of some other thing to tell. The time is not
   ripe for revealing this. Instead it must be hidden
   as far as possible, for, if I keep this secret,
   I shall escape my shameful bondage and my pain.

CHORUS: O never may Zeus, who holds the sway over all,
   set his might counter to my desire.
   Never may I be slow to approach the gods   530
   by the ever-flowing path of father Okeanos
   with the holy sacrifices of stricken bulls.
   Never may I in word
   fall into sin. O let
   this resolution stay
   fixed in my heart and never melt away.

Sweet it is to go through the length of life
   in confident hope, cheering the heart with bright
   shining of joy. But, oh, when I look on you
   wasting away in innumerable labours,
   I tremble at the sight I see, Prometheus.   540
   You have no fear of Zeus,
   but, following the way
   of a private judgment, you
   give honour in excess to mortal men.

O see what a gift that recoiled on the giver was that.
   What help is there anywhere, friend?
   What support from these things of a day? O did you not notice
   an impotent helplessness, weak as a dream,
   in which the blind tribe of mankind
   is fettered and bound?
   Never shall plans made by mortals   550
   go beyond the fixed pattern of Zeus.

This was the lesson, Prometheus, I learned when I saw
   this deadly disaster of yours.
   O how different the song that has leapt to my lips from the song
   I sang in delight at your wedding and bed

of your bride and ablutions, when you
won the heart of my sister
by your bride-gifts and brought her to be
the wife who would sleep at your side.   560

(*Enter* io.)

io: Where am I? Who lives here? Who shall I say
is this that I see in fetters of rock
exposed to the storm?
For what sin are you paying atonement?
Tell me where I have wandered,
poor wretch as I am.
Ah, ah,
again some biting fly stings my poor body.
It is the ghost of earth-born Argos. Keep,
keep him away, O Earth. I am afraid,
seeing the herdsman with his myriad eyes.
He stalks here with his cunning look, and even in death
Earth will not cover him; no, me, poor me   570
he rises from the dead to hunt, and drives me
wandering and hungry by the sand of the sea.

And meanwhile sounds the wax-made shrill
pipe a lullaby measure. O alas!
Where are they taking me, my far-wandering ways?
Whatever was it, O son of Kronos, I did?
When did you find me at fault that you tied me down,
Oh, to this pain,
and wear me away, poor thing, all crazy now   580
in fear of the stinging fly?
Burn me with fire, hide me in earth, and give me
for food to sea-monsters.
O hear my prayer, master!
My far-ranging courses
are discipline enough, nor can I tell
how to escape my pain.
Do you hear the voice of the girl with horns like a cow?
PROMETHEUS: I hear the maid who is driven by the stinging fly,
Inachos' daughter, she who melts the heart of Zeus   590
in love, and now, hated by Hera, violently
is disciplined in courses that have no ending.
io: How can you give my father's name?
Tell me, poor me, who can you be, O sad

sight that you are, to name so truly a poor
maid, and to tell of the sickness that wastes me away,
goading me on with its, ah! with its maddening stings.
Swiftly I came
sped to leap with the bitter hungry ache
and tamed by Hera's angry   600
plotting. O which of the wretched are there, which,
who suffer as I do?
But tell me now plainly
What more must I suffer,
or what help is there and relief from sickness.
Reveal it, if you know.
Speak, answer the girl who has wandered unhappily here.

PROMETHEUS: All that you wish to know I will tell you clearly,
not weaving riddles, but in a straight forward speech,   610
which is the right way to talk in front of one's friends.
You see the giver of fire to men — Prometheus.

IO: O poor Prometheus, you who showed yourself to be
a blessing shared by all men, why do you suffer so?

PROMETHEUS: Just now I ceased wailing over my sufferings.

IO: Will you not give me, then, this gift I ask of you?

PROMETHEUS: Say what it is you want. You will learn all from me.

IO: Tell who it was who nailed you in this mountain cleft.

PROMETHEUS: Zeus made the plan. Hephaistos carried out the work.

IO: What was the sin for which you are being punished?   620

PROMETHEUS: What I have said already is enough to say.

IO: Yet tell me more. Tell what the limit will be to
my wandering, and what the time set to my pain.

PROMETHEUS: It is better for you not to know this than to know it.

IO: Do not hide from me what I am going to suffer.

PROMETHEUS: Not that I grudge the giving of this gift to you.

IO: Why, then, do you hold back from telling me it all?

PROMETHEUS: Not from ill-feeling: but I shrink from maddening you.

IO: Take no more thought for me than I myself desire.

PROMETHEUS: Since you will have it so, then I must speak. Now listen.

CHORUS: Yet wait, and give to me my share of pleasure too.   631
First let us ask her of the sickness she suffers,
and let her tell herself of her destructive fate.
Then she may learn the rest of her trials from you.

PROMETHEUS: It is for you, Io, to do this kindness to them.
Remember, too, they are sisters of your father.
And time is well spent in grief and lamentation
over one's fortune in the kind of company
where one will win a tear from those who listen to you.

10: I do not see how I can fail to do your will.   640
  You will hear in plain words all that you wish to know,
  though even in speaking of it I feel the pain
  of the storm god launched upon me, and the change of shape,
  how it came suddenly on me, poor thing that I am.
  There were always visions haunting my virgin bed
  night after night, and speaking kindly in my ears
  with smooth words saying: 'O most fortunate maiden,
  why keep so long your maidenhood, when you might make
  the greatest match? Zeus is on fire with a shaft
  of longing for you, and wants to join in love with you.   650
  It is not for you, my child, to spurn aside the bed
  of Zeus. No, you must go out in the deep meadow
  of Lerna, to your father's herds and cattle stalls,
  so that the eye of Zeus may rest from its desire.'
  And I, poor I, by dreams like these through every hour
  of sleep was hard beset till the time I had courage
  to tell my father of the fears that came by night.
  Then he despatched to Pytho and to Dodona
  numerous messengers to find out what was right
  for him to do or say to suit the will of heaven.   660
  And they came back with messages of shifting speech,
  obscurely spoken oracles and hard to judge.
  Finally Inachos received a clear reply
  giving him a plain injunction and commanding him
  to thrust me out of my home and out of my land,
  and set me loose to wander to the ends of earth.
  And, if he would not do it, then from Zeus would come
  the fire-faced thunderbolt to wipe out all his race.
  By this reply of Loxias his mind was swayed:
  he drove me into exile, locked me out of home.   670
  It was against his will and mine, but Zeus's bridle
  put violent stress on him to do as he did.
  And immediately both my shape and my mind were changed.
  As you see, I grew horns. Stung by the sharp-mouthed fly
  I darted leaping madly onward till I came
  to the pleasant waters of the stream of Kerchneia,
  and to Lerna's fountain. And the earth-born cattle man,
  untempered in his anger, Argos, followed after,
  looking along my tracks with all his many eyes.
  There came on him a sudden unexpected fate   680
  and robbed him of his life. But I, stung by the fly,
  beneath the whip of heaven am forced from land to land.
  You have heard my story. Now, if you can tell what else

of future pain I have, reveal it. And do not
because of pity soothe me with false words. I say
insincere speeches are a most shameful malady.
CHORUS: Oh, cease, alas!
I had never thought, O never, that such strange words
would come to my hearing,
never that things so hard to be seen, so hard   690
to be borne would be hurting my heart with the double edge
of a goad, — desolation, distraction and terror.
O fate, fate, my blood runs cold
as I look on the fortunes of Io.
PROMETHEUS: Too soon you grieve and are like one that's full of fear.
Forbear till you have heard her future troubles too.
CHORUS: Speak, tell it all. For when one is sick it helps one
to know beforehand clearly what one must suffer.
PROMETHEUS: As for your first request, you have gained it from me
lightly, for first you wished to hear her own account   701
of the ordeal through which she has passed. Now listen
to the future, to the sufferings that this young girl
is fated still to undergo at Hera's hands.
And, child of Inachos, lay up these words of mine
within your heart, so you may learn your journey's end.
First, then, you must turn away from here to the rising
of the sun and go through lands that have not felt the plough.
You will reach the roving Scythians, who live raised up
above the ground in wattle huts that rest upon ·   710
the wheels of waggons. They are armed with long range bows.
Do not go near them. Turn your feet along the edge
of the salt-sounding shores and so go through their land.
Now on your left hand live the workers in iron,
the Chalybes, and of them too you must take care.
They are wild men, not fit for strangers to approach.
You will come to the river Hybristes, aptly named.
Do not cross over it, since it is hard to cross,
until you come to Caucasus itself, highest
of mountains, where the river pours away its might   720
from the very summit. And then you must pass over
star-neighbouring mountain tops, and set your foot upon
the road to the south, where you will reach the man-hating
host of the Amazons, who, in a time to come,
round Thermodon will inhabit Themiskyra
where Salmydessos lies, that rugged jaw of the sea,
no friend to sailors and to their ships a step-mother.
They will set you on your way and be glad to do it.

Then at the very narrows and gates of the sea
you will come to the Cimmerian strait. Leave this behind   730
bravely, and pass right out through the Maeotic channel.
And always among mortals there will be great talk
of your journey. The Bosporus will get its name
from you. So, when you have left the plain of Europe,
you will reach the land of Asia. Now, do you not think
that the dictator of the gods with all alike
deals violently? This mortal girl here he, a god,
craved for his love and laid these wanderings on her.
A bitter wooer you have found, my child, for this
marriage of yours. For the words which you have just heard   740
are to be thought of as hardly the beginning.

IO: Ah me! Alas! Ah me!

PROMETHEUS: Again you have cried out and sob away your breath.
What will you do when you have heard your future pain?

CHORUS: Can there be more pain for her that you will tell of?

PROMETHEUS: Indeed there can. A stormy sea of wicked woe.

IO: What then do I gain from living? Why did I not at once
throw myself headlong from this rugged rock, and so,
dashed to the earth, I might from all these pains of mine
have won my freedom. It is better to die once   750
than to suffer wretchedly throughout one's every day.

PROMETHEUS: It would be hard indeed for you to bear my pains,
since for me death is not permitted by the fates.
That would have been to find freedom from my trouble;
but now there lies before me no end to my labours
until the time Zeus falls from his dictatorship.

IO: Is it possible that Zeus will one day fall from power?

PROMETHEUS: You would be glad, I imagine, to see that happen.

IO: How should I not be, I who suffer ill from Zeus?

PROMETHEUS: What I say is true, and you may learn the truth of it.

IO: And who will take from Zeus the sceptre of his power?   761

PROMETHEUS: He will himself, he and his empty-headed plans.

IO: In what way? Tell me, if it does no harm to speak.

PROMETHEUS: He will make the sort of marriage that one day he'll rue.

IO: With a god or with a mortal? Say, if it may be told.

PROMETHEUS: What does it matter whom? I may not tell of this.

IO: Will it be by his wife that he will lose his throne?

PROMETHEUS: Yes. The son she'll bear will be better than his father.

IO: Has he no means by which to turn away this fate?

PROMETHEUS: No means at all, except if I were free from bondage.

IO: And who, against the will of Zeus, shall set you free?   771

PROMETHEUS: One of your children is destined to be my saviour.

IO: What's this? A child of mine will free you from your pain?
PROMETHEUS: Third in descent after ten generations more.
IO: This prophecy is now no longer plain to judge.
PROMETHEUS: And do not seek to know your own pains to the end.
IO: You must not offer me kindness and then withhold it.
PROMETHEUS: I have two tales to tell and I will tell you one.
IO: What are they? Say, and give me power to choose which one.
PROMETHEUS: I will. Choose then whether I shall tell you clearly   780
   of your future troubles or of him who will free me.
CHORUS: Be pleased to gratify her with one of your tales
   and me with the other. Do not grudge us your story.
   Tell her of the wandering she has still to do.
   and me of him who will free you. I long to hear.
PROMETHEUS: If this is what you wish for, I will not refuse
   to tell you everything of what you want to know.
   First, Io, I will tell of your sad wandering.
   Inscribe this in the mindful tablets of your heart.
   When you have passed the stream that bounds two continents   790
   go on towards the fire-faced and sun-trodden dawn,
   crossing the roaring of the sea, until you come
   to the Gorgon lowlands of Kisthene. Here there dwell
   the children of Phorkis, three old unmarried hags,
   swan shaped, and having a single eye between them,
   and a single tooth. On them the sun never looks down
   with rays from high, nor ever does the moon by night.
   And near to them are dwelling their three winged sisters,
   the Gorgons with their snaky hair, hated by men,
   for no mortal can see them and not cease to breathe.   800
   This is the sort of guard I say is set for you.
   Now here's another sight that's hard for you to face.
   You must beware of Zeus's sharp-beaked raging hounds,
   the griffins, and the one-eyed host of cavalry
   from Arimaspia who dwell beside a stream
   rolling with gold that is in the path of Pluto.
   Do not go near them. Afterwards you will arrive
   in a far land, among black people, those who dwell
   by the Aithiops and by the fountains of the sun.
   Go on along that river's bank until you come   810
   to a waterfall, where from the Bibline mountains down
   the Nile lets loose his holy and his pleasant stream.
   This stream will guide you to the triangular country
   of Nile-land. And here, Io, at last you are fated,
   you and your children, to found your far-off settlement.
   If any of this is indistinct and difficult for you,

go back to it again, and clearly learn it all.
I have more time to pass than I would like to have.
CHORUS: If you have any more to tell her or anything
    left out in your account of her heart-breaking way,   820
    then say it. But if you have told it all, then give
    to us the gift we asked and you, no doubt, recall.
PROMETHEUS: She has heard the whole of her journey to the end.
    But, to show her that she has not listened in vain,
    I will tell her of what she went through before she came here,
    and give this story as evidence for my account.
    I shall leave aside the greater part of the tale
    and come to what was the end of the path you trod.
    It was after you had come to the Molossian plains,
    then to Dodona of the craggy ridges, where   830
    are both Thesprotian Zeus's prophetic seat
    and, an incredible wonder, the talking oak trees.
    Beneath these trees, clearly and in no riddling words,
    you were declared one who, in the future, would be
    the famous wife of Zeus. Does this part stir your heart?
    Then driven by the fly, you darted on your way
    beside the sea and towards the great gulf of Rhea,
    from which you were driven back and forced to retrace
    your steps. But in the future that bay of the sea,
    you may be sure of it, will be called 'Ionian,'   840
    a memorial among all men of your journey.
    This I have said as a proof of my intelligence,
    how it sees rather further than what is evident.
    The rest I shall tell to you and to her alike,
    now back upon the path of what I said before.
    There is a city called Kanobos, at the end
    of the world, at the very mouth and bar of the Nile.
    And there at last Zeus gives you back your wits again,
    with just a touch and stroke of hand that brings no fear.
    Then, named from this manner of Zeus's impregnation,   850
    Your son will be black Epaphos,* and he will have
    the harvest of the land watered by Nile's broad stream.
    From him in the fifth generation comes a family
    of fifty women, who, against their will, will come
    once more to Argos, fleeing a kindred wedding
    with cousins, who, their hearts trembling with passion,
    falcons, not left far behind in the chase by doves,
    will come pursuing marriage that is not to be

---

* Derived from a verb meaning "to touch lightly."

pursued. God will grudge them the bodies of their wives.
Pelasgia will receive them with the kind of war   860
where women kill. ·They will be subdued by daring
that watches in the night. For every wife will take
her husband's life, and stain her two-edged sword in blood,
Such Love as this I pray may come upon my foes.
And yet desire will so melt one of these girls
as not to kill her bedfellow. Her purpose will be
made blunt, and, out of her two choices, she will wish
rather to be called irresolute than a murderess.
And she will give birth to a race of kings in Argos.
To tell of all this clearly would need many words;   870
however, from her family will come a child,
bold, famous for the bow, and he it is who will
free me from suffering. This, then, was the prophecy
my aged mother, Titan Themis, told to me.
How it will be fulfilled and by what means requires
long time to tell, nor would you gain by learning it.

IO: Away! Away!
Again it begins, sudden pain and a crazy
madness to urge me. The sting of the fly
burns without fire.   880
My heart in distraction beats at my breast.
With rolling eyes, my vision whirling,
out of my path by the raging breath
of madness driven, I lose control
of speech, and murky words go beating idly
on the waves of a doom I hate.

                                        (*Exit* IO.)

CHORUS: Wise, very wise was he
who first found this ring true within his judgment
and with his tongue gave out the word:
far the best thing is to wed within one's station,   890
and, if one works for one's living, not to long
for marriage with the glorious in wealth
or with the families whose pride is birth.

Never, O never, O
powerful Fates, may you behold me coming
to share the bed of Zeus. Let me
never be brought in marriage near to one of the
heavenly gods. I shrink as I see the loveless
maidenhood of Io, beaten down
by cruel wandering curse of pain from Hera.

For me, when marriage is well matched there is   900
nothing to fear. But let no eye of the gods
greater than I, ineluctable, perceive me.
That is a war when fighting does no good,
an arsenal of helplessness. I cannot tell
what would become of me. I do not see
how I could flee from what Zeus has devised.

PROMETHEUS: I swear to you that Zeus, for all his stubborn mind,
will yet be lowly; such a marriage is it that he plans
to make, one that will hurl him from his dictatorship,
a thing of nothing from his throne. The curse of Kronos   910
his father then indeed will come true utterly,
that curse he made when hurled from his established throne.
And from these troubles no one of the gods but I
can clearly show him how he can escape. I know
the means and how to accomplish it. And therefore now
let him sit confident, and in his airy noise
put faith, and brandish in his hands the fire-breathed bolt.
In no way will all this avail him to escape
falling into shame an intolerable fall.
So mighty is the wrestler that now he seeks   920
to equip against himself, an invincible wonder,
one that will find a mightier flame than the lightning,
and heavy crashes that go beyond the thunder.
And as for that plague of the sea that shakes the earth,
Poseidon's spear, the trident, he will brush it aside.
Zeus, stumbling on this misadventure, will find out
how far apart are supreme power and slavery.

CHORUS: What you would have yourself you mouth out against Zeus.
PROMETHEUS: I say what will come true and also what I wish.
CHORUS: Then must we look for one to hold power over Zeus?   930
PROMETHEUS: Yes, and pains for Zeus more hard to escape than these.
CHORUS: Do you not cower in fear when you let loose such words?
PROMETHEUS: What should I fear, I who am not fated to die?
CHORUS: Yet he might bring on you a trial still worse than this.
PROMETHEUS: Then let him. I can imagine all that's possible.
CHORUS: Those who bow down to Adrasteia show wisdom.
PROMETHEUS: Do honour, pray and fawn upon the powers that be.
As for me, Zeus matters to me less than nothing.
He is free to act and free to reign for this short time
just as he wills, since not for long he'll rule the gods.   940
But here I see coming the messenger of Zeus,
the agent of the newly-established dictator.
I am sure that he has come with something new to tell.

(*Enter* HERMES.)

HERMES: You there, the clever one, and too sharp in your sharpness,
the one who sinned against the gods by giving over
honour to creatures of a day, you thief of fire,
the father orders you to tell of that marriage
in which you boast and by which he will fall from power.
And also none of this must be said in riddles;
tell all of it straight out, and do not put on me,   950
Prometheus, a double journey back. You are aware
Zeus is not softened by such people as you are.

PROMETHEUS: Proud-mouthed indeed they are and full of arrogance
such words as these for a lackey of gods to speak.
You and your power are young, and so, no doubt, you think
you dwell in towers where grief can never come. And yet
have I not seen dictators twice hurled down from them?
Yes, and this third one, ruling now, I shall see fall
most sudden in dishonour. Do I look as though
I cowered and shrunk away in fear from these young gods?   960
I am far, yes, very far indeed from that. Now you
go back again over the road you came upon,
since you will hear from me none of the things you ask.

HERMES: Before now it was by a self-conceit like this
you brought and settled yourself among these sufferings.

PROMETHEUS: For your menial position I would not exchange
my own ill fortune. You may be sure of that.

HERMES: No doubt it is better to be a menial to this rock
than to be the trusted messenger of father Zeus.

PROMETHEUS: Insolent words are right where you find insolence.   970

HERMES: It seems that you take pride in what is happening to you.

PROMETHEUS: Take pride? I wish that I could see my enemies
take pride like this, and among them I reckon you.

HERMES: Me? Do you blame me at all for your disaster?

PROMETHEUS: Simply I am an enemy to all the gods.
I helped them, and they persecute me causelessly.

HERMES: You speak like a madman, brain-sick seriously.

PROMETHEUS: Yes, sick, if it is sickness to detest one's foes.

HERMES: You would not be tolerable if you were fortunate.

PROMETHEUS: Alas!

HERMES: That is a word Zeus does not understand.   980

PROMETHEUS: Yet Time, as Time grows old, instructs in everything.

HERMES: Though you do not yet know how to behave wisely.

PROMETHEUS: If I did, I would not have spoken to you, you lackey.

HERMES: It seems you will say nothing of what the father wants.

PROMETHEUS: I am his debtor and would like to pay him back.

HERMES: So then you laugh at me as if I was a child.

PROMETHEUS: Yes, are you not a child and still more foolish than a child,
if you expect to hear of anything from me?
There is no shame and no kind of device by which
Zeus can induce me ever to reveal these things, 990
until he loosens these despiteful chains of mine.
And so let all his burning flame be hurled at me,
and with the white-winged snow and subterranean
thunders let him confound and mingle everything.
None of all this will bend me so that I will tell
by whom he is bound to be thrown from his dictatorship.

HERMES: Now, look. Does this seem likely to be helpful to you?

PROMETHEUS: It has been looked to and decided long ago.

HERMES: You fool, have the courage, in the end have courage
to frame your thought correctly to your present ills. 1000

PROMETHEUS: Your soothing words beat on me vainly like a wave.
Let it not come into your head that I shall fear
ever the will of Zeus and have a woman's mind,
and be a suppliant to him I greatly hate,
with womanish up-turnings of the hands, that he
might loose me from these chains. I am wholly different.

HERMES: It seems that, speaking, I should speak a lot in vain.
You are neither soft at all nor melted by my prayers,
but, taking the bit between your teeth, like a colt 1010
not broken in, you try and fight against the rein.
Yet all this overkeenness comes from a weak design.
Stubbornness, in a mind whose thoughts have gone astray,
has in its simple self less strength than anything.
And now, if you are not persuaded by my words,
consider what a storm and hurricane of ill
will fall upon you past escape. For, first of all,
with thunder and with lightning flash the father will
tear up this rocky gully, will hide your body
beneath, and arms of stone will fold you round about.
And so you will pass through a lengthy stretch of time,
and then come back again into the light. And now 1020
Zeus's winged hound, the blood-red eagle, greedily
will tear into great rags the flesh of your body,
coming, although not asked, to dinner every day,
and he will feast upon and gnaw your liver black.
And do not look for any end to pains like these,
until a god appears to take upon himself
your load of suffering, and is willing to go down

to rayless Hades and the gloomy depths of Hell.
And now make up your mind. Be sure these words of mine   1030
are no pretended boasting, but too clearly true.
The mouth of Zeus does not know how to tell a lie:
no, he will bring his every word to act. Now you
look closely to yourself, reflect, and do not think
self-will can ever be a better thing than good advice.

CHORUS: To us it seems that Hermes' speech is to the point.
    What he commends to you is to relax from your
    self-will and seek the wisdom that's in good advice.
    Do as he says, since wrong is shameful in the wise.

PROMETHEUS: I tell you I know this news that he cries to me,   1040
    nor is there any shame in the suffering
    an enemy feels at the hands of his enemies.
    Therefore on me now let the double-edged
    curling of fire be loosed! Let air
    rage in anger with thunder and roaring
    of savage winds! Let a blast blow
    to make earth's depths totter down to their roots!
    In ungentle surge let it heap together
    waves of the sea in a mass and the paths of the
    heavenly stars! Let it raise my body   1050
    high and in whirlwind of strong compulsion,
    hurl it down into Hell! Zeus cannot
    any way put me to death.

HERMES: What is this but to listen to madmen's
    words and devices?
    This man's prayer is no different from raving.
    He cannot relax from his frenzy.
    You, then, at least, who sympathise with him
    in his suffering, take yourselves elsewhere,
    away from this place.   1060
    See that your wits are not driven crazy by
    terrible roaring of thunder.

CHORUS: Say something else, or give me advice
    that is able to move me. You cannot suppose
    I can endure this wild word you've spoken.
    How can you urge me to follow the coward's way?
    With him I am willing to suffer what must be,
    since I have learnt to hate all traitors;
    there exists no disease
    that I loathe more than that one.   1070

HERMES: Well, then, remember what I tell you
    and do not, when you are chased by destruction,
    find fault with fortune. Do not ever

say that Zeus has thrown you to suffering
unforeseen. It is not so. You brought it
all on yourselves. For with clear knowledge,
neither suddenly nor by deception,
you will be folded up by your folly
in an infinite net of destruction.

(*Thunder, lightning and earthquake.* PROMETHEUS *and the
rock to which he is bound gradually sink out of sight.*)

PROMETHEUS: Now it is fact, and no longer in words   1080
that the earth is convulsed.
Out of the deep the roaring of thunder
rolls past, and flickering fire of the lightning
flashes out, and the whirlwinds
roll up the dust, and the blasts of all storms
leap at each other, declaring
a war of the winds,
and the air and the sea are confounded.
These, most clearly, are strokes from Zeus
coming upon me to cause me fear.   1090
O my glorious mother, O Heaven
with circle of light that is common to everyone,
you see me and see this injustice.

AESCHYLUS

AGAMEMNON

Translated by Louis MacNeice

INTRODUCTION

(i) The Family Tree

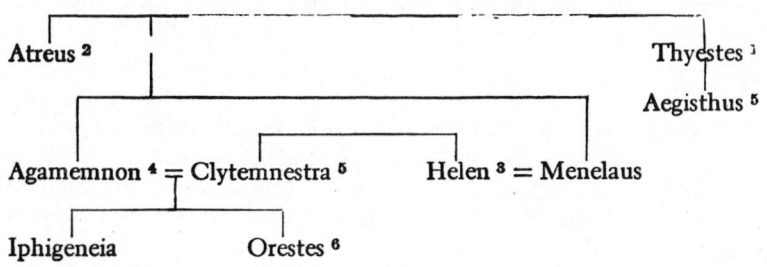

(ii) The Chain of Crimes

Two brothers, Agamemnon and Menelaus, were kings of Argos. They married two sisters, Clytemnestra and Helen; each married to his cost. On the Greek view Helen and Clytemnestra were not just bad women; they were agents rather than creators of evil. Nobody on this view is either simply a protagonist of evil or simply a victim of circumstance. The family is physically, and therefore morally, a unit: the same blood runs in all, and through it descends an inherited responsibility which limits, without wholly destroying, the power of choice in each. The sins of the fathers are visited on the children, so the children are victims of circumstance. But the children, because they are of the same blood, are tempted to sin in their turn. If a man holds such a view he will tend simultaneously to vindicate the ways of God and kick against the pricks of chance. It is this paradox that gives tension to a play like the Agamemnon. Here we have a chain of crimes, one leading on to another from generation to generation by a logic immanent in the blood and working through it. But the cause of the crimes, not only of the first link, the first crime, but present in every one of them, is the principle of Evil which logic cannot comprehend.

The chain of crimes in this play is as follows (see Family Tree above):

Past

(1) Thyestes seduced Atreus' wife.
(2) Atreus killed Thyestes' young children and gave him them as meat.
(3) Helen forsook her husband and went to Troy with Paris.

(4) Agamemnon, to promote the Trojan War, sacrificed his daughter Iphigeneia.

Present

(5) Aegisthus and Clytemnestra murder Agamemnon.

Future

(6) Orestes will kill Aegisthus and his mother Clytemnestra.

(iii)

I have written this translation primarily for the stage. I have consciously sacrificed certain things in the original — notably the liturgical flavor of the diction and the metrical complexity of the choruses. It is my hope that the play emerges as a play and not as a museum piece.

My thanks are very much due to my friend, Professor E. R. Dodds, who, with a tolerance rare among scholars and a sympathy rare in anyone, read through the whole of my unacademic version and pointed out to me its more culpable inadequacies. The translation of certain passages is our joint product; but for the faults which remain I alone am responsible.

LOUIS MACNEICE

AGAMEMNON

CHARACTERS

WATCHMAN

CHORUS *of old men of the city of Argos*

CLYTEMNESTRA, *wife of Agamemnon*

HERALD

AGAMEMNON, *king of Argos*

CASSANDRA, *a prophetess, daughter of King Priam of Troy*

AEGISTHUS, *the paramour or lover of Clytemnestra*

SCENE. *A space in front of the palace of Agamemnon in Argos. Night. A* WATCHMAN *on the roof of the palace.*

WATCHMAN: The gods it is I ask to release me from this watch
  A year's length now, spending my nights like a dog,
  Watching on my elbow on the roof of the sons of Atreus
  So that I have come to know the assembly of the nightly stars
  Those which bring storm and those which bring summer to men,
  The shining Masters riveted in the sky —
  I know the decline and rising of those stars.
  And now I am waiting for the sign of the beacon,
  The flame of fire that will carry the report from Troy,
  News of her taking. Which task has been assigned me   **10**
  By a woman of sanguine heart but a man's mind.
  Yet when I take my restless rest in the soaking dew,
  My night not visited with dreams —
  For fear stands by me in the place of sleep
  That I cannot firmly close my eyes in sleep —
  Whenever I think to sing or hum to myself

As an antidote to sleep, then every time I groan
And fall to weeping for the fortunes of this house
Where not as before are things well ordered now.
But now may a good chance fall, escape from pain,   20
The good news visible in the midnight fire.

> (*Pause. A light appears, gradually increasing, the light of the beacon.*)

Ha! I salute you, torch of the night whose light
Is like the day, an earnest of many dances
In the city of Argos, celebration of Peace.
I call to Agamemnon's wife; quickly to rise
Out of her bed and in the house to raise
Clamor of joy in answer to this torch
For the city of Troy is taken —
Such is the evident message of the beckoning flame.   30
And I myself will dance my solo first
For I shall count my master's fortune mine
Now that this beacon has thrown me a lucky throw.
And may it be when he comes, the master of this house,
That I grasp his hand in my hand.
As to the rest, I am silent. A great ox, as they say,
Stands on my tongue. The house itself, if it took voice,
Could tell the case most clearly. But I will only speak
To those who know. For the others I remember nothing.

> (*Enter* CHORUS *of old men. During the following chorus the day begins to dawn.*)

CHORUS: The tenth year it is since Priam's high   40
Adversary, Menelaus the king
And Agamemnon, the double-throned and sceptred
Yoke of the sons of Atreus
Ruling in fee from God,
From this land gathered an Argive army
On a mission of war a thousand ships,
Their hearts howling in boundless bloodlust
In eagles' fashion who in lonely   50
Grief for nestlings above their homes hang
Turning in cycles
Beating the air with the oars of their wings,
   Now to no purpose
   Their love and task of attention.

But above there is One,
Maybe Pan, maybe Zeus or Apollo,
Who hears the harsh cries of the birds
Guests in his kingdom,
Wherefore, though late, in requital
He sends the Avenger.
Thus Zeus our master
Guardian of guest and of host   60
Sent against Paris the sons of Atreus
For a woman of many men
Many the dog-tired wrestlings
Limbs and knees in the dust pressed —
   For both the Greeks and Trojans
   An overture of breaking spears.

Things are where they are, will finish
In the manner fated and neither
Fire beneath nor oil above can soothe
The stubborn anger of the unburnt offering.   70
As for us, our bodies are bankrupt,
The expedition left us behind
And we wait supporting on sticks
Our strength — the strength of a child;
For the marrow that leaps in a boy's body
Is no better than that of the old
For the War God is not in his body;
While the man who is very old
And his leaf withering away   80
Goes on the three-foot way
No better than a boy, and wanders
A dream in the middle of the day.

But you, daughter of Tyndareus,
Queen Clytemnestra,
What is the news, what is the truth, what have you learnt,
On the strength of whose word have you thus
Sent orders for sacrifice round?
All the gods, the gods of the town,
Of the worlds of Below and Above,
By the door, in the square,   90
Have their altars ablaze with your gifts,
From here, from there, all sides, all corners.
Sky-high leap the flame-jets fed
By gentle and undeceiving

Persuasion of sacred unguent,
Oil from the royal stores.
Of these things tell
That which you can, that which you may,
Be healer of this our trouble
Which at times torments with evil   100
Though at times by propitiations
A shining hope repels
The insatiable thought upon grief
Which is eating away our hearts.
Of the omen which powerfully speeded
That voyage of strong men, by God's grace even I
Can tell, my age can still
Be galvanized to breathe the strength of song,
To tell how the kings of all the youth of Greece
Two-throned by one in mind   110
Were launched with pike and punitive hand
Against the Trojan shore by angry birds.
Kings of the birds to our kings came,
One with a white rump, the other black,
Appearing near the palace on the spear-arm side
Where all could see them,
Tearing a pregnant hare with the unborn young
Foiled of their courses.   120
    Cry, cry upon Death; but may the good prevail.

But the diligent prophet of the army seeing the sons
Of Atreus twin in temper knew
That the hare-killing birds were the two
Generals, explained it thus —
"In time this expedition sacks the town
Of Troy before whose towers
By Fate's force the public
Wealth will be wasted.   130
Only let not some spite from the gods benight the bulky battalions,
The bridle of Troy, nor strike them untimely;
For the goddess feels pity, is angry
With the winged dogs of her father
Who killed the cowering hare with her unborn young;
Artemis hates the eagles' feast."
    Cry, cry upon Death; but may the good prevail.

"But though you are so kind, goddess,   140
To the little cubs of lions

And to all the suckling young of roving beasts
In whom your heart delights,
Fulfil us the signs of these things,
The signs which are good but open to blame,
And I call on Apollo the Healer
That his sister raise not against the Greeks
Unremitting gales to baulk their ships,
Hurrying on another kind of sacrifice, with no feasting,   150
Barbarous building of hates and disloyalties
Grown on the family. For anger grimly returns
Cunningly haunting the house, avenging the death
    of a child, never forgetting its due."
So cried the prophet — evil and good together,
Fate that the birds foretold to the king's house.
In tune with this
    Cry, cry upon Death; but may the good prevail.
Zeus, whoever He is, if this   160
Be a name acceptable,
By this name I will call him.
There is no one comparable
When I reckon all of the case
Excepting Zeus, if ever I am to jettison
The barren care which clogs my heart.

Not He who formerly was great *
With brawling pride and mad for broils   170
Will even be said to have been.
And He who was next has met †
His match and is seen no more,
But Zeus is the name to cry in your triumph-song
And win the prize for wisdom.

Who setting us on the road
Made this a valid law —
    "That men must learn by suffering."
Drop by drop in sleep upon the heart
Falls the laborious memory of pain,   180
Against one's will comes wisdom;
The grace of the gods is forced on us
    Throned inviolably.

So at that time the elder
Chief of the Greek ships

---

* Ouranos.   † Cronos.

Would not blame any prophet
Nor face the flail of fortune;
For unable to sail, the people
Of Greece were heavy with famine
Waiting in Aulis where the tides
   Flow back, opposite Chalcis.   190

But the winds that blew from the Strymon,
Bringing delay, hunger, evil harborage,
Crazing men, rotting ships and cables,
By drawing out the time
Were shredding into nothing the flower of Argos,
When the prophet screamed a new
Cure for that bitter tempest
And heavier still for the chiefs,   200
Pleading the anger of Artemis so that the sons of Atreus
Beat the ground with their sceptres and shed tears.
Then the elder king found voice and answered:
"Heavy is my fate, not obeying,
And heavy it is if I kill my child, the delight of my house,
And with a virgin's blood upon the altar   210
Make foul her father's hands.
Either alternative is evil.
How can I betray the fleet
And fail the allied army?
It is right they should passionately cry for the winds to be lulled
By the blood of a girl. So be it. May it be well."

But when he had put on the halter of Necessity
Breathing in his heart a veering wind of evil
Unsanctioned, unholy, from that moment forward   220
He changed his counsel, would stop at nothing.
For the heart of man is hardened by infatuation,
A faulty adviser, the first link of sorrow.
Whatever the cause, he brought himself to slay
His daughter, an offering to promote the voyage
To a war for a runaway wife.

Her prayers and her cries of father,
Her life of a maiden,
Counted for nothing with those militarists;   230
But her father, having duly prayed, told the attendants
To lift her, like a goat, above the altar
With her robes falling about her,

To lift her boldly, her spirit fainting,
And hold back with a gag upon her lovely mouth
By the dumb force of a bridle
The cry which would curse the house.
Then dropping on the ground her saffron dress,
Glancing at each of her appointed   240
Sacrificers a shaft of pity,
Plain as in a picture she wished
To speak to them by name, for often
At her father's table where men feasted
She had sung in celebration for her father
With a pure voice, affectionately, virginally,
The hymn for happiness at the third libation.
The sequel to this I saw not and tell not
But the crafts of Calchas gained their object.
To learn by suffering is the equation of Justice; the Future   250
Is known when it comes, let it go till then.
To know in advance is to sorrow in advance.
The facts will appear with the shining of the dawn.

    (*Enter* CLYTEMNESTRA.)

But may good, at the least, follow after
As the queen here wishes, who stands
Nearest the throne, the only
    Defence of the land of Argos.
LEADER OF THE CHORUS: I have come, Clytemnestra, reverencing your
    authority.
For it is right to honor our master's wife
When the man's own throne is empty.   260
But you, if you have heard good news for certain, or if
You sacrifice on the strength of flattering hopes,
I would gladly hear. Though I cannot cavil at silence.
CLYTEMNESTRA: Bearing good news, as the proverb says, may Dawn
Spring from her mother Night.
You will hear something now that was beyond your hopes.
The men of Argos have taken Priam's city.
LEADER: What! I cannot believe it. It escapes me.
CLYTEMNESTRA: Troy in the hands of the Greeks. Do I speak plain?
LEADER: Joy creeps over me, calling out my tears.   270
CLYTEMNESTRA: Yes. Your eyes proclaim your loyalty.
LEADER: But what are your grounds? Have you a proof of it?
CLYTEMNESTRA: There is proof indeed — unless God has cheated us.
LEADER: Perhaps you believe the inveigling shapes of dreams?
CLYTEMNESTRA: I would not be credited with a dozing brain!

LEADER: Or are you puffed up by Rumor, the wingless flyer?

CLYTEMNESTRA: You mock my common sense as if I were a child.

LEADER: But at what time was the city given to sack?

CLYTEMNESTRA: In this very night that gave birth to this day.

LEADER: What messenger could come so fast? 280

CLYTEMNESTRA: Hephaestus, launching a fine flame from Ida,
  Beacon forwarding beacon, despatch-riders of fire,
  Ida relayed to Hermes' cliff in Lemnos
  And the great glow from the island was taken over third
  By the height of Athos that belongs to Zeus,
  And towering then to straddle over the sea
  The might of the running torch joyfully tossed
  The gold gleam forward like another sun,
  Herald of light to the heights of Mount Macistus,
  And he without delay, nor carelessly by sleep 290
  Encumbered, did not shirk his intermediary role,
  His farflung ray reached the Euripus' tides
  And told Messapion's watchers, who in turn
  Sent on the message further
  Setting a stack of dried-up heather on fire.
  And the strapping flame, not yet enfeebled, leapt
  Over the plain of Asopus like a blazing moon
  And woke on the crags of Cithaeron
  Another relay in the chain of fire.
  The light that was sent from far was not declined 300
  By the look-out men, who raised a fiercer yet,
  A light which jumped the water of Gorgopis
  And to Mount Aegiplanctus duly come
  Urged the reveille of the punctual fire.
  So then they kindle it squanderingly and launch
  A beard of flame big enough to pass
  The headland that looks down upon the Saronic gulf,
  Blazing and bounding till it reached at length
  The Arachnaean steep, our neighbouring heights;
  And leaps in the latter end on the roof of the sons of Atreus 310
  Issue and image of the fire on Ida.
  Such was the assignment of my torch-racers,
  The task of each fulfilled by his successor,
  And victor is he who ran both first and last.
  Such is the proof I offer you, the sign
  My husband sent me out of Troy.

LEADER: To the gods, queen, I shall give thanks presently.
  But I would like to hear this story further,
  To wonder at it in detail from your lips.

CLYTEMNESTRA: The Greeks hold Troy upon this day.   320
  The cries in the town I fancy do not mingle.
  Pour oil and vinegar into the same jar,
  You would say they stand apart unlovingly;
  Of those who are captured and those who have conquered
  Distinct are the sounds of their diverse fortunes,
  For *these* having flung themselves about the bodies
  Of husbands and brothers, or sons upon the bodies
  Of aged fathers from a throat no longer
  Free, lament the fate of their most loved.
  But *those* a night's marauding after battle   330
  Sets hungry to what breakfast the town offers
  Not billeted duly in any barracks order
  But as each man has drawn his lot of luck.
  So in the captive homes of Troy already
  They take their lodging, free of the frosts
  And dews of the open. Like happy men
  They will sleep all night without sentry.
  But if they respect duly the city's gods,
  Those of the captured land and the sanctuaries of the gods,
  They need not, having conquered, fear reconquest.   340
  But let no lust fall first upon the troops
  To plunder what is not right, subdued by gain,
  For they must still, in order to come home safe,
  Get round the second lap of the doubled course.
  So if they return without offence to the gods
  The grievance of the slain may learn at last
  A friendly talk — unless some fresh wrong falls.
  Such are the thoughts you hear from me a woman.
  But may the good prevail for all to see.
  We have much good. I only ask to enjoy it.   350
LEADER: Woman, you speak with sense like a prudent man.
  I, who have heard your valid proofs, prepare
  To give the glory to God.
  Fair recompense is brought us for our troubles.

    (CLYTEMNESTRA *goes back into the palace.*)

CHORUS: O Zeus our king and Night our friend
  Donor of glories,
  Night who cast on the towers of Troy
  A close-clinging net so that neither the grown
  Nor any of the children can pass
  The enslaving and huge   360
  Trap of all-taking destruction.

Great Zeus, guardian of host and guest,
I honor who has done his work and taken
A leisured aim at Paris so that neither
Too short nor yet over the stars
He might shoot to no purpose.

From Zeus is the blow they can tell of,
This at least can be established,
They have fared according to his ruling. For some
Deny that the gods deign to consider those among men   370
Who trample on the grace of inviolate things;
It is the impious man says this,
For Ruin is revealed the child
Of not to be attempted actions
When men are puffed up unduly
And their houses are stuffed with riches.
Measure is the best. Let danger be distant,
This should suffice a man
With a proper part of wisdom.   380
For a man has no protection
Against the drunkenness of riches
Once he has spurned from his sight
The high altar of Justice.

Sombre Persuasion compels him,
Intolerable child of calculating Doom;
All cure is vain, there is no glozing it over,
But the mischief shines forth with a deadly light
And like bad coinage   390
By rubbings and frictions
He stands discolored and black
Under the test — like a boy
Who chases a winged bird
He has branded his city for ever.
His prayers are heard by no god;
Who makes such things his practice
The gods destroy him.
   This way came Paris
   To the house of the sons of Atreus   400
   And outraged the table of friendship
   Stealing the wife of his host.
Leaving to her countrymen clanging of
Shields and of spears and
Launching of warships

And bringing instead of a dowry destruction to Troy
Lightly she was gone through the gates daring
Things undared. Many the groans
Of the palace spokesmen on this theme —
"O the house, the house, and its princes,　　　　　410
O the bed and the imprint of her limbs;
One can see him crouching in silence
Dishonored and unreviling."
Through desire for her who is overseas, a ghost
Will seem to rule the household.
　　And now her husband hates
　　The grace of shapely statues;
　　In the emptiness of their eyes
　　All their appeal is departed.

But appearing in dreams persuasive　　　　　420
Images come bringing a joy that is vain,
Vain for when in fancy he looks to touch her —
Slipping through his hands the vision
Rapidly is gone
Following on wings the walks of sleep.
Such as these and worse than these,
But everywhere through the land of Greece which men have left
Are mourning women with enduring hearts　　　　　430
To be seen in all houses; many
Are the thoughts which stab their hearts;
　　For those they sent to war
　　They know, but in place of men
　　That which comes home to them
　　Is merely an urn and ashes.

But the money-changer War, changer of bodies,
Holding his balance in the battle
Home from Troy refined by fire　　　　　440
Sends back to friends the dust
That is heavy with tears, stowing
A man's worth of ashes
In an easily handled jar.
And they wail speaking well of the men how that one
Was expert in battle, and one fell well in the carnage —
But for another man's wife.
Muffled and muttered words;
And resentful grief creeps up against the sons
Of Atreus and their cause.　　　　　450

But others there by the wall
Entombed in Trojan ground
Lie, handsome of limb,
Holding and hidden in enemy soil.

Heavy is the murmur of an angry people
Performing the purpose of a public curse;
There is something cowled in the night
That I anxiously wait to hear. 460
For the gods are not blind to the
Murderers of many and the black
Furies in time
When a man prospers in sin
By erosion of life reduce him to darkness,
Who, once among the lost, can no more
Be helped. Over-great glory
Is a sore burden. The high peak
Is blasted by the eyes of Zeus. 470
 I prefer an unenvied fortune,
 Not to be a sacker of cities
 Nor to find myself living at another's
 Ruling, myself a captive.

AN OLD MAN: From the good news' beacon a swift
 Rumor is gone through the town.
 Who knows if it be true
 Or some deceit of the gods?
ANOTHER OLD MAN: Who is so childish or broken in wit
 To kindle his heart at a new-fangled message of flame 480
 And then be downcast
 At a change of report?
ANOTHER OLD MAN: It fits the temper of a woman
 To give her assent to a story before it is proved.
ANOTHER OLD MAN: The over-credulous passion of women expands
 In swift conflagration but swiftly declining is gone
 The news that a woman announced.
LEADER OF THE CHORUS: Soon we shall know about the illuminant
  torches,
 The beacons and the fiery relays, 490
 Whether they were true or whether like dreams
 That pleasant light came here and hoaxed our wits.
 Look: I see, coming from the beach, a herald
 Shadowed with olive shoots; the dust upon him,
 Mud's thirsty sister and colleague, is my witness

That he will not give dumb news nor news by lighting
A flame of fire with the smoke of mountain timber;
In words he will either corroborate our joy —
But the opposite version I reject with horror.
To the good appeared so far may good be added.   500
ANOTHER SPEAKER: Whoever makes other prayers for this our city,
  May he reap himself the fruits of his wicked heart.

(*Enter the* HERALD, *who kisses the ground before speaking.*)

HERALD: Earth of my fathers, O the earth of Argos,
  In the light of the tenth year I reach you thus
  After many shattered hopes achieving one,
  For never did I dare to think that here in Argive land
  I should win a grave in the dearest soil of home;
  But now hail, land, and hail, light of the sun,
  And Zeus high above the country and the Pythian king —
  May he no longer shoot his arrows at us   510
  (Implacable long enough beside Scamander)
  But now be savior to us and be healer,
  King Apollo. And all the Assembly's gods
  I call upon, and him my patron, Hermes,
  The dear herald whom all heralds adore,
  And the Heroes who sped our voyage, again with favor
  Take back the army that has escaped the spear.
  O cherished dwelling, palace of royalty,
  O august thrones and gods facing the sun,
  If ever before, now with your bright eyes   520
  Gladly receive your king after much time,
  Who comes bringing light to you in the night time,
  And to all these as well — King Agamemnon.
  Give him a good welcome as he deserves,
  Who with the axe of judgment-awarding God
  Has smashed Troy and levelled the Trojan land;
  The altars are destroyed, the seats of the gods,
  And the seed of all the land is perished from it.
  Having cast this halter round the neck of Troy
  The King, the elder son of Atreus, a blessed man,   530
  Comes, the most worthy to have honor of all
  Men that are now. Paris nor his guilty city
  Can boast that the crime was greater than the atonement.
  Convicted in a suit for rape and robbery
  He has lost his stolen goods and with consummate ruin
  Mowed down the whole country and his father's house.
  The sons of Priam have paid their account with interest.

LEADER OF THE CHORUS: Hail and be glad, herald of the Greek army.
HERALD: Yes. Glad indeed! So glad that at the gods' demand
    I should no longer hesitate to die.
LEADER: Were you so harrowed by desire for home? 540
HERALD: Yes. The tears come to my eyes for joy.
LEADER: Sweet then is the fever which afflicts you.
HERALD: What do you mean? Let me learn your drift.
LEADER: Longing for those whose love came back in echo.
HERALD: Meaning the land was homesick for the army?
LEADER: Yes. I would often groan from a darkened heart.
HERALD: This sullen hatred — how did it fasten on you?
LEADER: I cannot say. Silence is my stock prescription.
HERALD: What? In your masters' absence were there some you feared?
LEADER: Yes. In your phrase, death would now be a gratification.
HERALD: Yes, for success is ours. These things have taken time. 551
    Some of them we could say have fallen well,
    While some we blame. Yet who except the gods
    Is free from pain the whole duration of life?
    If I were to tell of our labors, our hard lodging,
    The sleeping on crowded decks, the scanty blankets,
    Tossing and groaning, rations that never reached us —
    And the land too gave matter for more disgust,
    For our beds lay under the enemy's walls.
    Continuous drizzle from the sky, dews from the marshes, 560
    Rotting our clothes, filling our hair with lice.
    And if one were to tell of the bird-destroying winter
    Intolerable from the snows of Ida
    Or of the heat when the sea slackens at noon
    Waveless and dozing in a depressed calm —
    But why make these complaints? The weariness is over;
    Over indeed for some who never again
    Need even trouble to rise.
    Why make a computation of the lost? 570
    Why need the living sorrow for the spites of fortune?
    I wish to say a long goodbye to disasters.
    For us, the remnant of the troops of Argos,
    The advantage remains, the pain cannot outweigh it;
    So we can make our boast to this sun's light,
    Flying on words above the land and sea:
    "Having taken Troy the Argive expedition
    Has nailed up throughout Greece in every temple
    These spoils, these ancient trophies."
    Those who hear such things must praise the city 580
    And the generals. And the grace of God be honored
    Which brought these things about. You have the whole story.

LEADER: I confess myself convinced by your report.
Old men are always young enough to learn.

(*Enter* CLYTEMNESTRA *from the palace.*)

This news belongs by right first to the house
And Clytemnestra — though I am enriched also.
CLYTEMNESTRA: Long before this I shouted at joy's command
At the coming of the first night-messenger of fire
Announcing the taking and capsizing of Troy.
And people reproached me saying, "Do mere beacons   590
Persuade you to think that Troy is already down?
Indeed a woman's heart is easily exalted."
Such comments made me seem to be wandering but yet
I began my sacrifices and in the women's fashion
Throughout the town they raised triumphant cries
And in the gods' enclosures
Lulling the fragrant, incense-eating flame.
And now what need is there for you to tell me more?
From the King himself I shall learn the whole story.
But how the best to welcome my honored lord   600
I shall take pains when he comes back — For what
Is a kinder light for a woman to see than this,
To open the gates to her man come back from war
When God has saved him? Tell this to my husband,
To come with all speed, the city's darling;
May he returning find a wife as loyal
As when he left her, watchdog of the house,
Good to *him* but fierce to the ill-intentioned,
And in all other things as ever, having destroyed
No seal or pledge at all in the length of time.   610
I know no pleasure with another man, no scandal,
More than I know how to dye metal red.
Such is my boast, bearing a load of truth,
A boast that need not disgrace a noble wife.

(*Exit.*)

LEADER: Thus has she spoken; if you take her meaning,
Only a specious tale to shrewd interpreters.
But do you, herald, tell me; I ask after Menelaus
Whether he will, returning safe preserved,
Come back with you, our land's loved master.
HERALD: I am not able to speak the lovely falsehood   620
To profit you, my friends, for any stretch of time.
LEADER: But if only the true tidings could be also good!
It is hard to hide a division of good and true.

HERALD: The prince is vanished out of the Greek fleet,
Himself and ship. I speak no lie.
LEADER: Did he put forth first in the sight of all from Troy,
Or a storm that troubled all sweep him apart?
HERALD: You have hit the target like a master archer,
Told succinctly a long tale of sorrow.
LEADER: Did the rumors current among the remaining ships   630
Represent him as alive or dead?
HERALD: No one knows so as to tell for sure
Except the sun who nurses the breeds of earth.
LEADER: Tell me how the storm came on the host of ships
Through the divine anger, and how it ended.
HERALD: Day of good news should not be fouled by tongue
That tells ill news. To each god his season.
When, despair in his face, a messenger brings to a town
The hated news of a fallen army —   640
One general wound to the city and many men
Outcast, outcursed, from many homes
By the double whip which War is fond of,
Doom with a bloody spear in either hand,
One carrying such a pack of grief could well
Recite this hymn of the Furies at your asking.
But when our cause is saved and a messenger of good
Comes to a city glad with festivity,
How am I to mix good news with bad, recounting
The storm that meant God's anger on the Greeks?   650
For they swore together, those inveterate enemies,
Fire and sea, and proved their alliance, destroying
The unhappy troops of Argos.
In night arose ill-waved evil,
Ships on each other the blasts from Thrace
Crashed colliding, which butting with horns in the violence
Of big wind and rattle of rain were gone
To nothing, whirled all ways by a wicked shepherd.
But when there came up the shining light of the sun
We saw the Aegean sea flowering with corpses
Of Greek men and their ships' wreckage.   660
But for us, our ship was not damaged,
Whether someone snatched it away or begged it off,
Some god, not a man, handling the tiller;
And Saving Fortune was willing to sit upon our ship
So that neither at anchor we took the tilt of waves
Nor ran to splinters on the crag-bound coast.
But then having thus escaped death on the sea,

In the white day, not trusting our fortune,
We pastured this new trouble upon our thoughts,
The fleet being battered, the sailors weary,   670
And now if any of *them* still draw breath,
They are thinking no doubt of us as being lost
And we are thinking of them as being lost.
May the best happen. As for Menelaus
The first guess and most likely is a disaster.
But still — if any ray of sun detects him
Alive, with living eyes, by the plan of Zeus
Not yet resolved to annul the race completely,
There is some hope then that he will return home.
So much you have heard. Know that it is the truth.   680

(*Exit.*)

CHORUS: Who was it named her thus
   In all ways appositely
   Unless it was Someone whom we do not see,
   Fore-knowing fate
   And plying an accurate tongue?
   Helen, bride of spears and conflict's
   Focus, who as was befitting
   Proved a hell to ships and men,
   Hell to her country, sailing
   Away from delicately-sumptuous curtains,   690
   Away on the wind of a giant Zephyr,
   And shielded hunters mustered many
   On the vanished track of the oars,
   Oars beached on the leafy
   Banks of a Trojan river
   For the sake of bloody war.

   But on Troy was thrust a marring marriage
   By the Wrath that working to an end exacts   700
   In time a price from guests
   Who dishonored their host
   And dishonored Zeus of the Hearth,
   From those noisy celebrants
   Of the wedding hymn which fell
   To the brothers of Paris
   To sing upon that day.
   But learning this, unlearning that,
   Priam's ancestral city now   710
   Continually mourns, reviling

Paris the fatal bridegroom.
The city has had much sorrow,
Much desolation in life,
From the pitiful loss of her people.

So in his house a man might rear
A lion's cub caught from the dam
In need of suckling,
In the prelude of its life   720
Mild, gentle with children,
For old men a playmate,
Often held in the arms
Like a new-born child,
Wheedling the hand,
Fawning at belly's bidding.

But matured by time he showed
The temper of his stock and paid
Thanks for his fostering
With disaster of slaughter of sheep   730
Making an unbidden banquet
And now the house is a shambles,
Irremediable grief to its people,
Calamitous carnage;
For the pet they had fostered was sent
By God as a priest of Ruin.

So I would say there came
To the city of Troy
A notion of windless calm,
Delicate adornment of riches,   740
Soft shooting of the eyes and flower
Of desire that stings the fancy.
But swerving aside she achieved
A bitter end to her marriage,
Ill guest and ill companion,
Hurled upon Priam's sons, convoyed
By Zeus, patron of guest and host,
Dark angel dowered with tears.

Long current among men an old saying   750
Runs that a man's prosperity
When grown to greatness
Comes to the birth, does not die childless —

His good luck breeds for his house
Distress that shall not be appeased.
I only, apart from the others,
Hold that the unrighteous action
Breeds true to its kind,
Leaves its own children behind it.   760
But the lot of a righteous house
Is a fair offspring always.

Ancient self-glory is accustomed
To bear to light in the evil sort of **men**
A new self-glory and madness,
Which sometime or sometime finds
The appointed hour for its birth,
And born therewith is the Spirit, intractaᴗle, unholy, irresistible.
The reckless lust that brings black Doom upon the house,   770
A child that is like its parents.

But Honest Dealing is clear
Shining in smoky homes,
Honors the god-fearing life.
Mansions gilded by filth of hands she leaves,
Turns her eyes elsewhere, visits the innocent house,
Not respecting the power
Of wealth mis-stamped with approval,   780
But guides all to the goal.

(*Enter* AGAMEMNON *and* CASSANDRA *on chariots.*)

CHORUS: Come then my King, stormer of Troy,
   Offspring of Atreus,
   How shall I hail you, how give you honor
   Neither overshooting nor falling short
     Of the measure of homage?
   There are many who honor appearance too **much**
   Passing the bounds that are right.
   To condole with the unfortunate man   790
   Each one is ready but the bite of the grief
     Never goes through to the heart.
   And they join in rejoicing, affecting to share **it**,
   Forcing their face to a smile.
   But he who is shrewd to shepherd his sheep
   Will fail not to notice the eyes of a man
   Which seem to be loyal but lie,
     Fawning with watery friendship.

Even you, in my thought, when you marshalled the troops
For Helen's sake, I will not hide it,   800
Made a harsh and ugly picture,
Holding badly the tiller of reason,
Paying with the death of men
   Ransom for a willing whore.
But now, not unfriendly, not superficially,
I offer my service, well-doers' welcome.
In time you will learn by inquiry
Who has done rightly, who transgressed
   In the work of watching the city.
AGAMEMNON: First to Argos and the country's gods   810
My fitting salutations, who have aided me
To return and in the justice which I exacted
From Priam's city. Hearing the unspoken case
The gods unanimously had cast their vote
Into the bloody urn for the massacre of Troy;
But to the opposite urn
Hope came, dangled her hand, but did no more.
Smoke marks even now the city's capture.
Whirlwinds of doom are alive, the dying ashes
Spread on the air the fat savor of wealth.   820
For these things we must pay some memorable return
To Heaven, having exacted enormous vengeance
For wife-rape; for a woman
The Argive monster ground a city to powder,
Sprung from a wooden horse, shield-wielding folk,
Launching a leap at the setting of the Pleiads,
Jumping the ramparts, a ravening lion,
Lapped its fill of the kingly blood.
To the gods I have drawn out this overture
But as for your concerns, I bear them in my mind   830
And say the same, you have me in agreement.
To few of men does it belong by nature
To congratulate their friends unenviously,
For a sullen poison fastens on the heart,
Doubling the pain of a man with this disease;
He feels the weight of his own griefs and when
He sees another's prosperity he groans.
I speak with knowledge, being well acquainted
With the mirror of comradeship — ghost of a shadow
Were those who seemed to be so loyal to me.   840
Only Odysseus, who sailed against his will,
Proved, when yoked with me, a ready tracehorse;

I speak of him not knowing if he is alive.
But for what concerns the city and the gods
Appointing public debates in full assembly
We shall consult. That which is well already
We shall take steps to ensure it remain well.
But where there is need of medical remedies,
By applying benevolent cautery or surgery
We shall try to deflect the dangers of disease. 850
But now, entering the halls where stands my hearth,
First I shall make salutation to the gods
Who sent me a far journey and have brought me back.
And may my victory not leave my side.

(*Enter* CLYTEMNESTRA, *followed by women slaves carrying purple tapestries.*)

CLYTEMNESTRA: Men of the city, you the aged of Argos,
I shall feel no shame to describe to you my love
Towards my husband. Shyness in all of us
Wears thin with time. Here are the facts first hand.
I will tell you of my own unbearable life
I led so long as this man was at Troy. 860
For first that the woman separate from her man
Should sit alone at home is extreme cruelty,
Hearing so many malignant rumors — First
Comes one, and another comes after, bad news to worse,
Clamor of grief to the house. If Agamemnon
Had had so many wounds as those reported
Which poured home through the pipes of hearsay, then —
Then he would be gashed fuller than a net has holes!
And if only he had died . . . as often as rumor told us,
He would be like the giant in the legend,
Three-bodied. Dying once for every body 870
He should have by now three blankets of earth above him —
All that above him; I care not how deep the mattress under!
Such are the malignant rumors thanks to which
They have often seized me against my will and undone
The loop of a rope from my neck.
And this is why our son is not standing here,
The guarantee of your pledges and mine,
As he should be, Orestes. Do not wonder;
He is being brought up by a friendly ally and host, 880
Strophius the Phocian, who warned me in advance
Of dubious troubles, both your risks at Troy
And the anarchy of shouting mobs that might

Overturn policy, for it is born in men
To kick the man who is down.
This is not a disingenuous excuse.
For me the outrushing wells of weeping are dried up,
There is no drop left in them.
My eyes are sore from sitting late at nights
Weeping for you and for the baffled beacons, 890
Never lit up. And, when I slept, in dreams
I have been waked by the thin whizz of a buzzing
Gnat, seeing more horrors fasten on you
Than could take place in the mere time of my dream.
Having endured all this, now, with unsorrowed heart
I would hail this man as the watchdog of the farm,
Forestay that saves the ship, pillar that props
The lofty roof, appearance of an only son
To a father or of land to sailors past their hope,
The loveliest day to see after the storm, 900
Gush of well-water for the thirsty traveller.
Such are the metaphors I think befit him,
But envy be absent. Many misfortunes already
We have endured. But now, dear head, come down
Out of that car, not placing upon the ground
Your foot, O King, the foot that trampled Troy.
Why are you waiting, slaves, to whom the task is assigned
To spread the pavement of his path with tapestries?
At once, at once let his way be strewn with purple 910
That Justice lead him toward his unexpected home.
The rest a mind, not overcome by sleep,
Will arrange rightly, with God's help, as destined.
AGAMEMNON: Daughter of Leda, guardian of my house,
You have spoken in proportion to my absence.
You have drawn your speech out long. Duly to praise me,
That is a duty to be performed by others.
And further — do not by women's methods make me
Effeminate nor in barbarian fashion
Gape ground-grovelling acclamations at me 920
Nor strewing my path with cloths make it invidious.
It is the gods should be honored in this way.
But being mortal to tread embroidered beauty
For me is no way without fear.
I tell you to honor me as a man, not god.
Footcloths are very well; embroidered stuffs
Are stuff for gossip. And not to think unwisely
Is the greatest gift of God. Call happy only him

Who has ended his life in sweet prosperity.
I have spoken. This thing I could not do with confidence.   930
CLYTEMNESTRA: Tell me now, according to your judgment.
AGAMEMNON: I tell you you shall not override my judgment.
CLYTEMNESTRA: Supposing you had feared something. . . .
Could you have vowed to God to do this thing?
AGAMEMNON: Yes. If an expert had prescribed that vow.
CLYTEMNESTRA: And how would Priam have acted in your place?
AGAMEMNON: He would have trod the cloths, I think, for certain.
CLYTEMNESTRA: Then do not flinch before the blame of men.
AGAMEMNON: The voice of the multitude is very strong.
CLYTEMNESTRA: But the man none envy is not enviable.
AGAMEMNON: It is not a woman's part to love disputing.   940
CLYTEMNESTRA: But it is a conqueror's part to yield upon occasion.
AGAMEMNON: You think such victory worth fighting for?
CLYTEMNESTRA: Give way. Consent to let me have the mastery.
AGAMEMNON: Well, if such is your wish, let someone quickly loose
My vassal sandals, underlings of my feet,
And stepping on these sea-purples may no god
Shoot me from far with the envy of his eye.
Great shame it is to ruin my house and spoil
The wealth of costly weavings with my feet.
But of this matter enough. This stranger woman here   950
Take in with kindness. The man who is a gentle master
God looks on from far off complacently.
For no one of his will bears the slave's yoke.
This woman, of many riches being the chosen
Flower, gift of the soldiers, has come with me.
But since I have been prevailed on by your words
I will go to my palace home, treading on purples.

> (*He dismounts from the chariot and begins to walk up the tapestried path. During the following speech he enters the palace.*)

CLYTEMNESTRA: There is the sea and who shall drain it dry? It breeds
Its wealth in silver of plenty of purple gushing
And ever-renewed, the dyeings of our garments.   960
The house has its store of these by God's grace, King.
This house is ignorant of poverty
And I would have vowed a pavement of many garments
Had the palace oracle enjoined that vow
Thereby to contrive a ransom for his life.
For while there is root, foliage comes to the house
Spreading a tent of shade against the Dog Star.

So now that you have reached your hearth and home
You prove a miracle — advent of warmth in winter;
And further this — even in the time of heat
When God is fermenting wine from the bitter grape,   970
Even then it is cool in the house if only
Its master walk at home, a grown man, ripe.
O Zeus the Ripener, ripen these my prayers;
Your part it is to make the ripe fruit fall.

    (*She enters the palace.*)

CHORUS: Why, why at the doors
    Of my fore-seeing heart
    Does this terror keep beating its wings?
    And my song play the prophet
    Unbidden, unhired —
    Which I cannot spit out   980
    Like the enigmas of dreams
    Nor plausible confidence
    Sit on the throne of my mind?
    It is long time since
    The cables let down from the stern
    Were chafed by the sand when the sea-
        faring army started for Troy.

    And I learn with my eyes
    And witness myself their return;
    But the hymn without lyre goes up,   990
    The dirge of the Avenging Fiend,
    In the depths of my self-taught heart
    Which has lost its dear
    Possession of the strength of hope.
    But my guts and my heart
    Are not idle which seethe with the waves
    Of trouble nearing its hour.
    But I pray that these thoughts
    May fall out not as I think
        And not be fulfilled in the end.   1000

    Truly when health grows much
    It respects not limit; for disease,
    Its neighbor in the next door room,
    Presses upon it.
    A man's life, crowding sail,
    Strikes on the blind reef:

But if caution in advance
Jettison part of the cargo
With the derrick of due proportion,   1010
The whole house does not sink,
Though crammed with a weight of woe
The hull does not go under.
The abundant bounty of God
And his gifts from the year's furrows
 Drive the famine back.

But when upon the ground there has fallen once
The black blood of a man's death,   1020
Who shall summon it back by incantations?
Even Asclepius who had the art
To fetch the dead to life, even to him
Zeus put a provident end.
But, if of the heaven-sent fates
One did not check the other,
Cancel the other's advantage,
My heart would outrun my tongue
In pouring out these fears.
But now it mutters in the dark,   1030
Embittered, no way hoping
To unravel a scheme in time
 From a burning mind.

 (CLYTEMNESTRA *appears in the door of the palace.*)

CLYTEMNESTRA: Go in too, you; I speak to you, Cassandra,
 Since God in his clemency has put you in this house
 To share our holy water, standing with many slaves
 Beside the altar that protects the house,
 Step down from the car there, do not be overproud.
 Heracles himself they say was once   1040
 Sold, and endured to eat the bread of slavery.
 But should such a chance inexorably fall,
 There is much advantage in masters who have long been rich.
 Those who have reaped a crop they never expected
 Are in all things hard on their slaves and overstep the line.
 From us you will have the treatment of tradition.
LEADER OF CHORUS: You, it is you she has addressed, and clearly.
 Caught as you are in these predestined toils
 Obey her if you can. But should you disobey ...
CLYTEMNESTRA: If she has more than the gibberish of the
 swallow,   1050

As unintelligible barbaric speech,
I hope to read her mind, persuade her reason.
LEADER: As things now stand for you, she says the best.
Obey her; leave that car and follow her.
CLYTEMNESTRA: I have no leisure to waste out here, outside the door.
Before the hearth in the middle of my house
The victims stand already, wait the knife.
You, if you will obey me, waste no time.
But if you cannot understand my language —   1060

> (*to* CHORUS LEADER)

You make it plain to her with the brute and voiceless hand.
LEADER: The stranger seems to need a clear interpreter.
She bears herself like a wild beast newly captured.
CLYTEMNESTRA: The fact is she is mad, she listens to evil thoughts,
Who has come here leaving a city newly captured
Without experience how to bear the bridle
So as not to waste her strength in foam and blood.
I will not spend more words to be ignored.

> (*She re-enters the palace.*)

CHORUS: But I, for I pity her, will not be angry.
Obey, unhappy woman. Leave this car.   1070
Yield to your fate. Put on the untried yoke.
CASSANDRA: Apollo! Apollo!
CHORUS: Why do you cry like this upon Apollo?
He is not the kind of god that calls for dirges.
CASSANDRA: Apollo! Apollo!
CHORUS: Once more her funereal cries invoke the god
Who has no place at the scene of lamentation.
CASSANDRA: Apollo! Apollo!   1080
God of the Ways! My destroyer!
Destroyed again — and this time utterly!
CHORUS: She seems about to predict her own misfortunes.
The gift of the god endures, even in a slave's mind.
CASSANDRA: Apollo! Apollo!
God of the Ways! My destroyer!
Where? To what house? Where, where have you brought me?
CHORUS: To the house of the sons of Atreus. If you do not know it,
I will tell you so. You will not find it false.
CASSANDRA: No, no, but to a god-hated, but to an accomplice   1090
In much kin-killing, murdering nooses,
Man-shambles, a floor asperged with blood.
CHORUS: The stranger seems like a hound with a keen scent,
Is picking up a trail that leads to murder.

CASSANDRA: Clues! I have clues! Look! They are these.
  These wailing, these children, butchery of children;
  Roasted flesh, a father sitting to dinner.
CHORUS: Of your prophetic fame we have heard before
  But in this matter prophets are not required.
CASSANDRA: What is she doing? What is she planning?   1100
  What is this new great sorrow?
  Great crime . . . within here . . . planning
  Unendurable to his folk, impossible
  Ever to be cured. For help
    Stands far distant.
CHORUS: This reference I cannot catch. But the children
  I recognized; that refrain is hackneyed.
CASSANDRA: Damned, damned, bringing this work to completion —
  Your husband who shared your bed
  To bathe him, to cleanse him, and then —
  How shall I tell of the end?
    The end comes hand over hand   1110
    Grasping in greed.
CHORUS: Not yet do I understand. After her former riddles
  Now I am baffled by these dim pronouncements.
CASSANDRA: Ah God, the vision! God, God, the vision!
  A net, is it? Net of Hell!
  But herself is the net; shared bed; shares murder.
  O let the pack ever-hungering after the family
  Howl for the unholy ritual, howl for the victim.
CHORUS: What black Spirit is this you call upon the house —
  To raise aloft her cries? Your speech does not lighten me.   1120
  Into my heart runs back the blood
  Yellow as when for men by the spear fallen
  The blood ebbs out with the rays of the setting life
  And death strides quickly.
CASSANDRA: Quick! Be on your guard! The bull —
  Keep him clear of the cow.
  Caught with a trick, the black horn's point,
  She strikes. He falls; lies in the water.
  Murder; a trick in a bath. I tell what I see.
CHORUS: I would not claim to be expert in oracles   1130
  But these, as I deduce, portend disaster.
  Do men ever get a good answer from oracles?
  No. It is only through disaster
  That their garrulous craft brings home
  The meaning of the prophet's panic.
CASSANDRA: And for me also, for me, chance ill-destined!
  My own now I lament, pour into the cup my own.

Where is this you have brought me in my misery?
Unless to die as well. What else is meant?
CHORUS: You are mad, mad, carried away by the god,   1140
Raising the dirge, the tuneless
Tune, for yourself. Like the tawny
Unsatisfied singer from her luckless heart
Lamenting 'Itys, Itys,' the nightingale
Lamenting a life luxuriant with grief.
CASSANDRA: Oh the lot of the songful nightingale!
The gods enclosed her in a winged body,
Gave her a sweet and tearless passing.
But for me remains the two-edged cutting blade.
CHORUS: From whence these rushing and God-inflicted   1150
Profitless pains?
Why shape with your sinister crying
The piercing hymn — fear-piercing?
How can you know the evil-worded landmarks
   On the prophetic path?
CASSANDRA: Oh the wedding, the wedding of Paris — death to his
   people!
O river Scamander, water drunk by my fathers!
When I was young, alas, upon your beaches
I was brought up and cared for.
But now it is the River of Wailing and the banks of Hell   1160
That shall hear my prophecy soon.
CHORUS: What is this clear speech, too clear?
A child could understand it.
I am bitten with fangs that draw blood
By the misery of your cries,
Cries harrowing the heart.
CASSANDRA: Oh trouble on trouble of a city lost, lost utterly!
My father's sacrifices before the towers,
Much killing of cattle and sheep,
No cure — availed not at all   1170
To prevent the coming of what came to Troy,
And I, my brain on fire, shall soon enter the trap.
CHORUS: This speech accords with the former.
What god, malicious, over-heavy, persistently pressing,
Drives you to chant of these lamentable
Griefs with death their burden?
But I cannot see the end.

   (CASSANDRA *now steps down from the car.*)

CASSANDRA: The oracle now no longer from behind veils
Will be peeping forth like a newly-wedded bride;

But I can feel it like a fresh wind swoop   1180
And rush in the face of the dawn and, wave-like, wash
Against the sun a vastly greater grief
Than this one. I shall speak no more conundrums.
And bear me witness, pacing me, that I
Am trailing on the scent of ancient wrongs.
For this house here a choir never deserts,
Chanting together ill. For they mean ill,
And to puff up their arrogance they have drunk
Men's blood, this band of revellers that haunts the house,
Hard to be rid of, fiends that attend the family.   1190
Established in its rooms they hymn their hymn
Of that original sin, abhor in turn
The adultery that proved a brother's ruin.
A miss? Or do my arrows hit the mark?
Or am I a quack prophet who knocks at doors, a babbler?
Give me your oath, confess I have the facts,
The ancient history of this house's crimes.

LEADER: And how could an oath's assurance, however finely assured,
    Turn out a remedy? I wonder, though, that you
    Being brought up overseas, of another tongue,   1200
    Should hit on the whole tale as if you had been standing by.

CASSANDRA: Apollo the prophet set me to prophesy.

LEADER: Was he, although a god, struck by desire?

CASSANDRA: Till now I was ashamed to tell that story.

LEADER: Yes. Good fortune keeps us all fastidious.

CASSANDRA: He wrestled hard upon me, panting love.

LEADER: And did you come, as they do, to child-getting?

CASSANDRA: No. I agreed to him. And I cheated him.

LEADER: Were you already possessed by the mystic art?

CASSANDRA: Already I was telling the townsmen all their future
    suffering.   1210

LEADER: Then how did you escape the doom of Apollo's anger?

CASSANDRA: I did not escape. No one ever believed me.

LEADER: Yet to us your words seem worthy of belief.

CASSANDRA: Oh misery, misery!
    Again comes on me the terrible labor of true
    Prophecy, dizzying prelude; distracts. . . .
    Do you see these who sit before the house,
    Children, like the shapes of dreams?
    Children who seem to have been killed by their kinsfolk,
    Filling their hands with meat, flesh of themselves,   1220
    Guts and entrails, handfuls of lament —
    Clear what they hold — the same their father tasted.

For this I declare someone is plotting vengeance —
A lion? Lion but coward, that lurks in bed,
Good watchdog truly against the lord's return —
My lord, for I must bear the yoke of serfdom.
Leader of the ships, overturner of Troy,
He does not know what plots the accursed hound
With the licking tongue and the pricked-up ear will plan
In the manner of a lurking doom, in an evil hour.   1230
A daring criminal! Female murders male.
What monster could provide her with a title?
An amphisbaena or hag of the sea who dwells
In rocks to ruin sailors —
A raving mother of death who breathes against her folk
War to the finish. Listen to her shout of triumph,
Who shirks no horrors, like men in a rout of battle.
And yet she poses as glad at their return.
If you distrust my words, what does it matter?
That which will come will come. You too will soon stand here 1240
And admit with pity that I spoke too truly.
LEADER: Thyestes' dinner of his children's meat
  I understood and shuddered, and fear grips me
  To hear the truth, not framed in parables.
  But hearing the rest I am thrown out of my course.
CASSANDRA: It is Agamemnon's death I tell you you shall witness.
LEADER: Stop! Provoke no evil. Quiet your mouth!
CASSANDRA: The god who gives me words is here no healer.
LEADER: Not if this shall be so. But may some chance avert it.
CASSANDRA: *You* are praying. But others are busy with murder.   1250
LEADER: What man is he promotes this terrible thing?
CASSANDRA: Indeed you have missed my drift by a wide margin!
LEADER: But I do not understand the assassin's method.
CASSANDRA: And yet too well I know the speech of Greece!
LEADER: So does Delphi but the replies are hard.
CASSANDRA: Ah what a fire it is! It comes upon me.
  Apollo, Wolf-Destroyer, pity, pity. . . .
  It is the two-foot lioness who beds
  Beside a wolf, the noble lion away,
  It is she will kill me. Brewing a poisoned cup   1260
  She will mix my punishment too in the angry draught
  And boasts, sharpening the dagger for her husband,
  To pay back murder for my bringing here.
  Why then do I wear these mockeries of myself,
  The wand and the prophet's garland round my neck?
  My hour is coming — but you shall perish first.

Destruction! Scattered thus you give me my revenge;
Go and enrich some other woman with ruin.
See: Apollo himself is stripping me
Of my prophetic gear, who has looked on   1276
When in this dress I have been a laughing-stock
To friends and foes alike, and to no purpose;
They call me crazy, like a fortune-teller,
A poor starved beggar-woman — and I bore it.
And now the prophet undoing his prophetess
Has brought me to this final darkness.
Instead of my father's altar the executioner's block
Waits me the victim, red with my hot blood.
But the gods will not ignore me as I die.
One will come after to avenge my death,   1280
A matricide, a murdered father's champion.
Exile and tramp and outlaw he will come back
To gable the family house of fatal crime;
His father's outstretched corpse shall lead him home.
Why need I then lament so pitifully?
For now that I have seen the town of Troy
Treated as she was treated, while her captors
Come to their reckoning thus by the gods' verdict,
I will go in and have the courage to die.   1290
Look, these gates are the gates of Death. I greet them.
And I pray that I may meet a deft and mortal stroke
So that without a struggle I may close
My eyes and my blood ebb in easy death.
LEADER: Oh woman very unhappy and very wise,
Your speech was long. But if in sober truth
You know your fate, why like an ox that the gods
Drive, do you walk so bravely to the altar?
CASSANDRA: There is no escape, strangers. No; not by postponement.
LEADER: But the last moment has the privilege of hope.   1300
CASSANDRA: The day is here. Little should I gain by flight.
LEADER: This patience of yours comes from a brave soul.
CASSANDRA: A happy man is never paid that compliment.
LEADER: But to die with credit graces a mortal man.
CASSANDRA: Oh my father! You and your noble sons!

(She approaches the door, then suddenly recoils.)

LEADER: What is it? What is the fear that drives you back?
CASSANDRA: Faugh.
LEADER: Why faugh? Or is this some hallucination?
CASSANDRA: These walls breathe out a death that drips with blood.

LEADER: Not so. It is only the smell of the sacrifice.   1310
CASSANDRA: It is like a breath out of a charnel-house.
LEADER: You think our palace burns odd incense then!
CASSANDRA: But I will go to lament among the dead
    My lot and Agamemnon's. Enough of life!
    Strangers,
    I am not afraid like a bird afraid of a bush
    But witness you my words after my death
    When a woman dies in return for me a woman
    And a man falls for a man with a wicked wife.
    I ask this service, being about to die.   1320
LEADER: Alas, I pity you for the death you have foretold.
CASSANDRA: One more speech I have; I do not wish to raise
    The dirge for my own self. But to the sun I pray
    In face of his last light that my avengers
    May make my murderers pay for this my death,
    Death of a woman slave, an easy victim.

      (*She enters the palace.*)

LEADER: Ah the fortunes of men! When they go well
    A shadow sketch would match them, and in ill-fortune
    The dab of a wet sponge destroys the drawing.
    It is not myself but the life of man I pity.   1330
CHORUS: Prosperity in all men cries
    For more prosperity. Even the owner
    Of the finger-pointed-at palace never shuts
    His door against her, saying "Come no more."
    So to our king the blessed gods had granted
    To take the town of Priam, and heaven-favored
    He reaches home. But now if for former bloodshed
    He must pay blood
    And dying for the dead shall cause
      Other deaths in atonement   1340
    What man could boast he was born
      Secure, who heard this story?
AGAMEMNON: (*within*) Oh! I am struck a mortal blow — within!
LEADER: Silence! Listen. Who calls out, wounded with a mortal
    stroke?
AGAMEMNON: Again — the second blow — I am struck again.
LEADER: You heard the king cry out. I think the deed is done.
    Let us see if we can concert some sound proposal.
2ND OLD MAN: Well, I will tell you my opinion —
    Raise an alarm, summon the folk to the palace.

3RD OLD MAN: I say burst in with all speed possible,   1350
  Convict them of the deed while still the sword is wet.
4TH OLD MAN: And I am partner to some such suggestion.
  I am for taking some course. No time to dawdle.
5TH OLD MAN: The case is plain. This is but the beginning.
  They are going to set up dictatorship in the state.
6TH OLD MAN: We are wasting time. The assassins tread to earth
  The decencies of delay and give their hands no sleep.
7TH OLD MAN: I do not know what plan I could hit on to propose.
  The man who acts is in the position to plan.
8TH OLD MAN: So I think, too, for I am at a loss   1360
  To raise the dead man up again with words.
9TH OLD MAN: Then to stretch out our life shall we yield thus
  To the rule of these profaners of the house?
10TH OLD MAN: It is not to be endured. To die is better.
  Death is more comfortable than tyranny.
11TH OLD MAN: And are we on the evidence of groans
  Going to give oracle that the prince is dead?
12TH OLD MAN: We must know the facts for sure and *then* be angry.
  Guesswork is not the same as certain knowledge.
LEADER: Then all of you back me and approve this plan —   1370
  To ascertain how it is with Agamemnon.

    (*The doors of the palace open, revealing the bodies of* AGA-
    MEMNON *and* CASSANDRA. CLYTEMNESTRA *stands above them.*)

CLYTEMNESTRA: Much having been said before to fit the moment,
  To say the opposite now will not outface me.
  How else could one serving hate upon the hated,
  Thought to be friends, hang high the nets of doom
  To preclude all leaping out?
  For me I have long been training for this match,
  I tried a fall and won — a victory overdue.
  I stand here where I struck, above my victims;
  So I contrived it — this I will not deny —   1380
  That he could neither fly nor ward off death;
  Inextricable like a net for fishes
  I cast about him a vicious wealth of raiment
  And struck him twice and with two groans he loosed
  His limbs beneath him, and upon him fallen
  I deal him the third blow to the God beneath the earth,
  To the safe keeper of the dead a votive gift,
  And with that he spits his life out where he lies
  And smartly spouting blood he sprays me with   1390

The somber drizzle of bloody dew and I
Rejoice no less than in God's gift of rain
The crops are glad when the ear of corn gives birth.
These things being so, you, elders of Argos,
Rejoice if rejoice you will. Mine is the glory.
And if I could pay this corpse his due libation
I should be right to pour it and more than right;
With so many horrors this man mixed and filled
The bowl — and, coming home, has drained the draught himself.

LEADER: Your speech astonishes us. This brazen boast
Above the man who was your king and husband! 1400

CLYTEMNESTRA: You challenge me as a woman without foresight
But I with unflinching heart to you who know
Speak. And you, whether you will praise or blame,
It makes no matter. Here lies Agamemnon,
My husband, dead, the work of this right hand,
An honest workman. There you have the facts.

CHORUS: Woman, what poisoned
Herb of the earth have you tasted
Or potion of the flowing sea
To undertake this killing and the people's curses?
You threw down, you cut off — The people will cast you out, 1410
Black abomination to the town.

CLYTEMNESTRA: Now your verdict — in my case — is exile
And to have the people's hatred, the public curses,
Though then in no way you opposed this man
Who carelessly, as if it were a head of sheep
Out of the abundance of his fleecy flocks,
Sacrificed his own daughter, to me the dearest
Fruit of travail, charm for the Thracian winds.
He was the one to have banished from this land,
Pay off the pollution. But when you hear what I 1420
Have done, you judge severely. But I warn you —
Threaten me on the understanding that I am ready
For two alternatives — Win by force the right
To rule me, but, if God brings about the contrary,
Late in time you will have to learn self-discipline.

CHORUS: You are high in the thoughts,
You speak extravagant things,
After the soiling murder your crazy heart
Fancies your forehead with a smear of blood.
Unhonored, unfriended, you must
Pay for a blow with a blow. 1430

CLYTEMNESTRA: Listen then to this — the sanction of my oaths:
By the Justice totting up my child's atonement,

By the Avenging Doom and Fiend to whom I killed this man,
For me hope walks not in the rooms of fear
So long as my fire is lit upon my hearth
By Aegisthus, loyal to me as he was before.
The man who outraged me lies here,
The darling of each courtesan at Troy,
And here with him is the prisoner clairvoyante,   1440
The fortune-teller that he took to bed,
Who shares his bed as once his bench on shipboard,
A loyal mistress. Both have their deserts.
He lies so, and she who like a swan
Sang her last dying lament
Lies his lover, and the sight contributes
An appetiser to my own bed's pleasure.
CHORUS: Ah would some quick death come not overpainful,
Not overlong on the sickbed,
Establishing in us the ever-   1450
Lasting unending sleep now that our guardian
Has fallen, the kindest of men,
Who suffering much for a woman
By a woman has lost his life.
      O Helen, insane, being one,
      One to have destroyed so many
      And many souls under Troy,
      Now is your work complete, blossomed not for oblivion,
      Unfading stain of blood. Here now, if in any home,   1460
      Is Discord, here is a man's deep-rooted ruin.
CLYTEMNESTRA: Do not pray for the portion of death
      Weighed down by these things, do not turn
      Your anger on Helen as destroyer of men,
      One woman destroyer of many
      Lives of Greek men,
         A hurt that cannot be healed.
CHORUS: O Evil Spirit, falling on the family,
      On the two sons of Atreus and using
      Two sisters in heart as your tools,   1470
      A power that bites to the heart —
      See on the body
      Perched like a raven he gloats
      Harshly croaking his hymn.
CLYTEMNESTRA: Ah, now you have amended your lips' opinion,
      Calling upon this family's three times gorged
      Genius — demon who breeds
      Blood-hankering lust in the belly:
      Before the old sore heals, new pus collects.   1480

CHORUS: It is a great spirit — great —
  You tell of, harsh in anger,
  A ghastly tale, alas,
  Of unsatisfied disaster
  Brought by Zeus, by Zeus,
  Cause and worker of all.
  For without Zeus what comes to pass among us?
  Which of these things is outside Providence?
    O my king, my king,
    How shall I pay you in tears,   1490
    Speak my affection in words?
    You lie in that spider's web,
    In a desecrating death breathe out your life,
    Lie ignominiously
    Defeated by a crooked death
    And the two-edged cleaver's stroke.

CLYTEMNESTRA: You say this is my work — mine?
  Do not cozen yourself that I am Agamemnon's wife.
  Masquerading as the wife   1500
  Of the corpse there the old sharp-witted Genius
  Of Atreus who gave the cruel banquet
  Has paid with a grown man's life
  The due for children dead.

CHORUS: That you are not guilty of
  This murder who will attest?
  No, but you may have been abetted
  By some ancestral Spirit of Revenge.
  Wading a millrace of the family's blood   1510
  The black Manslayer forces a forward path
  To make the requital at last
  For the eaten children, the blood-clot cold with time.
    O my king, my king,
    How shall I pay you in tears,
    Speak my affection in words?
    You lie in that spider's web,
    In a desecrating death breathe out your life,
    Lie ignominiously
    Defeated by a crooked death
    And the two-edged cleaver's stroke.   1520

CLYTEMNESTRA: Did he not, too, contrive a crooked
  Horror for the house? My child by him,
  Shoot that I raised, much-wept-for Iphigeneia,
  He treated her like this;
  So suffering like this he need not make

Any great brag in Hell having paid with death
Dealt by the sword for work of his own beginning.

CHORUS: I am at a loss for thought, I lack   1530
  All nimble counsel as to where
  To turn when the house is falling.
  I fear the house-collapsing crashing
  Blizzard of blood — of which these drops are earnest.
  Now is Destiny sharpening her justice
  On other whetstones for a new infliction.
    O earth, earth, if only you had received me
    Before I saw this man lie here as if in bed
      In a bath lined with silver.   1540
    Who will bury him? Who will keen him?
    Will you, having killed your own husband,
    Dare now to lament him
    And after great wickedness make
      Unamending amends to his ghost?
    And who above this godlike hero's grave
    Pouring praises and tears
    Will grieve with a genuine heart?   1550

CLYTEMNESTRA: It is not your business to attend to that.
  By my hand he fell low, lies low and dead,
  And I shall bury him low down in the earth,
  And his household need not weep him
  For Iphigeneia his daughter
  Tenderly, as is right,
  Will meet her father at the rapid ferry of sorrows,
  Put her arms round him and kiss him!

CHORUS: Reproach answers reproach,   1560
  It is hard to decide,
  The catcher is caught, the killer pays for his kill.
  But the law abides while Zeus abides enthroned
  That the wrongdoer suffers. That is established.
  Who could expel from the house the seed of the
    Curse?
  The race is soldered in sockets of Doom and
    Vengeance.

CLYTEMNESTRA: In this you say what is right and the will of God.
  But for my part I am ready to make a contract
  With the Evil Genius of the House of Atreus
  To accept what has been till now, hard though it is,   1570
  But that for the future he shall leave this house
  And wear away some other stock with deaths
  Imposed among themselves. Of my possessions

A small part will suffice if only I
Can rid these walls of the mad exchange of murder.

(*Enter* AEGISTHUS, *followed by soldiers.*)

AEGISTHUS: O welcome light of a justice-dealing day!
From now on I will say that the gods, avenging men,
Look down from above on the crimes of earth,
Seeing as I do in woven robes of the Furies   1580
This man lying here — a sight to warm my heart —
Paying for the crooked violence of his father.
For his father Atreus, when he ruled the country,
Because his power was challenged, hounded out
From state and home his own brother Thyestes.
My father — let me be plain — was this Thyestes,
Who later came back home a suppliant,
There, miserable, found so much asylum
As not to die on the spot, stain the ancestral floor.
But to show his hospitality godless Atreus   1590
Gave him an eager if not a loving welcome,
Pretending a day of feasting and rich meats
Served my father with his children's flesh.
The hands and feet, fingers and toes, he hid
At the bottom of the dish. My father sitting apart
Took unknowing the unrecognizable portion
And ate of a dish that has proved, as you see, expensive.
But when he knew he had eaten worse than poison
He fell back groaning, vomiting their flesh,
And invoking a hopeless doom on the sons of Pelops   1600
Kicked over the table to confirm his curse —
So may the whole race perish!
Result of this — you see this man lie here.
I stitched this murder together; it was my title.
Me the third son he left, an unweaned infant,
To share the bitterness of my father's exile.
But I grew up and Justice brought me back,
I grappled this man while still beyond his door,
Having pieced together the programme of his ruin.
So now would even death be beautiful to me   1610
Having seen Agamemnon in the nets of Justice.

LEADER: Aegisthus. I cannot respect brutality in distress.
You claim that you deliberately killed this prince
And that you alone planned this pitiful murder.
Be sure that in your turn your head shall not escape
The people's volleyed curses mixed with stones.

AEGISTHUS: Do you speak so who sit at the lower oar
    While those on the upper bench control the ship?
    Old as you are, you will find it is a heavy load
    To go to school when old to learn the lesson of tact.   1620
    For old age, too, gaol and hunger are fine
    Instructors in wisdom, second-sighted doctors.
    You have eyes. Cannot you see?
    Do not kick against the pricks. The blow will hurt you.
LEADER: You woman waiting in the house for those who return from
        battle
    While you seduce their wives! Was it you devised
    The death of a master of armies?
AEGISTHUS: And these words, too, prepare the way for tears.
    Contrast your voice with the voice of Orpheus: he
    Led all things after him bewitched with joy, but you   1630
    Having stung me with your silly yelps shall be
    Led off yourself, to prove more mild when mastered.
LEADER: Indeed! So you are now to be king of Argos,
    You who, when you had plotted the king's death,
    Did not even dare to do that thing yourself!
AEGISTHUS: No. For the trick of it was clearly woman's work.
    I was suspect, an enemy of old.
    But now I shall try with Agamemnon's wealth
    To rule the people. Any who is disobedient
    I will harness in a heavy yoke, no tracehorse work for him   1640
    Like barley-fed colt, but hateful hunger lodging
    Beside him in the dark will see his temper soften.
LEADER: Why with your cowardly soul did you yourself
    Not strike this man but left that work to a woman
    Whose presence pollutes our country and its gods?
    But Orestes — does he somewhere see the light
    That he may come back here by favor of fortune
    And kill this pair and prove the final victor?
AEGISTHUS (*summoning his guards*):
    Well, if such is your design in deeds and words, you will quickly
        learn —   1649
    Here my friends, here my guards, there is work for you at hand.
LEADER: Come then, hands on hilts, be each and all of us prepared.

    (*The old men and the guards threaten each other.*)

AEGISTHUS: Very well! I too am ready to meet death with sword in
    hand.
LEADER: We are glad you speak of dying. We accept your words for
    luck.

CLYTEMNESTRA: No, my dearest, do not so. Add no more to the train
of wrong.
To reap these many present wrongs is harvest enough of misery.
Enough of misery. Start no more. Our hands are red.
But do you, and you old men, go home and yield to fate in time,
In time before you suffer. We have acted as we had to act.
If only our afflictions now could prove enough, we should agree —
We who have been so hardly mauled in the heavy claws of the evil
god.   1660
So stands my word, a woman's if any man thinks fit to hear.
AEGISTHUS: But to think that these should thus pluck the blooms of an
idle tongue
And should throw out words like these, giving the evil god his
chance,
And should miss the path of prudence and insult their master so!
LEADER: It is not the Argive way to fawn upon a cowardly man.
AEGISTHUS: Perhaps. But I in later days will take further steps with
you.
LEADER: Not if the god who rules the family guides Orestes to his
home.
AEGISTHUS: Yes. I know that men in exile feed themselves on barren
hopes.   1668
LEADER: Go on, grow fat defiling justice . . . while you have your hour.
AEGISTHUS: Do not think you will not pay me a price for your stupidity.
LEADER: Boast on in your self-assurance, like a cock beside his hen.
CLYTEMNESTRA: Pay no heed, Aegisthus, to these futile barkings. You
and I,
Masters of this house, from now shall order all things well.   1673

(*They enter the palace.*)

SOPHOCLES

ANTIGONE

Translated by Shaemas O'Sheel

INTRODUCTION

CRITICISM of Sophocles' *Antigone* has since Hegel made much of the opposition between the rightful demands of the family versus those of the state, which led to the formulation of an abstract conflict between "divine" law, upheld by Antigone, and man-made law, represented by Creon. This is, of course, a useful dichotomy and may well introduce a discussion of the play; but it is by no means the only way in which to understand the complicated struggle of the chief players. The well-worn hamartia of Aristotle — the theory of a tragic flaw of character in a given character which brings about his downfall — likewise does not take us far, for it is difficult to attribute to Antigone any but the noblest motives for action. She is certainly not deliberately seeking martyrdom nor does she act through mere stubbornness or ignorance of the consequences. Hers is a supreme, completely voluntary courage which chooses the right and makes no compromise with reality; in fact, for her the true reality consists simply in the execution of her duty according to ancient Greek conventions: the burial of her brother.

Yet she does not self-consciously emphasize her religious duty; that theme is gradually subordinated to a more generalized and wholly feminine resistance to Creon which may be more reasonably interpreted in terms of an unavoidable clash between two strong personalities, both bent upon doing what, to each, seems right. Antigone has made her free choice within the framework of a situation which if left undisturbed would have become intolerable in its implications of personal dishonor.

Creon's arbitrary decree, although not without precedent or parallel in Greek tragedy, is on the other hand defended by him with desperate and sophistical arguments until his defense collapses completely into contrition and remorse. He sees his last son borne dead before him, his wife a suicide, and himself proven as blind as Oedipus, who, like Creon, had made the same accusations against the blind seer, Teiresias, — who could see better than both heroes into the realm of the spirit.

Creon's hybris — his fatal excess of behavior — lay in his unwillingness to yield to Antigone before it was too late, in his failure to see the sinister development of events and to withdraw with honor from a position which in the end became impossible for him to maintain. He himself states to the chorus the moral of his action: "It is hard to do — to retreat from a firm stand — but I yield, I will obey you. We must not wage a vain war with Fate." Antigone, although her action leads to death, has at least the comfort of having acted in a cause commended by all the Greek views of decent behavior toward gods and men. Creon's tragedy is further deepened by the overtones of political dissatisfaction with his government that is voiced by the people; he has mistaken firmness for harsh intolerance, a steadfast stand for hatred, since one cannot avoid the conclusion that much of his behavior is determined by his personal feeling against Polynices and not by governmental policy alone. Antigone is to some extent the symbol of national resistance to a tyrant, a name and a figure dreaded and feared by all the historic Greeks.

One may speak of the way Love must always conquer Hate, how man's wisdom is insufficient to solve the most crucial of moral problems such as the one Antigone faced, of the letter of the law which killeth and the spirit which giveth life. It is clear that Sophocles is praising the virtues of compassion, moderation, and sympathy in this profound analysis of human suffering, which he can neither justify nor explain. Kitto says that it is "the very core of Sophocles' philosophy, that virtue alone cannot assure happiness nor wickedness alone explain disaster." Further, there is certainly the curse on the house of Laius to reckon with, even the terrible harvest of the dragon's teeth that Cadmus sowed. Even the innocent must suffer under this curse, Ismene and Haemon as well as Antigone; for Creon the retribution brought upon himself by the wrong he has done the dead is clearly a dominant theme in the play.

These are all part of the lesson that *Antigone* teaches. Yet they are vague ideas indeed compared to the simple, unmistakable words of Antigone herself when she tells why she must bury her brother and thus bring ruin upon herself (904–912):

> "Not for my children, if I had been a mother, nor for my husband, if his dead body were rotting before me, would I have chosen to suffer like this in violent defiance of the citizens. For the sake of what law do I say this? If my husband had died, there would have been another man for me; I could have had a child from another husband if I had lost my first child. But with my mother and father both hidden away in Hades, no other brother could ever have come into being for me."

Nineteenth-century critics felt that this was a most un-romantic attitude for Antigone to take; Haemon, her fiancé, the pallid Romeo of this Greek drama, is not even mentioned in this speech, reminiscent in part of Alcestis' heart-rending farewell to her home and family. So, to repair this awkward and humiliating situation, a series of scholars headed by A. Jacob and including the great British Sophoclean scholar, R. C. Jebb, preferred to bracket these lines as spurious. Yet nothing in the play is better authenticated and more in keeping with the actual Greek feeling in such a crisis. Romance had a different meaning to the Greeks than it has for us. The fact is, Antigone is perfectly logical and correct in this statement.

The structure of the play does not have the smooth development of the *Oedipus Rex*, the same clear progress toward a remorseless goal. Antigone, for all her undeniable importance, disappears from the play before it is even two-thirds completed; her subsequent actions are reported by others and the focus of emotion turns irresistibly to Creon. We watch in fascinated horror as he stumbles from one blunder to another, hastening to bury Polynices at the very moment when Antigone in her sealed chamber is hanging herself, wheeling from the dead body of his son to the corpse of his wife in a sickening moment of indecision and despair. Despite the play's title it is hard to believe that Creon's fate was not at least equally significant to Sophocles.

A tragic and intolerable situation — a truly human situation — willfully and stubbornly brought to pass by two powerful and inflexible personalities — all other characters are foils for these two — set against the dark history of a luckless family makes this play one of Sophocles' greatest. It was presented at Athens before 442 B.C.; although it forms a trilogy with the *Oedipus Rex* and the *Oedipus at Colonus*, all three plays were produced at widely separate intervals and may not have formed a unity in the intention of Sophocles: the *Oedipus Rex* appeared about 430 B.C., the *Oedipus at Colonus* in 401. Whether *Antigone* won a prize or not is unknown. Creon was played by the third actor Sophocles introduced into drama. The messenger also played the parts of Ismene, Haemon, and the guard, apparently with the skill of a quick-change artist. The choruses are especially beautiful, full of sonorous and melancholy meditations about the nature of man, the victory of Thebes, the family curse, the mythological parallels to Antigone's fate, and Dionysus, the source of the woes of Cadmus' house. The play was often produced and hence quite popular. Euripides and the Roman playwright Accius wrote plays on the same theme. In our day the adaptation by the French author Jean Anouilh is now well-known, having even been produced on television with Claude Rains as Creon; Anouilh makes him as sympathetic as possible in his insistence upon political necessity and expedience as the reasons for his action: for, after all, he was a ruler required to make decisions and to back them up with force.

The play arises from the following circumstances. When Oedipus had discovered his crimes — the slaying of his father Laius and the marriage of his mother Jocasta — he tore out his eyes and in his blindness fled to Attica and the protection of Theseus, king of Athens, accompanied by his two daughters, Antigone and Ismene. The rule of Thebes passed to his sons, Eteocles and Polynices, who fell to quarreling. Eteocles, who refused to yield after his alternate year of rule, and Creon drove out Polynices, who attacked Thebes with six other prominent heroes he had enlisted from elsewhere in Greece. In the battle described by playwrights on the subject of *The Seven Against Thebes*, Polynices fell and his body was thrown out to rot and to be eaten by dogs, a ghastly fate for an ancient Greek; it was believed that unburied bodies could not send their souls safely into Hades. Creon has forbidden anyone on pain of death from offering burial to the body. It is at this point that the play opens.

L. R. LIND

ANTIGONE

CHARACTERS

ANTIGONE } *daughters of Oedipus*
ISMENE

CREON, *king of Thebes, brother of Jocasta*

HAEMON, *son of Creon*

TEIRESIAS, *a blind prophet*

A SENTRY

A MESSENGER

EURYDICE, *wife of Creon*

CHORUS *of Theban elders*

ATTENDANTS *of the king and queen*

SOLDIERS

A BOY *who leads Teiresias*

SCENE. *An open space before the house of Creon. The house is at the back, with gates opening from it. On the right, the city is to be supposed; to the left and in the distance, the Theban plain and the hills rising beyond it.* ANTIGONE *and* ISMENE *come from the middle door of three in the King's house.*

ANTIGONE: Ismene, O my dear, my little sister, of all the griefs bequeathed us by our father Oedipus, is there any that Zeus will spare us while we live? There is no sorrow and no shame we have not known. And now what is this new edict they tell about, that our Captain has published all through Thebes? Do you know? Have

you heard? Or is it kept from you that our friends are   10
threatened with the punishment due to foes?

ISMENE: I have heard no news, Antigone, glad or sad, about our
friends, since we two sisters lost two brothers at a single blow; and
since the Argive army fled last night, I do not know whether my
fortune is better or worse.

ANTIGONE: I know, I know it well. That is why I sent for you to
come outside the gates, to speak to you alone.

ISMENE: What is it? I can see that you are troubled.   20

ANTIGONE: Should I not be? — when Creon gives honors to one of
our brothers, but condemns the other to shame? Eteocles, they say,
he has laid in the earth with due observance of right and custom,
that all may be well with him among the shades below. But the
poor corpse of Polynices — it has been published to the city that
none shall bury him, none shall mourn him; but he shall be left
unwept and unsepulchred, and the birds are welcome to feast upon
him!   30

   Such, they say, are the orders the good Creon has given for you
and me — yes, for me! He is coming now to make his wishes clear;
and it is no light matter, for whoever disobeys him is condemned
to death by stoning before all the people. Now you know! — and
now you will show whether you are nobly bred, or the unworthy
daughter of a noble line.

ISMENE: Sister, sister! — if we are caught in this web, what could I
do to loose or tighten the knot?   40

ANTIGONE: Decide if you will share the work and the danger.

ISMENE: What are you planning? — what are you thinking of?

ANTIGONE: Will you help this hand to lift the dead?

ISMENE: Oh, you would bury him! — when it is forbidden to anyone
in Thebes?

ANTIGONE: He is still my brother, if he is not yours. No one shall say
I failed in my duty to him.

ISMENE: But how can you dare, when Creon has forbidden it?

ANTIGONE: He has no right to keep me from my own.

ISMENE: Alas, sister, remember how our father perished hated   50
and scorned, when he had struck out his eyes in horror of the sins
his own persistency had brought to light. Remember how she who
was both his mother and his wife hung herself with a twisted cord.
And only yesterday our two brothers came to their terrible end,
each by the other's hand. Now only we two are left, and we are
all alone. Think how we shall perish, more miserably than all the
rest, if in defiance of the law we brave the King's decree and   60
the King's power. No, no, we must remember we were born women,
not meant to strive with men. We are in the grip of those stronger

than ourselves, and must obey them in this and in things still more cruel. Therefore I will ask forgiveness of the gods and spirits who dwell below, for they will see that I yield to force, and I will hearken to our rulers. It is foolish to be too zealous even in a good cause.

ANTIGONE: I will not urge you. No, if you wished to join me now I would not let you. Do as you think best. As for me, I will 70 bury him; and if I die for that, I am content. I shall rest like a loved one with him whom I have loved, innocent in my guilt. For I owe a longer allegiance to the dead than to the living; I must dwell with them forever. You, if you wish, may dishonor the laws which the gods have established.

ISMENE: I would not dishonor them, but to defy the State — I am not strong enough for that!

ANTIGONE: Well, make your excuses — I am going now to heap the earth above the brother whom I love. 80

ISMENE: Oh, I fear something terrible will happen to you!

ANTIGONE: Fear not for me; but look to your own fate.

ISMENE: At least, then, tell no one what you intend, but hide it closely — and so too will I.

ANTIGONE: No, but cry it aloud! I will condemn you more if you are silent than if you proclaim my deed to all.

ISMENE: You have so hot a heart for deeds that make the blood run cold!

ANTIGONE: My deeds will please those they are meant to please.

ISMENE: Ah yes, if you can do what you plan — but you cannot. 90

ANTIGONE: When my strength fails, I shall confess my failure.

ISMENE: The impossible should not be tried at all.

ANTIGONE: If you say such things I will hate you, and the dead will haunt you! — But leave me, and the folly that is mine alone, to suffer what I must; for I shall not suffer anything so dreadful as an ignoble death.

ISMENE: Go then, if you must, though your errand is mad; and be sure of this, my love goes with you!

(ANTIGONE *goes toward the plain.* ISMENE *retires into the King's house. The* CHORUS, *being the elders of Thebes, comes into the place before the house.*)

CHORUS:

Over the waters, see! — over the stream of Dirke, the golden 100 eye of the dawn opens on the seven gates;

Terror crouched in the night, how welcome to Thebes is the morning, when the warriors of the white shields flee from the spears of the sun.

From Argos mailed they came, swords drawn for Polynices;   110
like eagles that scream in the air these plumed ones fell on our
land.
They ravened around our towers, and burst the doors of our dwellings; their spears sniffed at our blood — but they fled without
quenching that thirst.   120

They heaped the eager pine-boughs, flaming, against our bastions,
calling upon Hephaestos; but he the fire-god failed them.
The clash of battle was loud, the clamor beloved of the war-god;
but a thing they found too hard was to conquer the dragon's
brood.

And a thing abhorred by Zeus is the boastful tongue of the   130
haughty: one proud chief, armored in gold, with triumph in his
throat,
The stormy wave of the foe flung to the crest of our rampart —
the god, with a crooked bolt, smites-him crashing to earth.   140

At the seven gates of the city, seven of the host's grim captains
yielded to Zeus who turns the tide of battle, their arms of
bronze;
And woe to those two sons of the same father and mother, they
crossed their angry spears, and brought each other low.

But now since Victory, most desired of all men, to Thebes of the
many chariots has come scattering joy,   150
Let us forget the wars, and dance before the temples; and Bacchus
be our leader, loved by the land of Thebes!

But see, the King of this land comes yonder — Creon, son of
Menoekeus, our new ruler by virtue of the new turn the gods have
given things. What counsel is he pondering, that he has   160
called by special summons this gathering of the elders?
CREON: Sirs, our State has been like a ship tossed by stormy waves;
but thanks to the gods, it sails once more upon a steady keel. You
I have summoned here apart from all the people because I remember that of old you had great reverence for the royal power of
Laius; and I know how you upheld Oedipus when he ruled this
land, and, when he died, you loyally supported his two sons. Those
sons have fallen, both in one moment, each smitten by the other,
each stained with a brother's blood; now I possess the throne   170
and all its powers, since I am nearest kindred of the dead.
No man's worthiness to rule can be known until his mind and

soul have been tested by the duties of government and lawgiving. For my part, I have always held that any man who is the supreme guardian of the State, and who fails in his duty through fear, remaining silent when evil is done, is base and contemptible; 180 nor have I any regard for him who puts friendship above the common welfare. Zeus, who sees all things, be my witness that I will not be silent when danger threatens the people; nor will I ever call my country's foe my friend. For our country is the ship that bears us all, and he only is our friend who helps us sail a pros- 190 perous course.

Such are the rules by which I will guard this city's greatness; and in keeping with them is the edict I have published touching the sons of Oedipus. For Eteocles, who fell like a true soldier defending his native land, there shall be such funeral as we give the noblest dead. But as to his brother Polynices — he who came out of exile and sought to destroy with fire the city of his fathers and the shrines of his fathers' gods — he who thirsted for the 200 blood of his kin, and would have led into slavery all who escaped death — as to this man, it has been proclaimed that none shall honor him, none shall lament over him, but he shall lie unburied, a corpse mangled by birds and dogs, a gruesome thing to see. Such is my way with traitors. 210

CHORUS: Such is your way, Creon, son of Menoekeus, with the false and with the faithful; and you have power, I know, to give such orders as you please, both for the dead and for all of us who live.

CREON: Then look to it that my mandate is observed.

CHORUS: Call on some younger man for this hard task.

CREON: No, watchers of the corpse have been appointed.

CHORUS: What is this duty, then, you lay on us?

CREON: To side with no one breaking this command.

CHORUS: No man is foolish enough to go courting death. 220

CREON: That indeed shall be the penalty; but men have been lured even to death by the hope of gain.

(A GUARD, *coming from the direction of the plain, approaches* CREON.)

GUARD: Sire, I will not say that I am out of breath from hurrying, nor that I have come here on the run; for in fact my thoughts made me pause more than once, and even turn in my path, to go back. My mind was telling me two different things. "Fool," it said to me, "why do you go where you are sure to be condemned?" And then on the other hand, "Wretch, tarrying again? If Creon 230 hears of this from another, you'll smart for it." Torn between these fears, I came on slowly and unwillingly, making a short road long.

But at last I got up courage to come to you, and though there is little to my story, I will tell it; for I have got a good grip on one thought — that I can suffer nothing but what is my fate.

CREON: Well, and what is it that makes you so upset?

GUARD: First let me tell you that I did not do the deed and I did not see it done, so it would not be just to make me suffer for it. 240

CREON: You have a good care for your own skin, and armor yourself well against blame. I take it that you have news to tell?

GUARD: Yes, that I have, but bad news is nothing to be in a hurry about.

CREON: Tell it, man, will you? — tell it and be off.

GUARD: Well, this is it. The corpse — someone has done it funeral honors — sprinkled dust upon it, and other pious rites.

CREON: What — what do you say? What man has dared this deed?

GUARD: That I cannot tell you. There was no sign of a pick being used, no earth torn up the way it is by a mattock. The 250 ground was hard and dry; there was no track of wheels. Whoever did it left no trace; when the first day-watchman showed it to us, we were struck dumb. You couldn't see the dead man at all; not that he was in any grave, but dry dust was strewn that thick all over him. It was the hand of someone warding off a curse did that. There was no sign that any dog or wild beast had been at the body.

Then there were loud words, and hard words, among us of the guard, everyone accusing someone else, 'til we nearly came 260 to blows, and it's a wonder we didn't. Everyone was accused and no one was convicted, and each man stuck to it that he knew nothing about it. We were ready to take red-hot iron in our hands — to walk through fire — to swear by the gods that we did not do the deed and were not in the secret of whoever did it.

At last, when all our disputing got us nowhere, one of the men spoke up in a way that made us look down at the ground in silence and fear; for we could not see how to gainsay him, nor how 270 to escape trouble if we heeded him. What he said was, that this must be reported to you, it was no use hiding it. There was no doubt of it, he was right; so we cast lots, and it was my bad luck to win the prize. Here I am, then, as unwelcome as unwilling, I know; for no man likes the bearer of bad news.

CHORUS: O King, my thoughts have been whispering, could this deed perhaps have been the work of gods?

CREON: Silence, before your words fill me with anger, and you 280 prove yourself as foolish as you are old! You say what is not to be borne, that the gods would concern themselves with this corpse. What! — did they cover his nakedness to reward the reverence he paid them, coming to burn their pillared shrines and sacred treasures, to harry their land, to put scorn upon their laws? Do you think it is the way of the gods to honor the wicked? No! From the first there were some in this city who muttered against me, chafing at this edict, wagging their heads in secret; they would not   290 bow to the yoke, not they, like men contented with my rule.

I know well enough, it is such malcontents who have bribed and beguiled these guards to do this deed or let it be done. Nothing so evil as money ever arose among men. It lays cities low, drives peoples from their homes, warps honest souls 'til they give themselves to works of shame; it teaches men to practise villainies and grow familiar with impious deeds.   300

But the men who did this thing for hire, sooner or later they shall pay the price. Now, as Zeus still has my reverence, know this — I tell you on my oath: Unless you find the very man whose hand strewed dust upon that body, and bring him here before mine eyes, death alone shall not be enough for you, but you shall first be hung up alive until you reveal the truth about this outrage; that henceforth you may have a better idea about how to get money, and learn that it is not wise to grasp at it from any source. I will   310 teach you that ill-gotten gains bring more men to ruin than to prosperity.

GUARD: May I speak? Or shall I turn and go?

CREON: Can you not see that your voice offends me?

GUARD: Are your ears troubled, or your soul?

CREON: And why should you try to fix the seat of my pain?

GUARD: The doer of the deed inflames your mind, but I, only your ears.

CREON: Bah, you are a babbler born!   320

GUARD: I may be that, but I never did this deed.

CREON: You did, for silver; but you shall pay with your life.

GUARD: It is bad when a judge misjudges.

CREON: Prate about "judgment" all you like; but unless you show me the culprit in this crime, you will admit before long that guilty wages were better never earned.

(CREON *goes into his house.*)

GUARD: Well, may the guilty man be found, that's all I ask. But whether he's found or not — fate will decide that — you will not see me here again. I have escaped better than I ever hoped or thought — I owe the gods much thanks.   330

(*The* GUARD *departs, going toward the plain.*)

CHORUS:
Wonders are many in the world, and the wonder of all is man.

With his bit in the teeth of the storm and his faith in a fragile
prow,
Far he sails, where the waves leap white-fanged, wroth at his plan.
And he has his will of the earth by the strength of his hand on
the plough.   340

The birds, the clan of the light heart, he snares with his woven
cord,
And the beasts with wary eyes, and the stealthy fish in the sea;
That shaggy freedom-lover, the horse, obeys his word,
And the sullen bull must serve him, for cunning of wit   350
is he.

Against all ills providing, he tempers the dark and the light,
The creeping siege of the frost and the arrows of sleet and rain,
The grievous wounds of the daytime and the fever that steals in the
night;
Only against Death man arms himself in vain.   360

With speech and wind-swift thought he builds the State to his
mood,
Prospering while he honors the gods and the laws of the land.
Yet in his rashness often he scorns the ways that are good —
May such as walk with evil be far from my hearth and   370
hand!

(*The* GUARD *reappears leading* ANTIGONE.)

CHORUS: But what is this? — what portent from the gods is this? I
am bewildered, for surely this maiden is Antigone; I know her well.
O luckless daughter of a luckless father, child of Oedipus,   380
what does this mean? Why have they made you prisoner? Surely
they did not take you in the folly of breaking the King's laws?
GUARD: Here she is, the doer of the deed! We caught this girl burying
him. But where is Creon?
CHORUS: Look, he is coming from the house now.

(CREON *comes from the house.*)

CREON: What is it? What has happened that makes my coming
timely?
GUARD: Sire, a man should never say positively "I will do this" or
"I won't do that," for things happen to change the mind. I vowed
I would not soon come here again, after the way you   390
scared me, lashing me with your threats. But there's nothing so
pleasant as a happy turn when we've given up hope, so I have

broken my sworn oath to hurry back here with this girl, who was taken showing grace to the dead. This time there was no casting of lots; no, this is my good luck, no one else's. And now, Sire, take her yourself, question her, examine her, all you please; but I have a right to free and final quittance of this trouble. 400

CREON: Stay! — this prisoner — how and where did you take her?

GUARD: She was burying the man; that's all there is to tell you.

CREON: Do you mean what you say? Are you telling the truth?

GUARD: I saw her burying the corpse that you had forbidden to bury. Is that plain and clear?

CREON: What did you see? Did you take her in the act?

GUARD: It happened this way. When we came to the place where he lay, worrying over your threats, we swept away all the dirt, leaving the rotting corpse bare. Then we sat us down on the 410 brow of the hill to windward, so that the smell from him would not strike us. We kept wide awake frightening each other with what you would do to us if we didn't carry out your command. So it went until the sun was bright in the top of the sky, and the heat began to burn. Then suddenly a whirlwind came roaring down, making the sky all black, hiding the plain under clouds of choking dust and leaves torn from the trees. We closed our eyes and bore this plague from the gods. 420

And when, after a long while, the storm had passed, we saw this girl, and she crying aloud with the sharp cry of a bird in its grief; the way a bird will cry when it sees the nest bare and the nestlings gone, it was that way she lifted up her voice when she saw the corpse uncovered; and she called down dreadful curses on those that did it. Then straightway she scooped up dust in her hands, and she had a shapely ewer of bronze, and she held that 430 high while she honored the dead with three drink-offerings.

We rushed forward at this and closed on our quarry, who was not at all frightened at us. Then we charged her with the past and present offences, and she denied nothing — I was both happy and sorry for that. It is good to escape danger one's self, but hard to bring trouble to one's friends. However, nothing counts with me so much as my own safety. 440

CREON: You, then — you whose face is bent to the earth — do you confess or do you deny the deed?

ANTIGONE: I did it; I make no denial.

CREON (*to* GUARD): You may go your way, wherever you will, free and clear of a grave charge.

(*To* ANTIGONE): Now tell me — not in many words, but briefly — did you know of the edict that forbade what you did?

ANTIGONE: I knew it. How could I help knowing? — it was public.

CREON: And you had the boldness to transgress that law?

ANTIGONE: Yes, for it was not Zeus made such a law; such   450
is not the Justice of the gods. Nor did I think that your decrees
had so much force, that a mortal could override the unwritten and
unchanging statutes of heaven. For their authority is not of today
nor yesterday, but from all time, and no man knows when they were
first put forth.

Not through dread of any human power could I answer to the
gods for breaking these. That I must die I knew without your
edict. But if I am to die before my time, I count that a gain; for
who, living as I do in the midst of many woes, would not call
death a friend?   460

It saddens me little, therefore, to come to my end. If I had let
my mother's son lie in death an unburied corpse, that would have
saddened me, but for myself I do not grieve. And if my acts are
foolish in your eyes, it may be that a foolish judge condemns my
folly.   470

CHORUS: The maiden shows herself the passionate daughter of a passionate father, she does not know how to bend the neck.

CREON: Let me remind you that those who are too stiff and stubborn
are most often humbled; it is the iron baked too hard in the furnace
you will oftenest see snapped and splintered. But I have seen horses
that show temper brought to order by a little curb. Too much
pride is out of place in one who lives subject to another. This girl
was already versed in insolence when she transgressed the law that
had been published; and now, behold, a second insult —   480
to boast about it, to exult in her misdeed!

But I am no man, she is the man, if she can carry this off unpunished. No! She is my sister's child, but if she were nearer to
me in blood than any who worships Zeus at the altar of my house,
she should not escape a dreadful doom — nor her sister either, for
indeed I charge her too with plotting this burial.   490

And summon that sister — for I saw her just now within, raving and out of her wits. That is the way minds plotting evil in the
dark give away their secret and convict themselves even before they
are found out. But the most intolerable thing is that one who has
been caught in wickedness should glory in the crime.

ANTIGONE: Would you do more than slay me?

CREON: No more than that — no, and nothing less.

ANTIGONE: Then why do you delay? Your speeches give me no pleasure, and never will; and my words, I suppose, buzz hate-   500
fully in your ear. I am ready; for there is no better way I could
prepare for death than by giving burial to my brother. Everyone
would say so if their lips were not sealed by fear. But a king has
many advantages, he can do and say what he pleases.

CREON: You slander the race of Cadmus; not one of them shares your view of this deed.

ANTIGONE: They see it as I do, but their tails are between their legs.

CREON: They are loyal to their king; are you not ashamed 510 to be otherwise?

ANTIGONE: No; there is nothing shameful in piety to a brother.

CREON: Was it not a brother also who died in the good cause?

ANTIGONE: Born of the same mother and sired by the same father.

CREON: Why then do you dishonor him by honoring that other?

ANTIGONE: The dead will not look upon it that way.

CREON: Yes, if you honor the wicked equally with the virtuous.

ANTIGONE: It was his brother, not his slave, that died.

CREON: One perished ravaging his fatherland, the other defending it.

ANTIGONE: Nevertheless, Hades desires these rites.

CREON: Surely the good are not pleased to be made equal with the evil! 520

ANTIGONE: Who knows how the gods see good and evil?

CREON: A foe is never a friend — even in death.

ANTIGONE: It is not my nature to join in hating, but in loving.

CREON: Your place, then, is with the dead. If you must love, love them. While I live, no woman shall overbear me.

(ISMENE *is led from the King's house by two attendants.*)

CHORUS: See, Ismene comes through the gate shedding such tears as loving sisters weep. It seems as if a cloud gathers about her brow and breaks in rain upon her cheek. 530

CREON: And you, who lurked like a viper in my house, sucking the blood of my honor, while I knew not that I was nursing two reptiles ready to strike at my throne — come, tell me now, will you confess your part in this guilty burial, or will you swear you knew nothing of it?

ISMENE: I am guilty if she is, and share the blame.

ANTIGONE: No, no! Justice will not permit this. You did not consent to the deed, nor would I let you have part in it.

ISMENE: But now that danger threatens you, I am not ashamed to come to your side. 540

ANTIGONE: Who did the deed, the gods and the dead know; a friend in words is not the friend I love.

ISMENE: Sister, do not reject me, but let me die with you, and duly honor the dead.

ANTIGONE: Do not court death, nor claim a deed to which you did not put your hand. My death will suffice.

ISMENE: How could life be dear to me without you?

ANTIGONE: Ask Creon, you think highly of his word.

ISMENE: Why taunt me so, when it does you no good? 550

ANTIGONE: Ah, if I mock you, it is with pain I do it.

ISMENE: Oh tell me, how can I serve you, even now?

ANTIGONE: Save yourself; I do not grudge your escape.

ISMENE: Oh, my grief! Can I not share your fate?

ANTIGONE: You chose to live, and I to die.

ISMENE: At least I begged you not to make that choice.

ANTIGONE: This world approved your caution, but the gods my courage.

ISMENE: But now I approve, and so I am guilty too.

ANTIGONE: Ah little sister, be of good cheer, and live. My life has long
    been given to death, that I might serve the dead.   560

CREON: Behold, one of these girls turns to folly now, as the other one
    has ever since she was born.

ISMENE: Yes, Sire, such reason as nature gives us may break under mis-
    fortune, and go astray.

CREON: Yours did, when you chose to share evil deeds with the evil.

ISMENE: But I cannot live without her.

CREON: You mistake; she lives no more.

ISMENE: Surely you will not slay your own son's betrothed?

CREON: He can plough other fields.

ISMENE: But he cannot find such love again.   570

CREON: I will not have an evil wife for my son.

ANTIGONE: Ah, Haemon, my beloved! Dishonored by your father!

CREON: Enough! I'll hear no more of you and your marriage!

CHORUS: Will you indeed rob your son of his bride?

CREON: Death will do that for me.

CHORUS: It seems determined then, that she shall die.

CREON: Determined, yes — for me and for you. No more delay —
    servants, take them within. Let them know that they are women,
    not meant to roam abroad. For even the boldest seek to   580
    fly when they see Death stretching his hand their way.

(*Attendants lead* ANTIGONE *and* ISMENE *into the house.*)

CHORUS:

    Blest are they whose days have not tasted of sorrow:
    For if a house has dared the anger of heaven,
    Evil strikes at it down the generations,
    Wave after wave, like seas that batter a headland.   590

    I see how fate has harried the seed of Labdakos;
    Son cannot fly the curse that was laid on the sire,
    The doom incurred by the dead must fall on the living:
    When gods pursue, no race can find deliverance.

    And even these, the last of the children of Oedipus —   600

Because of the frenzy that rose in a passionate heart,
Because of a handful of blood-stained dust that was sprinkled —
The last of the roots is cut, and the light extinguished.

O Zeus, how vain is the mortal will that opposes
The Will Immortal that neither sleeps nor ages,
The Imperturbable Power that on Olympus
Dwells in unclouded glory, the All-Beholding!　　　　　　610

Wise was he who said that ancient saying:
Whom the gods bewilder, at last takes evil for virtue;
And let no man lament if his lot is humble —
No great things come to mortals without a curse.　　　　　620

But look, Sire: Haemon, the last of your sons, approaches. I
wonder if he comes grieving over the doom of his promised bride,
Antigone, and bitter that his marriage-hopes are baffled?　　630

(HAEMON *comes before his father.*)

CREON: We shall know soon, better than seers could tell us. My son,
you have heard the irrevocable doom decreed for your betrothed.
Do you come to rage against your father, or do you remember the
duty of filial love, no matter what I do?

HAEMON: Father, I am yours; and knowing you are wise, I follow the
paths you trace for me. No marriage could be more to me than
your good guidance.

CREON: Yes, my son, this should be your heart's first law, in all things
to obey your father's will. Men pray for dutiful children　　640
growing up about them in their homes, that such may pay their
father's foe with evil, and honor as their father does, his friend.
But if a man begets undutiful children, what shall we say that he
has sown, only sorrow for himself and triumph for his enemies? Do
not then, my son, thinking of pleasures, put aside reason for a
woman's sake. If you brought an evil woman to your bed and home,
you would find that such embraces soon grow hateful; and　　650
nothing can wound so deeply as to find a loved one false. No, but
with loathing, and as if she were your enemy, let this girl go to find
a husband in the house of Hades. For she alone in all the city
defied and disobeyed me; I have taken her in the act, and I will not
be a liar to my people — I will slay her.

Let her appeal all she pleases to the claims of kindred blood. If I
am to rear my own kin to evil deeds, certainly I must expect evil
among the people. Only a man who rules his own house-　　660

hold justly can do justice in the State. If anyone transgresses, and does violence to the laws, or thinks to dictate to the ruler, I will not tolerate it. No! — whoever the city shall appoint to rule, that man must be obeyed, in little things and great things, in just things and unjust; for the man who is a good subject is the one who would be a good ruler, and it is he who in time of war will stand his ground where he is placed, loyal to his comrades and without fear, 670 though the spears fall around him like rain in a storm.

But disobedience is the worst of evils. It desolates households; it ruins cities; it throws the ranks of allies into confusion and rout. On the other hand, note those whose lives are prosperous: they owe it, you will generally find, to obedience. Therefore we must uphold the cause of order; and certainly we must not let a woman defy us. It would be better to fall from power by a man's hand, than to be called weaker than a woman. 680

CHORUS: Unless the years have stolen our wits, all that you say seems wise.

HAEMON: Father, the gods implant reason in men, the highest of all things that we call our own. I have no skill to prove, and I would not wish to show, that you speak unwisely; and yet another man, too, might have some useful thought. I count it a duty to keep my ears alert for what men say about you, noting especially when they find fault. The people dare not say to your face what would displease you; but I can hear the things murmured in the dark, 690 and the whole city weeps for this maiden. "No woman ever," they say, "so little merited a cruel fate. None was ever doomed to a shameful death for deeds so noble as hers; who, when her brother lay dead from bloody wounds, would not leave him unburied for the birds and the dogs to mangle. Does not so pious an act deserve golden praise?"

Such is the way the people speak in secret. To me, father, 700 nothing is so precious as your welfare. What is there father or son can so rejoice in as the other's fair repute? I pray you therefore do not wear one mood too stubbornly, as if no one else could possibly be right. For the man who thinks he is the only wise man always proves hollow when we sound him. No, though a man be wise, it is no shame for him to learn many things, and to yield at the right time. When the streams rage and overflow in Winter, 710 you know how those trees that yield come safely through the flood; but the stubborn are torn up and perish, root and branch. Consider too, the sailor who keeps his sheet always taut, and never slackens it; presently his boat overturns and his keel floats uppermost.

So, though you are angry, permit reason to move you. If I, young as I am, may offer a thought, I would say it were best if 720 men were by nature always wise; but that being seldom so, it is prudent to listen to those who offer honest counsel.

CHORUS: Sire, it is fitting that you should weigh his words, if he speaks in season; and you, Haemon, should mark your father's words; for on both parts there has been wise speech.

CREON: What! Shall men of our age be schooled by youths like this?

HAEMON: In nothing that does not go with reason; but as to my youth, you should weigh my merits, not my years.

CREON: Is it your merit that you honor the lawless?   730

HAEMON: I could wish no one to respect evil-doers.

CREON: This girl — is she not tainted with that plague?

HAEMON: Our Theban folk deny it, with one voice.

CREON: Shall Thebes, then, tell me how to rule?

HAEMON: Now who speaks like a boy?

CREON: Tell me — am I to rule by my own judgment or the views of others?

HAEMON: That is no city which belongs to one man.

CREON: Is not the city held to be the ruler's?

HAEMON: That kind of monarchy would do well in a desert.

CREON: Ho, this boy, it seems, is the woman's champion!   740

HAEMON: Yes, if you are a woman, for my concern is for you.

CREON: Shameless, to bandy arguments with your father!

HAEMON: Only because I see you flouting justice.

CREON: Is it wrong for me to respect my royal position?

HAEMON: It is a poor way to respect it, trampling on the laws of the gods.

CREON: This is depravity, putting a woman foremost!

HAEMON: At least you will not find me so depraved that I fear to plead for justice.

CREON: Every word you speak is a plea for that girl.

HAEMON: And for you, and for me, and for the gods below.

CREON: Marry her you shall not, this side the grave.   750

HAEMON: She must die then, and in dying destroy others?

CREON: Ha, you go so far as open threats?

HAEMON: I speak no threats, but grieve for your fatal stubbornness.

CREON: You shall rue your unwise teaching of wisdom.

HAEMON: If you were not my father, I would call you unwise.

CREON: Slave of a woman, do not think you can cajole me.

HAEMON: Then no one but yourself may speak, you will hear no reason?

CREON: Enough of this — now, by Olympus, you shall smart for baiting me this way! Bring her here, that hateful rebel, that she   760 may die forthwith before his eyes — yes, at her bridegroom's side!

HAEMON: No, no, never think it, I shall not witness her death; but my face your eyes shall never see again. Give your passion its way before those who can endure you!

(HAEMON *rushes away*.)

CHORUS: He has gone, O King, in angry haste; a youthful mind, when stung, is impetuous.

CREON: Let him do what he will, let him dream himself more than a common man, but he shall not save those girls from their doom.

CHORUS: Are you indeed determined to slay them both?   770

CREON: Not the one whose hands are clean of the crime — you do well to remind me of that.

CHORUS: But how will you put the other one to death?

CREON: I will take her where the path is loneliest, and hide her, living, in a rocky vault, with only so much food as the pious laws require, that the city may avoid reproach. There she can pray to Hades, whose gods alone she worships; perhaps they will bargain with death for her escape. And if they do not, she will learn, too late, that it is lost labor to revere the dead.   780

(CREON *leaves*.)

CHORUS:

> Great is love, and what shall prevail against it,
> When from the deep and quiet eyes of a maiden
> Sallying forth, it mocks at our laws and powers,
> Pride and possessions?
>
> Wave of the sea is love, wind on the mountains:
> Neither deathless gods nor mortals escape it.
> The good it turns to evil, the wise to folly,   790
> All men to madness.
>
> And if a son is angered against his father,
> Blame him not, but see who has wrought this frenzy —
> She the goddess loveliest and most willful,
> Fierce Aphrodite!   800

(ANTIGONE *is led from the King's house*.)

But oh, this is a sight that shakes even my loyalty to the laws! I cannot stay my tears, when I see Antigone thus pass on her way to that bridal chamber where we shall all come at last.

ANTIGONE: See me, citizens of my fatherland, setting forth on my last journey, looking my last on the sunlight — soon for me it will be no more; but Death, who hides us all from the sun, is hasty   810 with me; soon I shall stand on Acheron's shore, I who have no portion in the song they sing for brides, nor the evening song before the bridal chamber; but the Lord of the Dark Lake will be my bridegroom.

CHORUS: Yet I would give it praise, the way of your going:
Neither did sickness waste nor violence smite you.
Mastering fate in this wise never has mortal   820
Gone down to Hades.

ANTIGONE: I have heard how in other days a terrible fate befell Niobe, daughter of Tantalus, and how on Mount Sipylos the rock grew around her as ivy grows on a wall. And they say that there on that desolate height, where rain and snow never cease, her tears   830 also never cease to flow beneath her stony lids. I think my doom is like hers.

CHORUS: She was a goddess, Niobe, born of immortals;
If one of the race of men that is born to perish
Fares like her whose sire had Zeus for father,
Great is the honor.

ANTIGONE: Oh, must you mock me? My city, my city, and   840 you her fortunate sons, in the name of our fathers' gods can you not wait 'til I am gone — must you taunt me to my face? Ah, river of Dirke, and sacred groves of Thebes, bear witness how no friend weeps for me as I near that rocky chamber, my prison and my tomb! — none weeps for me unhappy, who have no friend in the sun nor in the shadows, no home with the living or the dead.   850

CHORUS: All too rash was your deed, unhappy maiden,
Boldly daring even the throne of justice:
There you fell. Alas, you must pay to the utmost,
Doom of your father.

ANTIGONE: You touch the quick of all my grief, my bitterest thought — my father's sin and punishment, and how the implacable Fates still harry the famous house of Labdakos. Alas for the   860 horrors of that bed where a mother slept with her son — such parents gave me my miserable being, and now I go to them, accursed, unwed, to share their shadowy home. Alas my brother who married the Argive woman, your death has undone my life!   870

CHORUS: Reverence moved your hand, the deed I reverence,
Yet if a man have power over a city,
Scorn of that power he may not bear. O self-willed,
Your rashness slays you!

ANTIGONE: Then it is certain I must take this journey, for none befriends me. There will be no marriage-song; I may not longer even look on the sun. No one mourns my passing, none even   880 weeps.

   (CREON *returns.*)

CREON: Do you not know that if pleas and lamentations could save the doomed, they would never cease? Away with her, away! And when you have shut her in the vaulted tomb according to my word, leave her, leave her there alone. Let her choose whether she wishes to die, or to live buried in such a home. Our hands are clean as touching this maiden. Only this much is certain — she shall dwell no more in the light. 890

ANTIGONE: Tomb, my bridal-chamber, eternal prison in the caverned rock, when I come to you I shall find mine own, those many who have perished, who have seen Persephone. Last of all I take that way, and fare most miserably of all, my days so few! But I cherish good hope that my coming will be welcome to my father, and pleasant to my mother, and to you, my brother, pleasing too; for each of you in death I washed with my own hands, and dressed for your graves; and I poured drink-offerings over you. 900

And you too, Polynices; for you also in death I tended, and for that I win such recompense as this. Yet the just will say I did rightly in paying you these honors. Not for my children, if I had been a mother, nor for my husband, if his dead body were rotting before me, would I have chosen to suffer like this in violent defiance of the citizens. For the sake of what law do I say this? If my husband had died, there would have been another man for me; I could have had a child from another husband if I had lost my first child. But with my mother and father both hidden away in Hades, no other brother could ever have come into being for me.* For it was thus I saw the higher law; but Creon calls me guilty, brother, and leads me captive on the way to death. No bridal bed, no bridal song have been mine, no joy of marriage, no children at my breast; but thus forlorn and friendless I go living to the grave. 920

Yet what law of heaven did I offend? Ah, why should I look to the gods any more, for I see they do not hear me, but let me suffer the punishment of the impious for doing a pious deed. If my fate indeed is pleasing to the gods, when I have suffered my doom no doubt I shall learn my sin; but if the sin is with my judges, I wish them no measure of evil greater than they have measured out to me.

CHORUS: Still the same tempest vexes this maiden's soul. 930

CREON: Therefore her guards shall pay for their slowness.

ANTIGONE: Ah yes, your words tell death to hurry for me.

CREON: I cannot let you hope for any respite.

ANTIGONE: Land of my fathers, O my city, Thebes! O ye gods, eldest of our race! — they hurry me now, they are in haste to have done

---

* The passage beginning "Not for my children," omitted by the translator since he followed Jebb's text, has been added by the editor of this anthology.

with me. Behold me, princes of Thebes, the last of the   940
house of your kings — see what I suffer, and by whom — because
I feared to forget the fear of heaven!

(ANTIGONE *is led away by the guards, toward the plain.*)

CHORUS:
> Even thus in an older day was Danaë,
> Young and wistful, taken away from the sunlight.
> Noble of race was she, in a brass-walled prison
> Hid by her father.

> Yet the eye of the mighty god beheld her,
> Yet to her came Zeus in a golden shower;   950
> Well she bore the seed of the father immortal,
> Mothering a hero.

> Noble too was that Edonian chieftain,
> Rashly who scattered the Bacchanalian fires,
> Harried the Maenads, taunted Dionysus,
> Angered the Muses:

> Him the god made mad, and the godly power   960
> Thrust him, living, deep in a rocky dungeon;
> There he learned to know how impious frenzy
> Draws divine vengeance.

> Dire too was the plight of that grieving mother
> Who, where the Dark Rocks rise beyond Bosporus,
> Far away, in Thracian Salmydessos,   970
> Sacred to Ares,

> Saw the fierce implacable wife of Phineos
> Strike her children's eyes with the blinding shuttle —
> Their little faces turned toward heaven, unseeing,
> Tearless and bleeding: 980

> Noble that mother's race, sprung from Erechtheus —
> Daughter of Boreas she, reared in the wind's caves,
> Fleet her foot on the hills; yet upon her too,
> Hard bore the Fates.

> Dread indeed are the Fates, their ways mysterious:
> Neither by wealth nor war — neither by hiding

In strong-walled town, nor fleeing in ships sea-beaten —
Shall man evade them.

(TEIRESIAS, *led by a boy, appears before the King and the elders.*)

TEIRESIAS: Princes of Thebes, it is a hard journey for me to come here, for the blind must walk by another's steps and see with another's eyes; yet I have come. 990

CREON: And what, Teiresias, are your tidings?

TEIRESIAS: I shall tell you; and listen well to the seer.

CREON: I have never slighted your counsel.

TEIRESIAS: It is that way you have steered the city well.

CREON: I know, and bear witness, to the worth of your words.

TEIRESIAS: Then mark them now: for I tell you, you stand on fate's thin edge.

CREON: What do you mean? I snudder at your message.

TEIRESIAS: You will know, when you hear the signs my art has disclosed. For lately, as I took my place in my ancient seat of augury, where all the birds of the air gather about me, I heard 1000 strange things. They were screaming with feverish rage, their usual clear notes were a frightful jargon; and I knew they were rending each other murderously with their talons: the whir of their wings told an angry tale.

Straightway, these things filling me with fear, I kindled fire upon an altar, with due ceremony, and laid a sacrifice among the faggots; but Hephaestos would not consume my offering with flame. A moisture oozing out from the bones and flesh trickled upon the embers, making them smoke and sputter. Then the gall 1010 burst and scattered on the air, and the steaming thighs lay bared of the fat that had wrapped them.

Such was the failure of the rites by which I vainly asked a sign, as this boy reported them; for his eyes serve me, as I serve others. And I tell you, it is your deeds that have brought a sickness on the State. For the altars of our city and the altars of our hearths have been polluted, one and all, by birds and dogs who have fed on that outraged corpse that was the son of Oedipus. It is for this reason the gods refuse prayer and sacrifice at our hands, and will not consume the meat-offering with flame; nor does any bird give a clear sign by its shrill cry, for they have tasted the fatness of a 1020 slain man's blood.

Think then on these things, my son. All men are liable to err; but he shows wisdom and earns blessings who heals the ills his errors caused, being not too stubborn; too stiff a will is folly. Yield to the dead, I counsel you, and do not stab the fallen; what prowess is it

to slay the slain anew? I have sought your welfare, it is for 1030
your good I speak; and it should be a pleasant thing to hear a good
counsellor when he counsels for your own gain.

CREON: Old man, you all shoot your shafts at me, like archers at a butt
— you must practise your prophecies on me! Indeed, the tribe of
augurs has long trafficked in me and made me their merchandise!
Go, seek your price, drive your trade, if you will, in the precious
ore of Sardis and the gold of India; but you shall not buy that corpse
a grave! No, though the eagles of Zeus should bear their 1040
carrion dainties to their Master's throne — no, not even for dread
of that will I permit this burial! — for I know that no mortal can
pollute the gods. So, hoary prophet, the wisest come to a shameful
fall when they clothe shameful counsels in fair words to earn a
bribe.

TEIRESIAS: Alas! Does no man know, does none consider....

CREON: What pompous precept now?

TEIRESIAS: ... that honest counsel is the most priceless gift? 1050

CREON: Yes, and folly the most worthless.

TEIRESIAS: True, and you are infected with that disease.

CREON: This wise man's taunts I shall not answer in kind.

TEIRESIAS: Yet you slander me, saying I augur falsely.

CREON: Well, the tribe of seers always liked money.

TEIRESIAS: And the race of tyrants was ever proud and covetous.

CREON: Do you know you are speaking to your king?

TEIRESIAS: I know it: you saved the city when you followed my advice.

CREON: You have your gifts, but you love evil deeds.

TEIRESIAS: Ah, you will sting me to utter the dread secret I have kept
hidden in my soul. 1060

CREON: Out with it! — but if you hope to earn a fee by shaking my
purpose, you babble in vain.

TEIRESIAS: Indeed I think I shall earn no reward from you.

CREON: Be sure you shall not trade on my resolve.

TEIRESIAS: Know then — aye, know it well! — you will not live
through many days, seeing the sun's swift chariot coursing heaven,
'til one whose blood comes from your own heart shall be a corpse,
matching two other corpses; because you have given to the shadows
one who belongs to the sun, you have lodged a living soul in the
grave; yet in this world you detain one who belongs to the 1070
world below, a corpse unburied, unhonored and unblest. These
things outrage the gods; therefore those dread Erinyes, who serve
the fury of the gods, lie now in wait for you, preparing a vengeance
equal to your guilt.

And mark well if I speak these things as a hireling. A time not
long delayed will waken the wailing of men and women in your

house. But after these cries I hear a more dreadful tumult. For wrath and hatred will stir to arms against you every city whose mangled sons had the burial-rite from dogs and wild 1080 beasts, or from birds that will bear the taint of this crime even to the startled hearths of the unburied dead.

Such arrows I do indeed aim at your heart, since you provoke me — they will find their mark, and you shall not escape the sting. — Boy, lead me home, that he may spend his rage on younger men, or learn to curb his bitter tongue and temper his violent 1090 mind.

(TEIRESIAS *is led away.*)

CHORUS: The seer has gone, O King, predicting terrible things. And since the days when my white hair was dark, I know that he has never spoken false auguries for our city.

CREON: I know that too, I know it well, and I am troubled in soul. It is hard to yield; but if by stubbornness I bring my pride to ruin — that too would be hard.

CHORUS: Son of Menoekeus, it is time to heed good counsel.

CREON: What shall I do, then? Speak, and I will obey.

CHORUS: Go free the living maiden from her grave, and make 1100 a grave for the unburied dead.

CREON: Is this indeed your counsel? Do you bid me yield?

CHORUS: Yes, and without delay; for the swift judgments of the gods cut short the folly of men.

CREON: It is hard to do — to retreat from a firm stand — but I yield, I will obey you. We must not wage a vain war with Fate.

CHORUS: Go then, let your own hand do these things; do not leave them to others.

CREON: Even as I am I will go: come, servants, all of you, bring tools to raise one grave and open another. Since our judgment 1110 has taken this turn, I who buried the girl will free her myself. — My heart misgives me, it is best to keep the established laws, even to life's end.

(CREON *and his servants go toward the plain.*)

CHORUS: O god of many names,
          Fruit of the daughter of Cadmus
          Whom the loud-thundering Zeus
          Embraced amid lightnings,
          Ever your praise be sung
          From famed Italia's vineyards
          To the Eleusinian vale   1120
          Where Deo welcomes all;

But most, O Bacchus,
In Thebes where you dwell,
In Thebes, mother of Bacchants,
And by that stream Ismenus
Where the dragon's teeth were sown!

Where the two slender peaks
Of Muse-haunted Parnassus
Rise against the sky,
The torch-flames have revealed you;
And you have been seen
Where the Corycian nymphs
Dance for joy of you
Through the flowering meadows
Beside Castalia's stream.   1130

But from Nysa's hills,
With twining ivy mantled,
And from many a headland
Green with clustered vines,
Even while your name is lifted
In all men's song and prayer,
You turn to the dragon's land
And visit the ways of Thebes.

Thebes, where your mother
Conceived amid lightning,
First among cities
Stand always in your grace.
And now when the people
By this new plague are stricken,   1140
Swiftly from Parnassus
You come with healing tread!

O god with whom the stars,
The stars whose breath is fire,
Rejoice as they move in heaven —
O lord of the hymns of the night,
O Cadmean son of Zeus,
Amid the dancing maidens
Appear to us in majesty —   1150
O giver of all good gifts,
Iacchos, heed our prayer!

(A MESSENGER *appears, from the direction of the plain.*)

MESSENGER: Neighbors of the house of Cadmus, dwellers within Amphion's walls, there is no state of mortal life that I would praise or pity, for none is beyond swift change. Fortune raises men up and fortune casts them down from day to day, and no man can foretell the fate of things established. For Creon was blest in all 1160 that I count happiness: he had honor as our savior; power as our king; pride as the father of princely children. Now all is ended. For when a man is stripped of happiness, I count him not with the living — he is but a breathing corpse. Let a man have riches heaped in his house, and live in royal splendor; yet I would not 1170 give the shadow of a breath for all, if they bring no gladness.

CHORUS: What fearful news have you about our princes?

MESSENGER: Death; and the living are guilty of the dead.

CHORUS: Who is the slayer — who is slain?

MESSENGER: Haemon has perished, and it was no stranger shed his blood.

CHORUS: His father's hand, or his own?

MESSENGER: His own, maddened by his father's crime.

CHORUS: O prophet, how true your word has proved!

MESSENGER: This is the way things are: consider then, how to act.

CHORUS: Look! — the unhappy Eurydice, Creon's consort, 1180 comes from the house; is it by chance, or has she heard these tidings of her son?

(EURYDICE *comes from the house.*)

EURYDICE: I heard your words, citizens, as I was going to the shrine of Pallas with my prayers. As I loosed the bolts of the gate, the message of woe to my household smote my ear. I sank back, stricken with horror, into the arms of my handmaids, and my senses left me. Yet say again these tidings. I shall hear them as 1190 one who is no stranger to grief.

MESSENGER: Dear lady, I will tell you what I saw, I will hide nothing of the truth. I would gladly tell you a happier tale, but it would soon be found out false. Truth is the only way. — I guided your lord the King to the furthest part of the plain, where the body of Polynices, torn by dogs, still lay unpitied. There we prayed to the goddess of the roads, and to Pluto, in mercy to restrain their wrath. We washed the dead with holy rites, and all that was left 1200 of the mortal man we burned with fresh-plucked branches; and over the ashes at last we raised a mound of his native earth.

That done, we turned our steps toward those fearsome caves where in a cold nuptial chamber, with couch of stone, that maiden had been given as a bride of Death. But from afar off, one of us heard a voice wailing aloud, and turned to tell our master Creon.

And as the King drew nearer, the sharp anguish of broken cries came to his ears. Then he groaned and said like one in   1210 pain, "Can my sudden fear be true? Am I on the saddest road I ever went? That voice is my son's! Hurry, my servants, to the tomb, and through the gap where the stones have been torn out, look into the cell — tell me if it is Haemon's voice I hear, or if my wits are tortured by the gods."

At these words from our stricken master, we went to make that search; and in the dim furthest part of the tomb we saw   1220 Antigone hanging by the neck, her scarf of fine linen twisted into a cruel noose. And there too we saw Haemon — his arms about her waist, while he cried out upon the loss of his bride, and his father's deed, and his ill-starred love.

But now the King approached, and saw him, and cried out with horror, and went in and called with piteous voice, "Unhappy boy, what a deed have you done, breaking into this tomb! What purpose have you? Has grief stolen your reason? Come forth, my son! I pray you — I implore!" The boy answered no word, but   1230 glared at him with fierce eyes, spat in his face, and drew his cross-hilted sword. His father turned and fled, and the blow missed its mark. Then that maddened boy, torn between grief and rage, and penitence, straightway leaned upon his sword, and drove it half its length into his side; and in the little moment before death, he clasped the maiden in his arms, and her pale cheek was red where his blood gushed forth.

Corpse enfolding corpse they lie; he has won his bride,   1240 poor lad, not here but in the halls of Death; to all of us he has left a terrible witness that man's worst error is to reject good counsel.

(EURYDICE *goes into the house*.)

CHORUS: What does this mean? The lady turns and goes without a word.

MESSENGER: I too am startled; but I think it means she is too proud to cry out before the people. Within the house, with her hand-maids about her, the tears will flow. Life has taught her prudence.   1250

CHORUS: It may be; yet I fear. To me such silence seems more ominous than many lamentations.

MESSENGER: Then I will go into the house, and learn if some tragic purpose has formed in her tortured heart. Yes, you speak wisely; too much silence may hide terrible meanings.

(*The* MESSENGER *enters the house. As he goes,* CREON *comes into the open place before the house with attendants carrying the shrouded body of* HAEMON *on a bier.*)

CHORUS: See, the King himself draws near, with the sad proof of his folly; this tells a tale of no violence by strangers, but — if I may say it — of his own misdeeds.   1260

CREON: Woe for the sins of a darkened soul, the sins of a stubborn pride that played with death! Behold me, the father who has slain, behold the son who has perished! I am punished for the blindness of my counsels. Alas my son, cut down in youth untimely, woe is me! — your spirit fled — not yours the fault and folly, but my own!

CHORUS: Too late, too late your eyes are opened!   1270

CREON: I have learned that bitter lesson. But it was some god, I think, darkened my mind and turned me into ways of cruelty. Now my days are overthrown and my joys trampled. Alas, man's labors come but to foolish ends!

(*The* MESSENGER *comes from the house.*)

MESSENGER: Sire, one sees your hands are not empty, but there is more laid up in store for you. Woeful is the burden you bear, and you must look on further woes within your house.   1280

CREON: Why, how can there be more?

MESSENGER: Your queen is dead, the mother of that lad — unhappy lady! This is Fate's latest blow.

CREON: Death, Death, how many deaths will stay your hunger? For me is there no mercy? O messenger of evil, bearer of bitter tidings, what is this you tell me? I was already dead, but you smite me anew. What do you say? — what is this news you bring of slaughter heaped on slaughter?   1290

(*The doors of the King's house are opened, and the corpse of* EURYDICE *is disclosed.*)

CHORUS: Behold with your own eyes!

CREON: Oh, horror! — woe upon woe! Can any further dreadful thing await me? I have but now raised my son in these arms — and here again I see a corpse before me. Alas, unhappy mother — alas, alas my child!   1300

MESSENGER: At the altar of your house, self-stabbed with a keen knife, she suffered her darkening eyes to close, while she lamented that other son, Megareus, who died so nobly but a while ago, and then this boy whose corpse is here beside you. But with her last breath and with a bitter cry she invoked evil upon you, the slayer of your sons.

CREON: Will no one strike me to the heart with the two-edged sword? — miserable that I am, and plunged in misery!   1310

MESSENGER: Yes, both this son's death and that other son's, were charged to you by her whose corpse you see.

CREON: But how did she do this violence upon herself?

MESSENGER: Her own hand struck her to the heart, when she had heard how this boy died.

CREON: I cannot escape the guilt of these things, it rests on no other of mortal kind. I, only I, am the slayer, wretched that I am — I own the truth. Lead me away, my servants, lead me   1320 quickly hence, for my life is but death.

CHORUS: You speak well, if any speech is good amid so much evil. When all is trouble, the briefest way is best.

CREON: Oh let it come now, the fate most merciful for me, my last day — that will be the best fate of all. Oh let it come   1330 swiftly, that I may not look upon tomorrow's light!

CHORUS: That is hidden in the future. Present tasks claim our care. The ordering of the future does not rest with mortals.

CREON: Yet all my desire is summed up in that prayer.

CHORUS: Pray no more: no man evades his destiny.

CREON: Lead me away, I pray you; a rash, foolish man, who has slain you, O my son, unwittingly, and you too, my wife —   1340 unhappy that I am! Where can I find comfort, where can I turn my gaze? — for where I have turned my hand, all has gone wrong; and this last blow breaks me and bows my head.

(CREON *is led into his house as the* CHORUS *speaks.*)

CHORUS:
If any man would be happy, and not broken by Fate,
Wisdom is the thing he should seek, for happiness hides there.
Let him revere the gods and keep their words inviolate,   1350
For proud men who speak great words come in the end to despair,
And learn wisdom in sorrow, when it is too late.

SOPHOCLES

OEDIPUS REX

Translated by Albert Cook

INTRODUCTION

It is almost impossible to extricate from students' minds the inevitable conviction which they acquire at first sight of the *Oedipus Rex*, that man's fate is irrevocably fixed, that free will is an illusion, and that nothing can be done about it anyway. Aristotle, of course, shares part of the blame for this mesmerism of undergraduates. To him the *Oedipus* was the ideal play, and he admired most of all its recognition-scenes, its reversal of fortune (both of these narrowly defined), and its piot, smoothly achieved, marvellously engineered along the bright rails of an infernal machine, as Jean Cocteau also conceived it in his amusing adaptation, *La machine infernale*. One could, in fact, wish that Aristotle had chosen any other play but this one to mention eleven times in the *Poetics*.

Naturally students can, and usually do, reach the same conclusion without reading Aristotle. Before they come to Greek drama they have heard of fate, of the Oedipus complex, and of a few other unhelpful things. Sophocles does the rest for them: the Greek heroes turn into automata who walk around in a dream, helpless to determine their next move. Yet is it so easy to persuade them that Oedipus too, like all the other Greeks in epic and drama, possesses free will? One can say that fate is really the way life works out for a man, not how it was planned or foreordained for him from the beginning. One can say that the concept of retribution implies free will to act in a manner which calls for retribution, or else the concept becomes nonsense. One can quote Walter Agard, genial interpreter of "Three Themes in Classical Literature" (*The Humanities for Our Time*; University of Kansas Press, 1949): "even if everything is determined, we have no way of knowing what the total pattern is, so we must act on our own best judgment; free will is, therefore, a necessary illusion. Apparently wise men attain some insight into this pattern (or are given it by the gods), but all of us have the freedom to disregard such insight, follow our own desires, and suffer the consequences." The answers to the problem of fate given by Calvinists and both scientific and economic determinists do not help people who are resolved to believe in a fixed series of actions from which no man can escape. Perhaps the reason for this is that they have not read Zeno and Epicurus while reading too many modern materialistic novels.

The concept of human suffering as it is presented by Sophocles loses all meaning if his characters have no free will; as a matter of fact, they have more free will than most other characters in Greek drama. It is curious how the scholars agree (or repeat each other?) on Sophocles' view of suffering: "The central idea of a Sophoclean tragedy is that through suffering a man learns to be modest before the gods" (Bowra). "His Oedipus stands for human suffering, and he neither attempts, like Aeschylus, to justify the evil, nor presumes, like Euripides, to deny its divine origin" (J. T. Sheppard). "Sophocles' difficulty is the problem of suffering, as Aeschylus' is the problem of sin" (A. Zimmern).

Antigone, Hercules, Ajax, Electra, Philoctetes, Oedipus — none of these is forced to act in any way except the one he or she chooses. All Oedipus had to do to avoid his fate, if he had made the attempt to do so, was not to run away from Corinth, not to take the road to Thebes, not to kill an old man on that road even in self-defense, and certainly not to answer the riddle of the Sphinx. But I can see a hand raised in the back row and shall soon be set straight in my thinking.

Actually it is character that is fate: the Greeks themselves came to that conclusion. In Oedipus we have a headstrong, self-willed, impulsive, arrogant, and wholly sincere man who illustrates admirably Ibsen's frequently dramatized contention about the harm that good men do. Here is a man who will not let well enough alone, who will not let sleeping dogs lie, who wants to know the truth at all costs. Given such a character, almost any of the wrong choices he took along the way would have led to the subsequent series of wrong choices; you cannot keep a barroom brawler from doing harm to himself and others once he starts brawling except by knocking him out or locking him up. Reason cannot prevail with those who believe they are more right than anyone else in the world, who can even outguess the Sphinx.

Although the play poses the problems of fate and free will as though under the glaring light of a television stage, it has other aspects which enrich its themes and make it a far more subtle and intricate work of art than even Aristotle dreamed it was. Professor L. W. Daly in his authoritative articles and reviews on Oedipus has emphasized, for example, the abundant folklore material of its Sphinx-riddle, its contest for power, its marriage of the "princess" by the hero; the incest favorable to politicians if they dreamed of it (see Artemidorus, the Greek interpreter of dreams); the Sphinx herself, whom Cocteau represents in two aspects, a young girl and a male god, who is a female incubus from the underworld, like the Sirens and Lamiae: all these are fascinating elements in a brooding atmosphere of dark foreboding sufficient to raise the hair of any audience in fear and pity. The riddle itself is a deep folk saying whose answer is "Man":

"A thing there is whose voice is one,
Whose feet are two and four and three.
So mutable a thing is none
That moves in earth or sky or sea.
When on most feet this thing doth go
Its strength is weakest and its pace most slow!"

So J. T. Sheppard translates it from the argument of the Greek text.

There is the abundant, almost constant, irony of the play, its lines filled with the double meanings which critics call dramatic irony: the awesome gap between the one meaning known to the audience and the other known to the players, into which flows a stream of emotion so strong it chokes the very heart. Oedipus calls Teiresias blind, when he himself is blinder than any bat; Oedipus curses Laius' murderer and thus curses himself; Oedipus answers the Sphinx but finds no answer for his own dilemma; he tries to help his fellow men and merely harms himself, runs from danger only to find it, and so on.

There is further the obvious imagery of sight and blindness, of light and darkness, so obvious that many readers have to be told it is there. There are the choruses, not so grand as elsewhere in Sophocles, but outstanding all the same: objectively severe and conventional, as in the first stasimon; gradually more troubled and anxious, full of revulsion against the flaw of Oedipus (pride — as it was of Dante), as in the second stasimon; desolate and drowned in utter despair, as in the fourth stasimon "O generations of men, your lives add up to nothing!", to be contrasted with the ode in *Antigone* on the wonder of man. There is the final horror of the blinded Oedipus himself, inexorable executor of his own harsh decree, the blood streaming down his face; few scenes in literature are more horrible, not Dante's Ugolino gnawing his child's skull in the dungeon, Lear mad on the heath, Marlowe's Barabas in his caldron, the handmaidens hanging from the rafters in the *Odyssey*, or Ganelon drawn apart by horses in the *Song of Roland*.

The free spirit of inquiry reaches its saddest heights in this play; the Greek word for that — historia — occurs with a frequency which constitutes a major theme. It brings Oedipus blindness and exile, dragging his dreadful foot, both literally and allegorically dreadful, out of the land of Thebes, "now seeing straight, but then in shadow" (419), a line St. Paul might have had in mind as he reversed the effect in I Corinthians 13.12: "For now we see through a glass, darkly; but then face to face."

Francis Fergusson, in his *The Idea of a Theater* (1949), has made use of this theme in considering the *Oedipus Rex* as the archetype of drama. He discusses its meaning and form in terms of the hero's quest for himself as well as for the slayer of Laius in relation to what he calls "histrionic sensibility, i.e., our direct sense of the changing life of the psyche." He underlines the ambiguities of the play in its myth, ritual, chorus, and imitation of an action (Aristotle). His entire analysis is stimulating; but more important is his decision to make the play fundamental to his study of later drama from Racine to T. S. Eliot.

The *Oedipus Rex* is thus seen to be an immensely fruitful source for inspiration; one of its many influences appears in Gide's *Oedipe,* where among other innovations the incest of Oedipus' children is exaggerated. The ideas of the play are many; among them are the knowledge that comes through suffering, the responsibility of man for his own acts, the error of setting human reason above obedience to the gods, the myriad ironies of fate, the tragic consequences of excessive pride. To use the words of Joyce's *Ulysses* in another context, it is truly a play calculated to make men "reflect, ponder, excogitate, reply."

The date of its presentation is not certain; it may have been anywhere between 439 and 412 B.C.; perhaps 430–425 is a reasonable point. We do not know the names of the two other plays Sophocles presented at the same festival. The plot resembles some of Ibsen's plays in its use of "retrospective analysis," the revelation of past mistakes. The five choral odes are carefully arranged for the best effect.

The events before the play opens are described in the dialogue; the dialogue-prologue does not rehearse this information but plunges at once into the action. The story of the house of Laius has been most recently re-told by Robert Graves in his useful book, *The Greek Myths* II (1955). Laius of Thebes was told by the Delphic oracle that any child born to his childless wife Jocasta would murder his father. Thus he thrust her away, but she made him drunk and amorous once more: nine months later a child was born to the royal pair. Laius pierced the baby's feet with a nail — hence his name "Swollen Foot" — and exposed him on Mount Cithaeron. Here a shepherd found the child and brought him to Corinth, where he was adopted by King Polybus and Queen Periboea. The play then tells of the taunt offered Oedipus at a banquet and its consequences: his consultation of the oracle, the flight from Corinth, and his triumph and downfall at Thebes.

L. R. LIND

OEDIPUS REX

CHARACTERS

OEDIPUS, *king of Thebes*

A PRIEST

CREON, *brother-in-law of Oedipus*

CHORUS *of Theban elders*

TEIRESIAS, *a prophet*

JOCASTA, *sister of Creon, wife of Oedipus*

MESSENGER

SERVANT *of Laius, father of Oedipus*

SECOND MESSENGER

(*silent*) ANTIGONE *and* ISMENE, *daughters of Oedipus*

SCENE. *Before the palace of Oedipus at Thebes. In front of the large central doors, an altar; and an altar near each of the two side doors. On the altar steps are seated suppliants — old men, youths, and young boys — dressed in white tunics and cloaks, their hair bound with white fillets. They have laid on the altars olive branches wreathed with wool-fillets.*

The old PRIEST OF ZEUS *stands alone facing the central doors of the palace. The doors open, and* OEDIPUS, *followed by two attendants who stand at either door, enters and looks about.*

OEDIPUS: O children, last born stock of ancient Cadmus,
What petitions are these you bring to me
With garlands on your suppliant olive branches?
The whole city teems with incense fumes,
Teems with prayers for healing and with groans.

Thinking it best, children, to hear all this
Not from some messenger, I came myself,
The world renowned and glorious Oedipus.
But tell me, aged priest, since you are fit
To speak before these men, how stand you here,   10
In fear or want? Tell me, as I desire
To do my all; hard hearted I would be
To feel no sympathy for such a prayer.
PRIEST: O Oedipus, ruler of my land, you see
How old we are who stand in supplication
Before your altars here, some not yet strong
For lengthy flight, some heavy with age,
Priests, as I of Zeus, and choice young men.
The rest of the tribe sits with wreathed branches,
In market places, at Pallas' two temples,   20
And at prophetic embers by the river.
The city, as you see, now shakes too greatly
And cannot raise her head out of the depths
Above the gory swell. She wastes in blight,
Blight on earth's fruitful blooms and grazing flocks,
And on the barren birth pangs of the women.
The fever god has fallen on the city,
And drives it, a most hated pestilence
Through whom the home of Cadmus is made empty.
Black Hades is enriched with wails and groans.   30
Not that we think you equal to the gods
These boys and I sit suppliant at your hearth,
But judging you first of men in the trials of life,
And in the human intercourse with spirits: —
You are the one who came to Cadmus' city
And freed us from the tribute which we paid
To the harsh-singing Sphinx. And that you did
Knowing nothing else, unschooled by us.
But people say and think it was some god
That helped you to set our life upright.
Now Oedipus, most powerful of all,   40
We all are turned here toward you, we beseech you,
Find us some strength, whether from one of the gods
You hear an omen, or know one from a man.
For the experienced I see will best
Make good plans grow from evil circumstance.
Come, best of mortal men, raise up the state.
Come, prove your fame, since now this land of ours
Calls you savior for your previous zeal.

O never let our memory of your reign
Be that we first stood straight and later fell,   50
But to security raise up this state.
With favoring omen once you gave us luck;
Be now as good again; for if henceforth
You rule as now, you will be this country's king,
Better it is to rule men than a desert,
Since nothing is either ship or fortress tower
Bare of men who together dwell within.

OEDIPUS: O piteous children, I am not ignorant
Of what you come desiring. Well I know
You are all sick, and in your sickness none   6c
There is among you as sick as I,
For your pain comes to one man alone,
To him and to none other, but my soul
Groans for the state, for myself, and for you.
You do not wake a man who is sunk in sleep;
Know that already I have shed many tears,
And travelled many wandering roads of thought.
Well have I sought, and found one remedy;
And this I did: the son of Menoeceus,
Creon, my brother-in-law, I sent away   70
Unto Apollo's Pythian halls to find
What I might do or say to save the state.
The days are measured out that he is gone;
It troubles me how he fares. Longer than usual
He has been away, more than the fitting time.
But when he comes, then evil I shall be,
If all the god reveals I fail to do.

PRIEST: You speak at the right time. These men just now
Signal to me that Creon is approaching.

OEDIPUS: O Lord Apollo, grant that he may come   80
In saving fortune shining as in eye.

PRIEST: Glad news he brings, it seems, or else his head
Would not be crowned with leafy, berried bay.

OEDIPUS: We will soon know. He is close enough to hear. —
Prince, my kinsman, son of Menoeceus,
What oracle do you bring us from the god?

CREON: A good one. For I say that even burdens
If they chance to turn out right, will all be well.

OEDIPUS: Yet what is the oracle? Your present word
Makes me neither bold nor apprehensive.   90

CREON: If you wish to hear in front of this crowd
I am ready to speak, or we can go within.

OEDIPUS: Speak forth to all. The sorrow that I bear
Is greater for these men than for my life.
CREON: May I tell you what I heard from the god?
Lord Phoebus clearly bids us to drive out,
And not to leave uncured within this country,
A pollution we have nourished in our land.
OEDIPUS: With what purgation? What kind of misfortune?
CREON: Banish the man, or quit slaughter with slaughter   100
In cleansing, since this blood rains on the state.
OEDIPUS: Who is this man whose fate the god reveals?
CREON: Laius, my lord, was formerly the guide
Of this our land before you steered this city.
OEDIPUS: I know him by hearsay, but I never saw him.
CREON: Since he was slain, the god now plainly bids us
To punish his murderers, whoever they may be.
OEDIPUS: Where are they on the earth? How shall we find
This indiscernible track of ancient guilt?
CREON: In this land, said Apollo. What is sought   110
Can be apprehended; the unobserved escapes.
OEDIPUS: Did Laius fall at home on this bloody end?
Or in the fields, or in some foreign land?
CREON: As a pilgrim, the god said, he left his tribe
And once away from home, returned no more.
OEDIPUS: Was there no messenger, no fellow wayfarer
Who saw, from whom an inquirer might get aid?
CREON: They are all dead, save one, who fled in fear
And he knows only one thing sure to tell.
OEDIPUS: What is that? We may learn many facts from one   120
If we might take for hope a short beginning.
CREON: Robbers, Apollo said, met there and killed him
Not by the strength of one, but many hands.
OEDIPUS: How did the robber unless something from here
Was at work with silver, reach this point of daring?
CREON: These facts are all conjecture. Laius dead,
There rose in evils no avenger for him.
OEDIPUS: But when the king had fallen slain, what trouble
Prevented you from finding all this out?
CREON: The subtle-singing Sphinx made us let go   130
What was unclear to search at our own feet.
OEDIPUS: Well then, I will make this clear afresh
From the start. Phoebus was right, you were right
To take this present interest in the dead.
Justly it is you see me as your ally
Avenging alike this country and the god.

Not for the sake of some distant friends,
But for myself I will disperse this filth.
Whoever it was who killed that man
With the same hand may wish to do vengeance on me.   140
And so assisting Laius I aid myself.
But hurry quickly, children, stand up now
From the altar steps, raising these suppliant boughs.
Let someone gather Cadmus' people here
To learn that I will do all, whether at last
With Phoebus' help we are shown saved or fallen.

PRIEST: Come, children, let us stand. We came here
First for the sake of what this man proclaims.
Phoebus it was who sent these prophecies
And he will come to save us from the plague.   150

CHORUS:

    Strophe A

O sweet-tongued voice of Zeus, in what spirit do you come
From Pytho rich in gold
To glorious Thebes? I am torn on the rack, dread shakes my fearful
    mind,
Apollo of Delos, hail!
As I stand in awe of you, what need, either new
Do you bring to the full for me, or old in the turning times of the
    year?
Tell me, O child of golden Hope, undying Voice!

    Antistrophe A

First on you do I call, daughter of Zeus, undying Athene
And your sister who guards our land,   160
Artemis, seated upon the throne renowned of our circled Place,
And Phoebus who darts afar;
Shine forth to me, thrice warder-off of death;
If ever in time before when ruin rushed upon the state,
The flame of sorrow you drove beyond our bounds, come also now.

    Strophe B

O woe! Unnumbered that I bear
The sorrows are! My whole host is sick, nor is there a sword of
    thought
To ward off pain. The growing fruits   170
Of glorious earth wax not, nor women
Withstand in childbirth shrieking pangs.
Life on life you may see, which, like the well-winged bird,

Faster than stubborn fire, speed
To the strand of the evening god.

Antistrophe B

Unnumbered of the city die.   180
Unpitied babies bearing death lie unmoaned on the ground.
Grey-haired mothers and young wives
From all sides at the altar's edge
Lift up a wail beseeching, for their mournful woes.
The prayer for healing shines blent with a grieving cry;
Wherefore, O golden daughter of Zeus,
Send us your succour with its beaming face.

Strophe C

Grant that fiery Ares, who now with no brazen shield   190
Flames round me in shouting attack
May turn his back in running flight from our land,
May be borne with fair wind
To Amphitrite's great chamber
Or to the hostile port
Of the Thracian surge.
For even if night leaves any ill undone
It is brought to pass and comes to be in the day.
O Zeus who bear the fire   200
And rule the lightning's might,
Strike him beneath your thunderbolt with death!

Antistrophe C

O lord Apollo, would that you might come and scatter forth
Untamed darts from your twirling golden bow;
Bring succour from the plague; may the flashing
Beams come of Artemis,
With which she glances through the Lycian hills.
Also on him I call whose hair is held in gold,
Who gives a name to this land,   210
Bacchus of winy face, whom maidens hail!
Draw near with your flaming Maenad band
And the aid of your gladsome torch
Against the plague, dishonoured among the gods.

OEDIPUS: You pray; if for what you pray you would be willing
To hear and take my words, to nurse the plague,
You may get succour and relief from evils.
A stranger to this tale I now speak forth,

A stranger to the deed, for not alone 220
Could I have tracked it far without some clue,
But now that I am enrolled a citizen
Latest among the citizens of Thebes
To all you sons of Cadmus I proclaim
Whoever of you knows at what man's hand
Laius, the son of Labdacus, met his death,
I order him to tell me all, and even
If he fears, to clear the charge and he will suffer
No injury, but leave the land unharmed.
If someone knows the murderer to be an alien 230
From foreign soil, let him not be silent;
I will give him a reward, my thanks besides.
But if you stay in silence and from fear
For self or friend thrust aside my command,
Hear now from me what I shall do for this;
I charge that none who dwell within this land
Whereof I hold the power and the throne
Give this man shelter whoever he may be,
Or speak to him, or share with him in prayer
Or sacrifice, or serve him lustral rites, 240
But drive him, all, out of your homes, for he
Is this pollution on us, as Apollo
Revealed to me just now in oracle.
I am therefore the ally of the god
And of the murdered man. And now I pray
That the murderer, whether he hides alone
Or with his partners, may, evil coward,
Wear out in luckless ills his wretched life.
I further pray, that, if at my own hearth
He dwells known to me in my own home, 250
I may suffer myself the curse I just now uttered.
And you I charge to bring all this to pass
For me, and for the god, and for our land
Which now lies fruitless, godless, and corrupt.
Even if Phoebus had not urged this affair,
Not rightly did you let it go unpurged
When one both noble and a king was murdered!
You should have sought it out. Since now I reign
Holding the power which he had held before me,
Having the selfsame wife and marriage bed — 260
And if his seed had not met barren fortune
We should be linked by offspring from one mother;
But as it was, fate leapt upon his head.

Therefore in this, as if for my own father
I fight for him, and shall attempt all
Searching to seize the hand which shed that blood,
For Labdacus' son, before him Polydorus,
And ancient Cadmus, and Agenor of old.
And those who fail to do this, I pray the gods
May give them neither harvest from their earth   270
Nor children from their wives, but may they be
Destroyed by a fate like this one, or a worse.
You other Thebans, who cherish these commands,
May Justice, the ally of a righteous cause,
And all the gods be always on your side.

CHORUS: By the oath you laid on me, my king, I speak.
I killed not Laius, nor can show who killed him.
Phoebus it was who sent this question to us,
And he should answer who has done the deed.

OEDIPUS: Your words are just, but to compel the gods   280
In what they do not wish, no man can do.

CHORUS: I would tell what seems to me our second course.

OEDIPUS: If there is a third, fail not to tell it too.

CHORUS: Lord Teiresias I know, who sees this best
Like lord Apollo; in surveying this,
One might, my lord, find out from him most clearly.

OEDIPUS: Even this I did not neglect; I have done it already.
At Creon's word I twice sent messengers.
It is a wonder he has been gone so long.

CHORUS: And also there are rumors, faint and old.   290

OEDIPUS: What are they? I must search out every tale.

CHORUS: They say there were some travellers who killed him.

OEDIPUS: So I have heard, but no one sees a witness.

CHORUS: If his mind knows a particle of fear
He will not long withstand such curse as yours.

OEDIPUS: He fears no speech who fears not such a deed.

CHORUS: But here is the man who will convict the guilty.
Here are these men leading the divine prophet
In whom alone of men the truth is born.

OEDIPUS: O you who ponder all, Teiresias,   300
Both what is taught and what cannot be spoken,
What is of heaven and what trod on the earth,
Even if you are blind, you know what plague
Clings to the state, and, master, you alone
We find as her protector and her saviour.
Apollo, if the messengers have not told you,
Answered our question, that release would come

From this disease only if we make sure
Of Laius' slayers and slay them in return
Or drive them out as exiles from the land.
But you now, grudge us neither voice of birds   310
Nor any way you have of prophecy.
Save yourself and the state; save me as well.
Save everything polluted by the dead.
We are in your hands; it is the noblest task
To help a man with all your means and powers.

TEIRESIAS: Alas! Alas! How terrible to be wise,
Where it does the seer no good. Too well I know
And have forgot this, or would not have come here.

OEDIPUS: What is this? How fainthearted you have come!

TEIRESIAS: Let me go home; it is best for you to bear   320
Your burden, and I mine, if you will heed me.

OEDIPUS: You speak what is lawless, and hateful to the state
Which raised you, when you deprive her of your answer.

TEIRESIAS: And I see that your speech does not proceed
In season; I shall not undergo the same.

OEDIPUS: Don't by the gods turn back when you are wise,
When all we suppliants lie prostrate before you.

TEIRESIAS: And all unwise; I never shall reveal
My evils, so that I may not tell yours.

OEDIPUS: What do you say? You know, but will not speak?   330
Would you betray us and destroy the state?

TEIRESIAS: I will not hurt you or me. Why in vain
Do you probe this? You will not find out from me.

OEDIPUS: Worst of evil men, you would enrage
A stone itself. Will you never speak,
But stay so untouched and so inconclusive?

TEIRESIAS: You blame my anger and do not see that
With which you live in common, but upbraid me.

OEDIPUS: Who would not be enraged to hear these words
By which you now dishonor this our city?   340

TEIRESIAS: Of itself this will come, though I hide it in silence.

OEDIPUS: Then you should tell me what it is will come.

TEIRESIAS: I shall speak no more. If further you desire,
Rage on in wildest anger of your soul.

OEDIPUS: I shall omit nothing I understand
I am so angry. Know that you seem to me
Creator of the deed and worker too
In all short of the slaughter; if you were not blind,
I would say this crime was your work alone.

TEIRESIAS: Really? Abide yourself by the decree   350

You just proclaimed, I tell you! From this day
Henceforth address neither these men nor me.
You are the godless defiler of this land.
OEDIPUS: You push so bold and taunting in your speech;
And how do you think to get away with this?
TEIRESIAS: I have got away. I nurse my strength in truth.
OEDIPUS: Who taught you this? Not from your art you got it.
TEIRESIAS: From you. You had me speak against my will.
OEDIPUS: What word? Say again, so I may better learn.
TEIRESIAS: Didn't you get it before? Or do you bait me?   360
OEDIPUS: I don't remember it. Speak forth again.
TEIRESIAS: You are the slayer whom you seek, I say.
OEDIPUS: Not twice you speak such bitter words unpunished.
TEIRESIAS: Shall I speak more to make you angrier still?
OEDIPUS: Do what you will, your words will be in vain.
TEIRESIAS: I say you have forgot that you are joined
With those most dear to you in deepest shame
And do not see where you are in sin.
OEDIPUS: Do you think you will always say such things in joy?
TEIRESIAS: Surely, if strength abides in what is true.
OEDIPUS: It does, for all but you, this not for you   370
Because your ears and mind and eyes are blind.
TEIRESIAS: Wretched you are to make such taunts, for soon
All men will cast the selfsame taunts on you.
OEDIPUS: You live in entire night, could do no harm
To me or any man who sees the day.
TEIRESIAS: Not at my hands will it be your fate to fall.
Apollo suffices, whose concern it is to do this.
OEDIPUS: Are these devices yours, or are they Creon's?
TEIRESIAS: Creon is not your trouble; you are yourself.
OEDIPUS: O riches, empire, skill surpassing skill   380
In all the numerous rivalries of life,
How great a grudge there is stored up against you
If for this kingship, which the city gave,
Their gift, not my request, into my hands —
For this, the trusted Creon, my friend from the start
Desires to creep by stealth and cast me out
Taking a seer like this, a weaver of wiles,
A crooked swindler who has got his eyes
On gain alone, but in his art is blind.
Come, tell us, in what clearly are you a prophet?   390
How is it, when the weave-songed bitch was here
You uttered no salvation for these people?
Surely the riddle then could not be solved

By some chance comer; it needed prophecy.
You did not clarify that with birds
Or knowledge from a god; but when I came,
The ignorant Oedipus, I silenced her,
Not taught by birds, but winning by my wits,
Whom you are now attempting to depose,
Thinking to minister near Creon's throne.   **400**
I think that to your woe you and that plotter
Will purge the land, and if you were not old
Punishment would teach you what you plot.
CHORUS: It seems to us, O Oedipus our king,
  Both this man's words and yours were said in anger.
  Such is not our need, but to find out
  How best we shall discharge Apollo's orders.
TEIRESIAS: Even if you are king, the right to answer
  Should be free to all; of that I too am king.
  I live not as your slave, but as Apollo's.   **410**
  And not with Creon's wards shall I be counted.
  I say, since you have taunted even my blindness,
  You have eyes, but see not where in evil you are
  Nor where you dwell, nor whom you are living with.
  Do you know from whom you spring? And you forget
  You are an enemy to your own kin
  Both those beneath and those above the earth.
  Your mother's and father's curse, with double goad
  And dreaded foot shall drive you from this land.
  You who now see straight shall then be blind,
  And there shall be no harbour for your cry   **420**
  With which all Mount Cithaeron soon shall ring,
  When you have learned the wedding where you sailed
  At home, into no port, by voyage fair.
  A throng of other ills you do not know
  Shall equal you to yourself and to your children.
  Throw mud on this, on Creon, on my voice —
  Yet there shall never be a mortal man
  Eradicated more wretchedly than you.
OEDIPUS: Shall these unbearable words be heard from him?
  Go to perdition! Hurry! Off, away,   **430**
  Turn back again and from this house depart.
TEIRESIAS: If you had not called me, I should not have come.
OEDIPUS: I did not know that you would speak such folly
  Or I would not soon have brought you to my house.
TEIRESIAS: And such a fool I am, as it seems to you.
  But to the parents who bore you I seem wise.

OEDIPUS: What parents? Wait! What mortals gave me birth?
TEIRESIAS: This day shall be your birth and your destruction.
OEDIPUS: All things you say in riddles and unclear.
TEIRESIAS: Are you not he who best can search this out?   440
OEDIPUS: Mock, if you wish, the skill that made me great.
TEIRESIAS: This is the very fortune that destroyed you.
OEDIPUS: Well, if I saved the city, I do not care.
TEIRESIAS: I am going now. You, boy, be my guide.
OEDIPUS: Yes, let him guide you. Here you are in the way.
    When you are gone you will give no more trouble.
TEIRESIAS: I go when I have said what I came to say
    Without fear of your frown; you cannot destroy me.
    I say, the very man whom you long seek
    With threats and announcements about Laius' murder —   450
    This man is here. He seems an alien stranger,
    But soon he shall be revealed of Theban birth,
    Nor at this circumstance shall he be pleased.
    He shall be blind who sees, shall be a beggar
    Who now is rich, shall make his way abroad
    Feeling the ground before him with a staff.
    He shall be revealed at once as brother
    And father to his own children, husband and son
    To his mother, his father's kin and murderer.   460
    Go in and ponder that. If I am wrong,
    Say then that I know nothing of prophecy.

CHORUS:
    Strophe A
Who is the man the Delphic rock said with oracular voice
Unspeakable crimes performed with his gory hands?
It is time for him now to speed
His foot in flight, more strong
Than horses swift as the storm.
For girt in arms upon him springs
With fire and lightning, Zeus' son   470
And behind him, terrible,
Come the unerring Fates.

    Antistrophe A
From snowy Parnassus just now the word flashed clear
To track the obscure man by every way,
For he wanders under the wild
Forest, and into caves
And cliff rocks, like a bull,

Reft on his way, with care on care
Trying to shun the prophecy
Come from the earth's mid-navel,   480
But about him flutters the ever living doom.

Strophe B

Terrible, terrible things the wise bird-augur stirs.
I neither approve nor deny, at a loss for what to say,
I flutter in hopes and fears, see neither here nor ahead;
For what strife has lain
On Labdacus' sons or Polybus' that I have found ever before   490
Or now, whereby I may run for the sons of Labdacus
In sure proof against Oedipus' public fame
As avenger for dark death?

Antistrophe B

Zeus and Apollo surely understand and know
The affairs of mortal men, but that a mortal seer
Knows more than I, there is no proof. Though a man   500
May surpass a man in knowledge,
Never shall I agree, till I see the word true, when men blame
    Oedipus,
For there came upon him once clear the winged maiden
And wise he was seen, by sure test sweet for the state.   510
So never shall my mind judge him evil guilt.

CREON: Men of our city, I have heard dread words
　　That Oedipus our king accuses me.
　　I am here indignant. If in the present troubles
　　He thinks that he has suffered at my hands
　　One word or deed tending to injury
　　I do not crave the long-spanned age of life
　　To bear this rumor, for it is no simple wrong
　　The damage of this accusation brings me;   520
　　It brings the greatest, if I am called a traitor
　　To you and my friends, a traitor to the state.
CHORUS: Come now, for this reproach perhaps was forced
　　By anger, rather than considered thought.
CREON: And was the idea voiced that my advice
　　Persuaded the prophet to give false accounts?
CHORUS: Such was said. I know not to what intent.
CREON: Was this accusation laid against me
　　From straightforward eyes and straightforward mind?
CHORUS: I do not know. I see not what my masters do;   530

But here he is now, coming from the house.

OEDIPUS: How dare you come here? Do you own a face
So bold that you can come before my house
When you are clearly the murderer of this man
And manifestly pirate of my throne?
Come, say before the gods, did you see in me
A coward or a fool, that you plotted this?
Or did you think I would not see your wiles
Creeping upon me, or knowing, would not ward off?
Surely your machination is absurd   540
Without a crowd of friends to hunt a throne
Which is captured only by wealth and many men.

CREON: Do you know what you do? Hear answer to your charges
On the other side. Judge only what you know.

OEDIPUS: Your speech is clever, but I learn it ill
Since I have found you harsh and grievous toward me.

CREON: This very matter hear me first explain.

OEDIPUS: Tell me not this one thing: you are not false.

CREON: If you think stubbornness a good possession
Apart from judgment, you do not think right.   550

OEDIPUS: If you think you can do a kinsman evil
Without the penalty, you have no sense.

CREON: I agree with you. What you have said is just.
Tell me what you say you have suffered from me.

OEDIPUS: Did you, or did you not, advise my need
Was summoning that prophet person here?

CREON: And still is. I hold still the same opinion.

OEDIPUS: How long a time now has it been since Laius —

CREON: Performed what deed? I do not understand.

OEDIPUS: — Disappeared to his ruin at deadly hands.   560

CREON: Far in the past the count of years would run.

OEDIPUS: Was this same seer at that time practising?

CREON: As wise as now, and equally respected.

OEDIPUS: At that time did he ever mention me?

CREON: Never when I stood near enough to hear.

OEDIPUS: But did you not make inquiry of the murder?

CREON: We did, of course, and got no information.

OEDIPUS: How is it that this seer did not utter this then?

CREON: When I don't know, as now, I would keep still.

OEDIPUS: This much you know full well, and so should speak: —   570

CREON: What is that? If I know, I will not refuse.

OEDIPUS: This: If he had not first conferred with you
He never would have said that I killed Laius.

CREON: If he says this, you know yourself, I think;

I learn as much from you as you from me.
OEDIPUS: Learn then: I never shall be found a slayer.
CREON: What then, are you the husband of my sister?
OEDIPUS: What you have asked is plain beyond denial.
CREON: Do you rule this land with her in equal sway?
OEDIPUS: All she desires she obtains from me. 580
CREON: Am I with you two not an equal third?
OEDIPUS: In just that do you prove a treacherous friend.
CREON: No, if, like me, you reason with yourself.
Consider this fact first: would any man
Choose, do you think, to have his rule in fear
Rather than doze unharmed with the same power?
For my part I have never been desirous
Of being king instead of acting king.
Nor any other man has, wise and prudent.
For now I obtain all from you without fear. 590
If I were king, I would do much unwilling.
How then could kingship sweeter be for me
Than rule and power devoid of any pain?
I am not yet so much deceived to want
Goods besides those I profitably enjoy.
Now I am hailed and gladdened by all men.
Now those who want from you speak out to me,
Since all their chances' outcome dwells therein.
How then would I relinquish what I have
To get those gains? My mind runs not so bad. 600
I am prudent yet, no lover of such plots,
Nor would I ever endure others' treason.
And first as proof of this go on to Pytho;
See if I told you truly the oracle.
Next proof: see if I plotted with the seer;
If you find so at all, put me to death
With my vote for my guilt as well as yours.
Do not convict me just on unclear conjecture.
It is not right to think capriciously
The good are bad, nor that the bad are good. 610
It is the same to cast out a noble friend,
I say, as one's own life, which best he loves.
The facts, though, you will safely know in time,
Since time alone can show the just man just,
But you can know a criminal in one day.
CHORUS: A cautious man would say he has spoken well.
O king, the quick to think are never sure.
OEDIPUS: When the plotter, swift, approaches me in stealth

I too in counterplot must be as swift.
If I wait in repose, the plotter's ends   620
Are brought to pass and mine will then have erred.
CREON: What do you want then? To cast me from the land?
OEDIPUS: Least of all that. My wish is you should die,
  Not flee to exemplify what envy is.
CREON: Do you say this? Will you neither trust nor yield?
OEDIPUS: [No, for I think that you deserve no trust.]
CREON: You seem not wise to me
OEDIPUS: I am for me.
CREON: You should be for me too.
OEDIPUS: No, you are evil.
CREON: Yes, if you understand nothing.
OEDIPUS: Yet I must rule.
CREON: Not when you rule badly.
OEDIPUS: O city, city!
CREON: It is my city too, not yours alone.   630
CHORUS: Stop, princes. I see Jocasta coming
  Out of the house at the right time for you.
  With her you must settle the dispute at hand.
JOCASTA: O wretched men, what unconsidered feud
  Of tongues have you aroused? Are you not ashamed,
  The state so sick, to stir up private ills?
  Are you not going home? And you as well?
  Will you turn a small pain into a great?
CREON: My blood sister, Oedipus your husband
  Claims he will judge against me two dread ills: 640
  Thrust me from the fatherland or take and kill me.
OEDIPUS: I will, my wife; I caught him in the act
  Doing evil to my person with evil skill.
CREON: Now may I not rejoice but die accursed
  If ever I did any of what you accuse me.
JOCASTA: O, by the gods, believe him, Oedipus.
  First, in reverence for his oath to the gods,
  Next, for my sake and theirs who stand before you.
CHORUS: Hear my entreaty, lord. Consider and consent.
OEDIPUS: What wish should I then grant?   650
CHORUS: Respect the man, no fool before, who now in oath is strong.
OEDIPUS: You know what you desire?
CHORUS: I know.
OEDIPUS: Say what you mean.
CHORUS: Your friend who has sworn do not dishonour
  By casting guilt for dark report.
OEDIPUS: Know well that when you ask this grant from me,
  You ask my death or exile from the land.

CHORUS: No, by the god foremost among the gods, 660
    The Sun, may I perish by the utmost doom
    Godless and friendless, if I have this in mind.
    But ah, the withering earth wears down
    My wretched soul, if to these ills
    Of old are added ills from both of you.
OEDIPUS: Then let him go, though surely I must die
    Or be thrust dishonoured from this land by force. 670
    Your grievous voice I pity, not that man's;
    Wherever he may be, he will be hated.
CREON: Sullen you are to yield, as you are heavy
    When you exceed in wrath. Natures like these
    Are justly sorest for themselves to bear.
OEDIPUS: Will you not go and leave me?
CREON: I am on my way.
    You know me not, but these men see me just.
CHORUS: O queen, why do you delay to bring this man indoors?
JOCASTA: I want to learn what happened here. 680
CHORUS: Unknown suspicion rose from talk, and the unjust devours.
JOCASTA: In both of them?
CHORUS: Just so.
JOCASTA: What was the talk?
CHORUS: Enough, enough! When the land is pained
    It seems to me at this point we should stop.
OEDIPUS: Do you see where you have come? Though your intent
    Is good, you slacken off and blunt my heart.
CHORUS: O lord, I have said not once alone,
    Know that I clearly would be mad 690
    And wandering in mind, to turn away
    You who steered along the right,
    When she was torn with trouble, our beloved state.
    O may you now become in health her guide.
JOCASTA: By the gods, lord, tell me on what account
    You have set yourself in so great an anger.
OEDIPUS: I shall tell you, wife; I respect you more than these men.
    Because of Creon, since he has plotted against me. 701
JOCASTA: Say clearly, if you can; how started the quarrel?
OEDIPUS: He says that I stand as the murderer of Laius.
JOCASTA: He knows himself, or learned from someone else?
OEDIPUS: No, but he sent a rascal prophet here.
    He keeps his own mouth clean in what concerns him.
JOCASTA: Now free yourself of what you said, and listen.
    Learn from me, no mortal man exists
    Who knows prophetic art for your affairs,
    And I shall briefly show you proof of this: 710

An oracle came once to Laius. I do not say
From Phoebus himself, but from his ministers
That his fate would be at his son's hand to die —
A child, who would be born from him and me.
And yet, as the rumor says, they were strangers,
Robbers who killed him where three highways meet.
But three days had not passed from the child's birth
When Laius pierced and tied together his ankles,
And cast him by others' hands on a pathless mountain.
Therein Apollo did not bring to pass   720
That the child murder his father, nor for Laius
The dread he feared, to die at his son's hand.
Such did prophetic oracles determine.
Pay no attention to them. For the god
Will easily make clear the need he seeks.

OEDIPUS: What wandering of soul, what stirring of mind
Holds me, my wife, in what I have just heard!

JOCASTA: What care has turned you back that you say this?

OEDIPUS: I thought I heard you mention this, that Laius
Was slaughtered at the place where three highways meet.   730

JOCASTA: That was the talk. The rumour has not ceased.

OEDIPUS: Where is this place where such a sorrow was?

JOCASTA: The country's name is Phocis. A split road
Leads to one place from Delphi and Daulia.

OEDIPUS: And how much time has passed since these events?

JOCASTA: The news was heralded in the city scarcely
A little while before you came to rule.

OEDIPUS: O Zeus, what have you planned to do to me?

JOCASTA: What passion is this in you, Oedipus?

OEDIPUS: Don't ask me that yet. Tell me about Laius.   740
What did he look like? How old was he when murdered?

JOCASTA: A tall man, with his hair just brushed with white.
His shape and form differed not far from yours.

OEDIPUS: Alas! Alas! I think unwittingly
I have just laid dread curses on my head.

JOCASTA: What are you saying? I shrink to behold you, lord.

OEDIPUS: I am terribly afraid the seer can see.
That will be clearer if you say one thing more.

JOCASTA: Though I shrink, if I know what you ask, I will answer.

OEDIPUS: Did he set forth with few attendants then,   750
Or many soldiers, since he was a king?

JOCASTA: They were five altogether among them.
One was a herald. One chariot bore Laius.

OEDIPUS: Alas! All this is clear now. Tell me, my wife,
   Who was the man who told these stories to you?
JOCASTA: One servant, who alone escaped, returned.
OEDIPUS: Is he by chance now present in our house?
JOCASTA: Not now. Right from the time when he returned
   To see you ruling and Laius dead,
   Touching my hand in suppliance, he implored me   760
   To send him to fields and to pastures of sheep
   That he might be farthest from the sight of this city.
   So I sent him away, since he was worthy
   For a slave, to bear a greater grant than this.
OEDIPUS: How then could he return to us with speed?
JOCASTA: It can be done. But why would you order this?
OEDIPUS: O lady, I fear I have said too much.
   On this account I now desire to see him.
JOCASTA: Then he shall come. But I myself deserve
   To learn what it is that troubles you, my lord.   770
OEDIPUS: And you shall not be prevented, since my fears
   Have come to such a point. For who is closer
   That I may speak to in this fate than you?
   Polybus of Corinth was my father,
   My mother, Dorian Merope. I was held there
   Chief citizen of all, till such a fate
   Befell me — as it is, worthy of wonder,
   But surely not deserving my excitement.
   A man at a banquet overdrunk with wine
   Said in drink I was a false son to my father.   780
   The weight I held that day I scarcely bore,
   But on the next day I went home and asked
   My father and mother of it. In bitter anger
   They took the reproach from him who had let it fly.
   I was pleased at their actions; nevertheless
   The rumour always rankled; and spread abroad.
   In secret from mother and father I set out
   Toward Delphi. Phoebus sent me away ungraced
   In what I came for, but other wretched things
   Terrible and grievous, he revealed in answer;   790
   That I must wed my mother and produce
   An unendurable race for men to see,
   That I should kill the father who begot me.
   When I heard this response, Corinth I fled
   Henceforth to measure her land by stars alone.
   I went where I should never see the disgrace

Of my evil oracles be brought to pass,
And on my journey to that place I came
At which you say this king had met his death.
My wife, I shall speak the truth to you. My way   800
Led to a place close by the triple road.
There a herald met me, and a man
Seated on colt-drawn chariot, as you said.
There both the guide and the old man himself
Thrust me with driving force out of the path.
And I in anger struck the one who pushed me,
The driver. Then the old man, when he saw me,
Watched when I passed, and from his chariot
Struck me full on the head with double goad.
I paid him back and more. From this very hand   810
A swift blow of my staff rolled him right out
Of the middle of his seat onto his back.
I killed them all. But if relationship
Existed between this stranger and Laius,
What man now is wretcheder than I?
What man is cursed by a more evil fate?
No stranger or citizen could now receive me
Within his home, or even speak to me,
But thrust me out; and no one but myself
Brought down these curses on my head.   820
The bed of the slain man I now defile
With hands that killed him. Am I evil by birth?
Am I not utterly vile if I must flee
And cannot see my family in my flight
Nor tread my homeland soil, or else be joined
In marriage to my mother, kill my father,
Polybus, who sired me and brought me up?
Would not a man judge right to say of me
That this was sent on me by some cruel spirit?
O never, holy reverence of the gods,   830
May I behold that day, but may I go
Away from mortal men, before I see
Such a stain of circumstance come to me.
CHORUS: My lord, for us these facts are full of dread.
Until you hear the witness, stay in hope.
OEDIPUS: And just so much is all I have of hope,
Only to wait until the shepherd comes.
JOCASTA: What, then, do you desire to hear him speak?
OEDIPUS: I will tell you, if his story is found to be
The same as yours, I would escape the sorrow.   840

JOCASTA: What unusual word did you hear from me?
OEDIPUS: You said he said that they were highway robbers
  Who murdered him. Now, if he still says
  The selfsame number, I could not have killed him,
  Since one man does not equal many men.
  But if he speaks of a single lonely traveller,
  The scale of guilt now clearly falls to me.
JOCASTA: However, know the word was set forth thus
  And it is not in him now to take it back;
  This tale the city heard, not I alone.   850
  But if he diverges from his previous story,
  Even then, my lord, he could not show Laius' murder
  To have been fulfilled properly. Apollo
  Said he would die at the hands of my own son.
  Surely that wretched child could not have killed him,
  But he himself met death some time before.
  Therefore, in any prophecy henceforth
  I would not look to this side or to that.
OEDIPUS: Your thoughts ring true, but still let someone go
  To summon the peasant. Do not neglect this.   860
JOCASTA: I shall send without delay. But let us enter.
  I would do nothing that did not please you.

CHORUS:
    Strophe A
  May fate come on me as I bear
  Holy pureness in all word and deed,
  For which the lofty striding laws were set down,
  Born through the heavenly air
  Whereof the Olympian sky alone the father was;
  No mortal spawn of mankind gave them birth,
  Nor may oblivion ever lull them down;   870
  Mighty in them the god is, and he does not age.

    Antistrophe A
  Pride breeds the tyrant.
  Pride, once overfilled with many things in vain,
  Neither in season nor fit for man,
  Scaling the sheerest height
  Hurls to a dire fate
  Where no foothold is found.
  I pray the god may never stop the rivalry   880
  That works well for the state.
  The god as my protector I shall never cease to hold.

Strophe B

But if a man goes forth haughty in word or deed
With no fear of the Right
Nor pious to the spirits' shrines,
May evil doom seize him
For his ill-fated pride,
If he does not fairly win his gain
Or works unholy deeds,   890
Or, in bold folly lays on the sacred profane hands.
For when such acts occur, what man may boast
Ever to ward off from his life darts of the gods?
If practices like these are in respect,
Why then must I dance the sacred dance?

Antistrophe B

Never again in worship shall I go
To Delphi, holy navel of the earth,
Nor to the temple at Abae,
Nor to Olympia,   900
If these prophecies do not become
Examples for all men.
O Zeus, our king, if so you are rightly called,
Ruler of all things, may they not escape
You and your forever deathless power.
Men now hold light the fading oracles
Told about Laius long ago
And nowhere is Apollo clearly honored;
Things divine are going down to ruin.   910

JOCASTA: Lords of this land, the thought has come to me
To visit the spirits' shrines, bearing in hand
These suppliant boughs and offerings of incense.
For Oedipus raises his soul too high
With all distresses; nor, as a sane man should,
Does he confirm the new by things of old,
But stands at the speaker's will if he speaks terrors.
And so, because my advice can do no more,
To you, Lycian Apollo — for you are nearest —
A suppliant, I have come here with these prayers,   920
That you may find some pure deliverance for us:
We all now shrink to see him struck in fear,
That man who is the pilot of our ship.
MESSENGER: Strangers, could I learn from one of you
Where is the house of Oedipus the king?
Or best, if you know, say where he is himself.

CHORUS: This is his house, stranger; he dwells inside;
    This woman is the mother of his children.
MESSENGER: May she be always blessed among the blest,
    Since she is the fruitful wife of Oedipus.   930
JOCASTA: So may you, stranger, also be. You deserve
    As much for your graceful greeting. But tell me
    What you have come to search for or to show.
MESSENGER: Good news for your house and your husband, lady.
JOCASTA: What is it then? And from whom have you come?
MESSENGER: From Corinth. And the message I will tell
    Will surely gladden you — and vex you, perhaps.
JOCASTA: What is it? What is this double force it holds?
MESSENGER: The men who dwell in the Isthmian country
    Have spoken to establish him their king.   940
JOCASTA: What is that? Is not old Polybus still ruling?
MESSENGER: Not he. For death now holds him in the tomb.
JOCASTA: What do you say, old man? Is Polybus dead?
MESSENGER: If I speak not the truth, I am ready to die.
JOCASTA: O handmaid, go right away and tell your master
    The news. Where are you, prophecies of the gods?
    For this man Oedipus has trembled long,
    And shunned him lest he kill him. Now the man
    Is killed by fate and not by Oedipus.
OEDIPUS: O Jocasta, my most beloved wife,   950
    Why have you sent for me within the house?
JOCASTA: Listen to this man, and while you hear him, think
    To what have come Apollo's holy prophecies.
OEDIPUS: Who is this man? Why would he speak to me?
JOCASTA: From Corinth he has come, to announce that your father
    Polybus no longer lives, but is dead.
OEDIPUS: What do you say, stranger? Tell me this yourself.
MESSENGER: If I must first announce my message clearly,
    Know surely that the man is dead and gone.
OEDIPUS: Did he die by treachery or chance disease?   960
MESSENGER: A slight scale tilt can lull the old to rest.
OEDIPUS: The poor man, it seems, died by disease.
MESSENGER: And by the full measure of lengthy time.
OEDIPUS: Alas, alas! Why then do any seek
    Pytho's prophetic art, my wife, or hear
    The shrieking birds on high, by whose report
    I was to slay my father? Now he lies
    Dead beneath the earth, and here am I
    Who have not touched the blade. Unless in longing
    For me he died, and in this sense was killed by me.   970

Polybus has packed away these oracles
In his rest in Hades. They are now worth nothing.
JOCASTA: Did I not tell you that some time ago?
OEDIPUS: You did, but I was led astray by fear.
JOCASTA: Henceforth put nothing of this on your heart.
OEDIPUS: Why must I not still shrink from my mother's bed?
JOCASTA: What should man fear, whose life is ruled by fate,
 For whom there is clear foreknowledge of nothing?
 It is best to live by chance, however you can.
 Be not afraid of marriage with your mother;   980
 Already many mortals in their dreams
 Have shared their mother's bed. But he who counts
 This dream as nothing, easiest bears his life.
OEDIPUS: All that you say would be indeed propitious,
 If my mother were not alive. But since she is,
 I still must shrink, however well you speak.
JOCASTA: And yet your father's tomb is a great eye.*
OEDIPUS: A great eye indeed. But I fear her who lives.
MESSENGER: Who is this woman that you are afraid of?
OEDIPUS: Merope, old man, with whom Polybus lived.   990
MESSENGER: What is it in her that moves you to fear?
OEDIPUS: A dread oracle, stranger, sent by the god.
MESSENGER: Can it be told, or must no other know?
OEDIPUS: It surely can. Apollo told me once
 That I must join in intercourse with my mother
 And shed with my own hands my father's blood.
 Because of this, long since I have kept far
 Away from Corinth — and happily — but yet
 It would be most sweet to see my parents' faces.
MESSENGER: Was this your fear in shunning your own city?   1000
OEDIPUS: I wished, too, old man, not to slay my father.
MESSENGER: Why then have I not freed you from this fear,
 Since I have come with friendly mind, my lord?
OEDIPUS: Yes, and take thanks from me, which you deserve.
MESSENGER: And this is just the thing for which I came,
 That when you got back home I might fare well.
OEDIPUS: Never shall I go where my parents are.
MESSENGER: My son, you clearly know not what you do.
OEDIPUS: How is that, old man? By the gods, let me know.
MESSENGER: If for these tales you shrink from going home   1010
OEDIPUS: I tremble lest what Phoebus said comes true.
MESSENGER: Lest you incur pollution from your parents?

---

* That is, a bright comfort.

OEDIPUS: That is the thing, old man, that always haunts me.
MESSENGER: Well, do you know that surely you fear nothing?
OEDIPUS: How so? If I am the son of those who bore me.
MESSENGER: Since Polybus was no relation to you.
OEDIPUS: What do you say? Was Polybus not my father?
MESSENGER: No more than this man here but just so much.
OEDIPUS: How does he who begot me equal nothing?
MESSENGER: That man was not your father, any more than I am.
OEDIPUS: Well then, why was it he called me his son? 1021
MESSENGER: Long ago he got you as a gift from me.
OEDIPUS: Though from another's hand, yet so much he loved me!
MESSENGER: His previous childlessness led him to that.
OEDIPUS: Had you bought or found me when you gave me to him?
MESSENGER: I found you in Cithaeron's folds and glens.
OEDIPUS: Why were you travelling in those regions?
MESSENGER: I guarded there a flock of mountain sheep.
OEDIPUS: Were you a shepherd, wandering for pay?
MESSENGER: Yes, and your saviour too, child, at that time 1030
OEDIPUS: What pain gripped me, that you took me in your arms?
MESSENGER: The ankles of your feet will tell you that.
OEDIPUS: Alas, why do you mention that old trouble?
MESSENGER: I freed you when your ankles were pierced together.
OEDIPUS: A terrible shame from my swaddling clothes I got.
MESSENGER: Your very name you got from this misfortune.
OEDIPUS: By the gods, did my mother or father do it? Speak.
MESSENGER: I know not. He who gave you knows better than I.
OEDIPUS: You didn't find me, but took me from another?
MESSENGER: That's right. Another shepherd gave you to me. 1040
OEDIPUS: Who was he? Can you tell me who he was?
MESSENGER: Surely. He belonged to the household of Laius.
OEDIPUS: The man who ruled this land once long ago?
MESSENGER: Just so. He was a herd in that man's service.
OEDIPUS: Is this man still alive, so I could see him?
MESSENGER: You dwellers in this country should know best.
OEDIPUS: Is there any one of you who stand before me
    Who knows the shepherd of whom this man speaks?
    If you have seen him in the fields or here,
    Speak forth; the time has come to find this out. 1050
CHORUS: I think the man you seek is no one else
    Than the shepherd you were so eager to see before.
    Jocasta here might best inform us that.
OEDIPUS: My wife, do you know the man we just ordered
    To come here? Is it of him that this man speaks?
JOCASTA: Why ask of whom he spoke? Think nothing of it.

Brood not in vain on what has just been said.

OEDIPUS: It could not be that when I have got such clues,
    I should not shed clear light upon my birth.

JOCASTA: Don't, by the gods, investigate this more   1060
    If you care for your own life. I am sick enough.

OEDIPUS: Take courage. Even if I am found a slave
    For three generations, your birth will not be base.

JOCASTA: Still, I beseech you, hear me. Don't do this.

OEDIPUS: I will hear of nothing but finding out the truth.

JOCASTA: I know full well and tell you what is best.

OEDIPUS: Well, then, this best, for some time now, has given me pain.

JOCASTA: O ill-fated man, may you never know who you are.

OEDIPUS: Will someone bring the shepherd to me here?
    And let this lady rejoice in her opulent birth.   1070

JOCASTA: Alas, alas, hapless man. I have this alone
    To tell you, and nothing else forevermore.

CHORUS: O Oedipus, where has the woman gone
    In the rush of her wild grief? I am afraid
    Evil will break forth out of this silence.

OEDIPUS: Let whatever will break forth. I plan to see
    The seed of my descent, however small.
    My wife, perhaps, because a noblewoman
    Looks down with shame upon my lowly birth.
    I would not be dishonoured to call myself
    The son of Fortune, giver of the good.   1080
    She is my mother. The years, her other children,
    Have marked me sometimes small and sometimes great.
    Such was I born! I shall prove no other man,
    Nor shall I cease to search out my descent.

CHORUS:
    Strophe
    If I am a prophet and can know in mind,
    Cithaeron, by tomorrow's full moon   1090
    You shall not fail, by mount Olympus,
    To find that Oedipus, as a native of your land,
    Shall honour you for nurse and mother.
    And to you we dance in choral song because you bring
    Fair gifts to him our king.
    Hail, Phoebus, may all this please you.

    Antistrophe
    Who, child, who bore you in the lengthy span of years?
    One close to Pan who roams the mountain woods,   1100

One of Apollo's bedfellows?
For all wild pastures in mountain glens to him are dear.
Was Hermes your father, who Cyllene sways,
Or did Bacchus, dwelling on the mountain peaks,
Take you a foundling from some nymph
Of those by springs of Helicon, with whom he sports the most?

OEDIPUS: If I may guess, although I never met him, 1110
    I think, elders, I see that shepherd coming
    Whom we have long sought, as in the measure
    Of lengthy age he accords with him we wait for.
    Besides, the men who lead him I recognize
    As servants of my house. You may perhaps
    Know better than I if you have seen him before.
CHORUS: Be assured, I know him as a shepherd
    As trusted as any other in Laius' service.
OEDIPUS: Stranger from Corinth, I will ask you first,
    Is this the man you said?
MESSENGER: You are looking at him. 1120
OEDIPUS: You there, old man, look here and answer me
    What I shall ask you. Were you ever with Laius?
SERVANT: I was a slave, not bought but reared at home.
OEDIPUS: What work concerned you? What was your way of life?
SERVANT: Most of my life I spent among the flocks.
OEDIPUS: In what place most of all was your usual pasture?
SERVANT: Sometimes Cithaeron, or the ground nearby.
OEDIPUS: Do you know this man before you here at all?
SERVANT: Doing what? And of what man do you speak?
OEDIPUS: The one before you. Have you ever had congres with
    him? 1130
SERVANT: Not to say so at once from memory.
MESSENGER: That is no wonder, master, but I shall remind him,
    Clearly, who knows me not; yet well I know
    That he knew once the region of Cithaeron.
    He with a double flock and I with one
    Dwelt there in company for three whole years
    During the six months' time from spring to fall.
    When winter came, I drove into my fold
    My flock, and he drove his to Laius' pens.
    Do I speak right, or did it not happen so? 1140
SERVANT: You speak the truth, though it was long ago.
MESSENGER: Come now, do you recall you gave me then
    A child for me to rear as my own son?
SERVANT: What is that? Why do you ask me this?

MESSENGER: This is the man, my friend, who then was young.

SERVANT: Go to destruction! Will you not be quiet?

OEDIPUS: Come, scold him not, old man. These words of yours
Deserve a scolding more than this man's do.

SERVANT: In what, most noble master, do I wrong?

OEDIPUS: Not to tell of the child he asks about.   1150

SERVANT: He speaks in ignorance, he toils in vain.

OEDIPUS: If you will not speak freely, you will under torture.

SERVANT: Don't, by the gods, outrage an old man like me.

OEDIPUS: Will someone quickly twist back this fellow's arms?

SERVANT: Alas, what for? What do you want to know?

OEDIPUS: Did you give this man the child of whom he asks?

SERVANT: I did. Would I had perished on that day!

OEDIPUS: You will come to that unless you tell the truth.

SERVANT: I come to far greater ruin if I speak.

OEDIPUS: This man, it seems, is trying to delay.   1160

SERVANT: Not I. I said before I gave it to him.

OEDIPUS: Where did you get it? At home or from someone else?

SERVANT: It was not mine. I got him from a man.

OEDIPUS: Which of these citizens? Where did he live?

SERVANT: O master, by the gods, ask me no more.

OEDIPUS: You are done for if I ask you this again.

SERVANT: Well then, he was born of the house of Laius.

OEDIPUS: One of his slaves, or born of his own race?

SERVANT: Alas, to speak I am on the brink of horror.

OEDIPUS: And I to hear. But still it must be heard.   1170

SERVANT: Well, then, they say it was his child. Your wife
Who dwells within could best say how this stands.

OEDIPUS: Was it she who gave him to you?

SERVANT: Yes, my lord.

OEDIPUS: For what intent?

SERVANT: So I could put it away.

OEDIPUS: When she bore him, the wretch.

SERVANT: She feared bad oracles.

OEDIPUS: What were they?

SERVANT: They said he should kill his father.

OEDIPUS: Why did you give him up to this old man?

SERVANT: I pitied him, master, and thought he would take him away
To another land, the one from which he came.
But he saved him for greatest woe. If you are he   1180
Whom this man speaks of, you were born curst by fate.

OEDIPUS: Alas, alas! All things are now come true.
O light, for the last time now I look upon you;
I am shown to be born from those I ought not to have been.

I married the woman I should not have married,
I killed the man whom I should not have killed.

CHORUS:
  Strophe A
Alas, generations of mortal men!
How equal to nothing do I number you in life!
Who, O who, is the man
Who bears more of bliss   1190
Than just the seeming so,
And then, like a waning sun, to fall away?
When I know your example,
Your guiding spirit, yours, wretched Oedipus,
I call no mortal blest.

  Antistrophe A
He is the one, O Zeus,
Who peerless shot his bow and won well-fated bliss,
Who destroyed the hook-clawed maiden,
The oracle-singing Sphinx,   1200
And stood a tower for our land from death;
For this you are called our king,
Oedipus, are highest-honoured here,
And over great Thebes hold sway.

  Strophe B
And now who is more wretched for men to hear,
Who so lives in wild plagues, who dwells in pains,
In utter change of life?
Alas for glorious Oedipus!
The selfsame port of rest
Was gained by bridegroom father and his son,   1210
How, O how did your father's furrows ever bear you, suffering
   man?
How have they endured silence for so long?

  Antistrophe B
You are found out, unwilling, by all seeing Time.
It judges your unmarried marriage where for long
Begetter and begot have been the same.
Alas, child of Laius,
Would I had never seen you.
As one who pours from his mouth a dirge I wail,
To speak the truth, through you I breathed new life,   1220
And now through you I lulled my eye to sleep.

SECOND MESSENGER: O men most honoured always of this land
What deeds you shall hear, what shall you behold!
What grief shall stir you up, if by your kinship
You are still concerned for the house of Labdacus!
I think neither Danube nor any other river
Could wash this palace clean, so many ills
Lie hidden there which now will come to light.
They were done by will, not fate; and sorrows hurt   **1230**
The most when we ourselves appear to choose them.
CHORUS: What we heard before causes no little sorrow.
What can you say which adds to that a burden?
SECOND MESSENGER: This is the fastest way to tell the tale;
Hear it: Jocasta, your divine queen, is dead.
CHORUS: O sorrowful woman! From what cause did she die?
SECOND MESSENGER: By her own hand. The most painful of the action
Occurred away, not for your eyes to see.
But still, so far as I have memory
You shall learn the sufferings of that wretched woman: **1240**
How she passed on through the door enraged
And rushed straight forward to her nuptial bed,
Clutching her hair's ends with both her hands.
Once inside the doors she shut herself in
And called on Laius, who has long been dead,
Having remembrance of their seed of old
By which he died himself and left her a mother
To bear an evil brood to his own son.
She moaned the bed on which by double curse
She bore husband to husband, children to child.   **1250**
How thereafter she perished I do not know,
For Oedipus burst in on her with a shriek,
And because of him we could not see her woe.
We looked on him alone as he rushed around.
Pacing about, he asked us to give him a sword,
Asked where he might find the wife no wife,
A mother whose plowfield bore him and his children.
Some spirit was guiding him in his frenzy,
For none of the men who are close at hand did so.
With a horrible shout, as if led on by someone,   **1260**
He leapt on the double doors, from their sockets
Broke hollow bolts aside, and dashed within.
There we beheld his wife hung by her neck
From twisted cords, swinging to and fro.
When he saw her, wretched man, he terribly groaned
And slackened the hanging noose. When the poor woman

Lay on the ground, what happened was dread to see.
He tore the golden brooch pins from her clothes,
And raised them up, and struck his own eyeballs,   **1270**
Shouting such words as these "No more shall you
Behold the evils I have suffered and done.
Be dark from now on, since you saw before
What you should not, and knew not what you should."
Moaning such cries, not once but many times
He raised and struck his eyes. The bloody pupils
Bedewed his beard. The gore oozed not in drops,
But poured in a black shower, a hail of blood.
From both of them these woes have broken out,   **1280**
Not for just one, but man and wife together.
The bliss of old that formerly prevailed
Was bliss indeed, but now upon this day
Lamentation, madness, death, and shame —
No evil that can be named is not at hand.
CHORUS: Is the wretched man in any rest now from pain?
SECOND MESSENGER: He shouts for someone to open up the doors
    And show to all Cadmeans his father's slayer,
    His mother's — I should not speak the unholy word.
    He says he will hurl himself from the land, no more   **1290**
    To dwell cursed in the house by his own curse.
    Yet he needs strength and someone who will guide him.
    His sickness is too great to bear. He will show it to you
    For the fastenings of the doors are opening up,
    And such a spectacle you will soon behold
    As would make even one who abhors it take pity.
CHORUS: O terrible suffering for men to see,
    Most terrible of all that I
    Have ever come upon. O wretched man,
    What madness overcame you, what springing daimon   **1300**
    Greater than the greatest for men
    Has caused your evil-daimoned fate?
    Alas, alas, grievous one,
    But I cannot bear to behold you, though I desire
    To ask you much, much to find out,
    Much to see,
    You make me shudder so!
OEDIPUS: Alas, alas, I am grieved!
    Where on earth, so wretched, shall I go?
    Where does my voice fly through the air,   **1310**
    O Fate, where have you bounded?
CHORUS: To dreadful end, not to be heard or seen.

Strophe A

OEDIPUS: O cloud of dark
That shrouds me off, has come to pass, unspeakable,
Invincible, that blows no favoring blast.
Woe,
O woe again, the goad that pierces me,
Of the sting of evil now, and memory of before.
CHORUS: No wonder it is that among so many pains
You should both mourn and bear a double evil.   1320

Antistrophe A

OEDIPUS: Ah, friend,
You are my steadfast servant still,
You still remain to care for me, blind.
Alas! Alas!
You are not hid from me; I know you clearly,
And though in darkness, still I hear your voice.
CHORUS: O dreadful doer, how did you so endure
To quench your eyes? What daimon drove you on?

Strophe B

OEDIPUS: Apollo it was, Apollo, friends
Who brought to pass these evil, evil woes of mine.   1330
The hand of no one struck my eyes but wretched me.
For why should I see,
When nothing sweet there is to see with sight?
CHORUS: This is just as you say.
OEDIPUS: What more is there for me to see,
My friends, what to love,
What joy to hear a greeting?
Lead me at once away from here,   1340
Lead me away, friends, wretched as I am,
Accursed, and hated most
Of mortals to the gods.
CHORUS: Wretched alike in mind and in your fortune,
How I wish that I had never known you.

Antistrophe B

OEDIPUS: May he perish, whoever freed me
From fierce bonds on my feet,   1350
Snatched me from death and saved me, doing me no joy.
For if then I had died, I should not be
So great a grief to friends and to myself.

CHORUS: This also is my wish.
OEDIPUS: I would not have come to murder my father,
    Nor have been called among men
    The bridegroom of her from whom I was born.
    But as it is I am godless, child of unholiness,   1360
    Wretched sire in common with my father.
    And if there is any evil older than evil left,
    It is the lot of Oedipus.
CHORUS: I know not how I could give you good advice,
    For you would be better dead than living blind.

OEDIPUS: That how things are was not done for the best —
    Teach me not this, or give me more advice.   1370
    If I had sight, I know not with what eyes
    I could ever face my father among the dead,
    Or my wretched mother. What I have done to them
    Is too great for a noose to expiate.
    Do you think the sight of my children would be a joy
    For me to see, born as they were to me?
    No, never for these eyes of mine to see.
    Nor the city, nor the tower, nor the sacred
    Statues of gods; of these I deprive myself,
    Noblest among the Thebans, born and bred,   1380
    Now suffering everything. I tell you all
    To exile me as impious, shown by the gods
    Untouchable and of the race of Laius.
    When I uncovered such a stain on me,
    Could I look with steady eyes upon the people?
    No, No! And if there were a way to block
    The spring of hearing, I would not forbear
    To lock up wholly this my wretched body.
    I should be blind and deaf. — For it is sweet
    When thought can dwell outside our evils.   1390
    Alas, Cithaeron, why did you shelter me?
    Why did you not take and kill me at once, so I
    Might never reveal to men whence I was born?
    O Polybus, O Corinth, O my father's halls,
    Ancient in fable, what an outer fairness,
    A festering of evils, you raised in me.
    For now I am evil found, and born of evil.
    O the three paths! Alas the hidden glen,
    The grove of oak, the narrow triple roads
    That drank from my own hands my father's blood.   1400
    Do you remember any of the deeds

I did before you then on my way here
And what I after did? O wedlock, wedlock!
You gave me birth, and then spawned in return
Issue from the selfsame seed; you revealed
Father, brother, children, in blood relation,
The bride both wife and mother, and whatever
Actions are done most shameful among men.
But it is wrong to speak what is not good to do.
By the gods, hide me at once outside our land,   1410
Or murder me, or hurl me in the sea
Where you shall never look on me again.
Come, venture to lay your hands on this wretched man.
Do it. Be not afraid. No mortal man
There is, except myself, to bear my evils.
CHORUS: Here is Creon, just in time for what you ask
To work and to advise, for he alone
Is left in place of you to guard the land.
OEDIPUS: Alas, what word, then, shall I tell this man?
What righteous ground of trust is clear in me,   1420
As in the past in all I have done him evil?
CREON: Oedipus, I have not come to laugh at you,
Nor to reproach you for your former wrongs.

(To the attendants)

If you defer no longer to mortal offspring,
Respect at least the all-nourishing flame
Of Apollo, lord of the sun. Fear to display
So great a pestilence, which neither earth
Nor holy rain nor light will well receive.
But you, conduct him to the house at once.
It is most pious for the kin alone   1430
To hear and to behold the family sins.
OEDIPUS: By the gods, since you have plucked me from my fear,
Most noble, facing this most vile man,
Hear me one word — I will speak for you, not me.
CREON: What desire do you so persist to get?
OEDIPUS: As soon as you can, hurl me from this land
To where no mortal man will ever greet me.
CREON: I would do all this, be sure. But I want first
To find out from the god what must be done.
OEDIPUS: His oracle, at least, is wholly clear;   1440
Leave me to ruin, an impious parricide.
CREON: Thus spake the oracle. Still, as we stand
It is better to find out sure what we should do.

OEDIPUS: Will you inquire about so wretched a man?
CREON: Yes. You will surely put trust in the god.
OEDIPUS: I order you and beg you, give the woman
  Now in the house such burial as you yourself
  Would want. Do last rites justly for your kin.
  But may this city never be condemned —
  My father's realm — because I live within.   **1450**
  Let me live in the mountains where Cithaeron
  Yonder has fame of me, which father and mother
  When they were alive established as my tomb.
  There I may die by those who sought to kill me.
  And yet this much I know, neither a sickness
  Nor anything else can kill me. I would not
  Be saved from death, except for some dread evil.
  Well, let my fate go wherever it may.
  As for my sons, Creon, assume no trouble;
  They are men and will have no difficulty   **1460**
  Of living wherever they may be.
  O my poor grievous daughters, who never knew
  Their dinner table set apart from me,
  But always shared in everything I touched —
  Take care of them for me, and first of all
  Allow me to touch them and bemoan our ills.
  Grant it, lord,
  Grant it, noble. If with my hand I touch them
  I would think I had them just as when I could see.   **1470**

    (*Creon's attendants bring in* ANTIGONE *and* ISMENE.)

  What's that?
  By the gods, can it be I hear my dear ones weeping?
  And have you taken pity on me, Creon?
  Have you had my darling children sent to me?
  Do I speak right?
CREON: You do. For it was I who brought them here,
  Knowing this present joy your joy of old.
OEDIPUS: May you fare well. For their coming may the spirit
  That watches over you be better than mine.
  My children, where are you? Come to me, come   **1480**
  Into your brother's hands, that brought about
  Your father's eyes, once bright, to see like this.
  Your father, children, who, seeing and knowing nothing,
  Became a father whence he was got himself.
  I weep also for you — I cannot see you —
  To think of the bitter life in days to come

Which you will have to lead among mankind.
What citizens' gatherings will you approach?
What festivals attend, where you will not cry   1490
When you go home, instead of gay rejoicing?
And when you arrive at marriageable age,
What man, my daughters, will there be to chance you,
Incurring such reproaches on his head,
Disgraceful to my children and to yours?
What evil will be absent, when your father
Killed his own father, sowed seed in her who bore him,
From whom he was born himself, and equally
Has fathered you whence he himself was born.
Such will be the reproaches. Who then will wed you?   1500
My children, there is no one for you. Clearly
You must decay in barrenness, unwed.
Son of Menoeceus — since you are alone
Left as a father to them, for we who produced them
Are both in ruin — see that you never let
These girls wander as beggars without husbands,
Let them not fall into such woes as mine.
But pity them, seeing how young they are
To be bereft of all except your aid.
Grant this, my noble friend, with a touch of your hand.   1510
My children, if your minds were now mature,
I would give you much advice. But, pray this for me,
To live as the time allows, to find a life
Better than that your siring father had.
CREON: You have wept enough here, come, and go inside the house.
OEDIPUS: I must obey, though nothing sweet.
CREON: All things are good in their time.
OEDIPUS: Do you know in what way I go?
CREON: Tell me, I'll know when I hear.
OEDIPUS: Send me outside the land.
CREON: You ask what the god will do.
OEDIPUS: But to the gods I am hated.
CREON: Still, it will soon be done.
OEDIPUS: Then you agree?
CREON: What I think not I would not say in vain.   1520
OEDIPUS: Now lead me away.
CREON: Come then, but let the children go.
OEDIPUS: Do not take them from me.
CREON: Wish not to govern all,
    For what you ruled will not follow you through life.
CHORUS: Dwellers in native Thebes, behold this Oedipus

Who solved the famous riddle, was your mightiest man.
What citizen on his lot did not with envy gaze?
See to how great a surge of dread fate he has come!
So I would say a mortal man, while he is watching
To see the final day, can have no happiness
Till he pass the bound of life, nor be relieved of pain.   1530

SOPHOCLES

PHILOCTETES

Translated by Kathleen Freeman

INTRODUCTION

IT IS striking to note how many of the Greek dramas are connected in some way, directly or indirectly, with warfare. This is a natural consequence not only of the chronic conditions of ancient Greek life but of the sources of Greek drama in the great mythological sagas which deal essentially with wars: the sagas of Troy, the house of Tantalus (Argos), the house of Laius (Thebes), the line of Aegeus of Athens (Theseus and others), Hercules, the Argonauts, Perseus, and Dionysus. The playwrights often choose for their plays a remote and more intimate aspect of these wars; certainly one of the most charming as well as touching of them is the *Philoctetes*. It is part of the largest body of play-subjects, the story of the Trojan war, and is briefly told in the *Iliad*, 2.721–725, just after the mention of Alcestis.

Philoctetes the Malian led seven ships to Troy from Meliboea in Thessaly and from Olizon. When the fleet touched at Lemnos to take on fresh water Philoctetes was bitten by a snake; the wound festered and became offensively odorous. The Greeks decided to leave him on that deserted shore, with the bow and arrows Hercules had given him for his service in lighting that great hero's funeral pyre when no one else would do so. It was these splendid weapons which according to the prophecy of Helenus, son of Priam, were needed for the capture of Troy. Hera, jealous of Zeus's reception of his son, Hercules, into Olympus at his death, had arranged to have a snake bite Philoctetes.

After nine years of indecisive war at Troy the Greeks concluded that they could not succeed without the talisman of Philoctetes' weapons. Accordingly, Diomedes (in the epic version) and Odysseus were sent to bring them back together with their owner. Sophocles, in a stroke of dramatic genius, substituted Neoptolemus, son of Achilles, for Diomedes in his telling of the story. Euripides and Aeschylus wrote plays on the same subject; Dio Chrysostom in Oration 52 discussed the treatment of the theme by the three dramatists. The *Little Iliad* and the *Iliu persis*, among the epic poems after Homer, told of the exploits of Philoctetes, who upon his return to Troy shot Paris with his arrow and thus avenged the death of Achilles.

Since Odysseus, who had many enemies, had also made an enemy of Philoctetes by leading the plan to steal his magic weapons and to force him to come back to Troy, he enlisted the naïve young Neoptolemus to persuade the stranded Greek Robinson Crusoe. Actually a sailor disguised as a merchant prevails on Philoctetes to believe the prophecy that his presence at Troy was necessary for Greek success. Odysseus stays in the background, craftily egging on his young companion as he makes the final attempt to break down the stubborn refusal of Philoctetes to leave his island home, to which he has become genuinely attached.

Actually, Philoctetes has only a bitter choice between maintaining his obstinate pride and dying a slow death (presumably from gangrene, although there is an obvious discrepancy in the fact that he had not yet died in the nine years of his abandonment) and returning to Troy. His hatred for the Greeks and particularly for Odysseus struggles with his patriotic instincts. The rôle in which character-change is most apparent, however, is that of Neoptolemus; he will not carry further the deception which Odysseus had persuaded him to undertake when he discovers the cynical cruelty of his elder comrade, willing to leave Philoctetes behind if only he can take his weapons back to Troy.

Neoptolemus is tempted by the opportunity Odysseus offers him of winning renown by successfully completing his mission. Yet his essential nobility of character inherited from his famous father will not allow him to win glory at the expense of the wretched Philoctetes. He almost comes to blows with Odysseus, but faces him down and takes both Philoctetes and the weapons with him to Troy. The ghost of the dead Hercules appears to his one-time benefactor as a "god from the machine" at the end of the play to solve the problem of breaking down the still unswerving resolution of the castaway.

The pathetic joy of Philoctetes as he learns the identity of his young visitor; his bitter rage and despair at the slow revelation of the callous plot against him; his paroxysm of physical pain which almost prevents his departure after all; and his final calm determination to repress his hatred and to help his fellow-warriors who had so mistreated him — these are the highlights of his performance.

The *Philoctetes* is a play of intrigue with a high ethical purpose. The disclosure of Odysseus' villainy to Neoptolemus and its effect upon him is its central purpose. There is no true tragedy in the Aristotelian sense but a kind of morality show presented in realistic form. It is possible that the play marks a late stage in the development of Sophocles' art and certainly comes very late in his career; its political implications may be too vague to be employed for any plausible theory as to the playwright's views in reference to actual contemporary events. There is a strong Euripidean influence on the play.

The *Philoctetes* was presented in 409 B.C. and won the first prize. Its dialogue-language is closer to conversational Greek than is that of any other Greek tragedy, as Professor Harsh points out. It has a happy ending like several other Greek plays. Romantic scenery is used in it for great effect, as also in Aeschylus' *Prometheus Bound.* The chorus of old Greek sailors (so called by the writer of the argument which precedes the Greek text), the sea-coast setting and the cave of Philoctetes, his final lyrical farewell to the haunts he had come to know so well, give the play an unusual and most attractive atmosphere. The chorus speeches are cleverly and consistently integrated with the character-dialogue; the chorus becomes, in fact, an active participant in the action.

The play has been used for a modern adaptation, as the present-day French writers have used so many Greek plays, by André Gide. Edmund Wilson, the American critic, has written a stimulating essay on the *Philoctetes,* which he makes the title-piece of his book, *The Wound and the Bow,* 1941. It should be noted that Miss Freeman's translation is an acting version designed for speaking on a stage as well as for silent reading; many contemporary translations of Greek drama are not fitted for utterance upon the stage but make their appeal to the eye and the reason instead of the ear.

L. R. LIND

PHILOCTETES

CHARACTERS

ODYSSEUS *of Ithaca*
NEOPTOLEMUS, *son of Achilles*
PHILOCTETES, *son of Poeas*
SAILOR, *disguised as a Merchant Captain*
HERACLES, *son of Zeus and Alcmene of Thebes*
SAILORS *as chorus from the crew of Neoptolemus*
    (*not less than six, not more than fourteen*)
MATE *of the ship*

TIME: *Towards the end of the ten years' war against Troy.*
SCENE: *A wild place on the north-east coast of Lemnos, an island off Asia Minor. A great rock rises steeply in the background; in it, part of the way up, is the entrance to a cave. The rock rises up from the seashore; a path winding round the face of the rock would lead round to a point overlooking the sea.*

Enter Right, ODYSSEUS *and* NEOPTOLEMUS. *The former is a man of about forty, well-built, but sturdy rather than tall, with a fine head and broad shoulders. The latter is a young man, tall and strong, with a direct glance; not too clever-looking, but honest, fearless and of free bearing. He is not at all in awe of his companion, though* ODYSSEUS *is greatly his superior in experience and resourcefulness. They stand at one side, not immediately seeing the entrance to the cave.*

ODYSSEUS: This is the shore, Neoptolemus. This is the island of
    Lemnos. There are no inhabitants: you will find no footprints

here. Yet here is the very spot where once, years ago, I myself
put ashore this man, Philoctetes the Malian. I was the one com-
missioned by the commanders to do it. The reason was, he was
sick; he had a suppurating wound in his foot, and as a result, it
had become impossible for us to pour a libation or perform a
sacrifice in peace. His screams were blood-curdling: they filled the
whole camp, as he shouted and groaned with the pain of   10
his agonizing wound. But there's no need to tell you the story.
We haven't much time for talking. I don't want him to find out
I'm here: that would certainly upset the whole plan — my scheme
to get hold of him here and now.

Now it's your job to see to the rest. What you are to look for
is a place where there is a cave with two entrances — the sort of
place where in cold weather one has a chance of sitting in the
sun twice a day, and where in summer a breeze blows through the
tunnel, making sleep easy. Just below, on the left, you will probably see a spring of fresh water, if it is still intact. I want   20
you to go up quietly, and signal to me whether he still lives in this
same place, or whether he has moved off somewhere else. Then
you can hear the rest of my plans, which I will explain to you so
that we can both do our share in forwarding them.

NEOPTOLEMUS (*who has listened carefully, now begins looking round*):
Well, Prince Odysseus, I shan't have far to go for this task you
set me, for I think I see the sort of cave you mention.

ODYSSEUS: Above, or below? I don't see it.

NEOPTOLEMUS (*pointing*): Here. (*He goes up to the mouth of the
cave, and listens.*) I don't hear any footsteps.

ODYSSEUS: Take care! He may be inside, asleep.   30

NEOPTOLEMUS (*going in a little way*): I see an empty dwelling: there
are no inmates.

ODYSSEUS: And is there no sign of food, or human occupation?

NEOPTOLEMUS: Yes, there is a bed of leaves pressed down, as if someone were camping here.

ODYSSEUS (*advancing cautiously*): And otherwise it's bare? There's
nothing else under the roof?

NEOPTOLEMUS: Yes, there's a cup of unpolished wood — the work of
a very poor craftsman! — and here, close by, is some firewood.

ODYSSEUS (*laughs unkindly*): The treasure you describe is undoubtedly
his.

NEOPTOLEMUS (*pursuing his investigations*): Aha! Here's something
else! Yes, some rags drying in the sun. (*Recoiling.*) They're reek-
ing with matter from some terrible sore.

ODYSSEUS (*coming forward with satisfaction*): The man ob-   40
viously lives round these parts; and he must be somewhere not far

off. How could a man with such a long-standing disease of the foot
go far afield? No: he has either gone off to bring in something to
eat, or else he has somewhere discovered some kind of plant which
relieves pain. Send your man to keep watch, in case Philoctetes falls
upon me unawares. He would rather catch *me* than all the rest of
the Greeks put together.

NEOPTOLEMUS (*makes a sign to his man off-stage Right*): All right,
he's going. He will watch the path. — Now, if you have anything
further to tell me, go on again.

ODYSSEUS (*speaking with great force, though quietly*):

Son of Achilles,   50
    The task which brings you here needs courage.
    Oh, not physical courage merely;
    But — if some new thing you have never heard comes out,
    Your part is service.
    You are here to serve the cause.

NEOPTOLEMUS: What are your orders?

ODYSSEUS:

    You are to deceive the mind of Philoctetes with your story.
    When he asks "Who are you? Where from?" you may reply
    "Achilles' son." *That* need not be concealed.
    You are sailing home, you'll say;
    You have left the fleet and army of the Greeks, in furious anger,
    Because these men, who brought you with their prayers from
        home,   60
    — Their only hope of taking Troy —
    Refused to give you, when you came, your due:
    Your father's armour.
    But instead (you'll tell him)
    They gave it to Odysseus.
    — At that point
    Say all the vilest things you can against me.
    I shall not mind.
    But if you will not do it,
    You'll bring distress on all the Greeks.
    You see,
Unless his bow and arrows first are captured,
    You cannot sack the land of Troy.

    (*Goes up to him.*)

Now listen:
I cannot meet or talk with him,
But you can safely do so.   70
I will tell you why.

You brought your ships to Troy without compulsion,
Not under oath to any man.
You came later, not with the first contingent.
I — well,
I must own to the reverse, on every count.
So if, while he is armed, he catches sight of me,
I'm done for,
And I cause your death as well.
This is the thing you have to scheme for:

(NEOPTOLEMUS *comes forward.*)

How to get by *robbery* his invincible arms.

(NEOPTOLEMUS *makes a gesture of disgust.* ODYSSEUS *continues:*)

Oh, I know, I know, my son:
You are not built to utter lies, to plan another's harm.   80
But — there is something sweet about success,
So dare it!
We will shine as honest men another time.
Meanwhile, to-day, for a little shameless hour
Give yourself to me.
Then, for ever more,
You shall be called most virtuous of mortals.
NEOPTOLEMUS (*sternly*): Son of Laertes,
When I hear suggestions painful to me,
I hate to act upon them.
I was not made to act with evil cunning.
(In that, they tell me, I am like my father.)
Instead, I am ready to bring this man along by force,   90
Not trickery.
Surely, lame as he is,
He cannot cope with us, who are so many.
— Oh, I know I was sent to help you.
And I shrink from being called a traitor.
But I'd rather have defeat with fair means than success with foul.
ODYSSEUS (*indulgently*): Brave words!

(*Steps forward.*)

You are like your father Achilles.
He was by far the noblest of the Greeks.
— Yes, I too, when young, was slow of speech and quick of hand,
But now, experience has taught me,
Words, not deeds, rule over men in everything.

NEOPTOLEMUS: What else do you command me, besides lying? 100
ODYSSEUS: I say you are to capture Philoctetes
> By cunning.

NEOPTOLEMUS: Why cunning? Why not by persuasion?
ODYSSEUS: Persuasion's useless.
> And you cannot take him by force.

NEOPTOLEMUS (*scornfully*):
> What *strength* can he rely on, to frighten me?

ODYSSEUS (*gravely, very clearly*):
> *Arrows, that cannot miss — death-dealing always.*

NEOPTOLEMUS: Then it's true!
> He cannot even be approached with safety?

ODYSSEUS:
> No, as I've told you: not unless you use cunning.

NEOPTOLEMUS:
> And do you really not find it shameful to tell lies?

ODYSSEUS: No, not if lying brings escape from danger.
NEOPTOLEMUS:
> But how can one have the face to lie so brazenly? 110

ODYSSEUS: When one stands to gain, scruples are out of place.
NEOPTOLEMUS: What do *I* gain if this man goes to Troy?
ODYSSEUS: His bow is the only weapon that can take Troy.
NEOPTOLEMUS:
> Then have you lied? Am *I* not destined to take it?

ODYSSEUS (*goes to him*): Both you and he will fail without the other.
NEOPTOLEMUS: Well, then, I suppose it's worth trying, if that's so.
ODYSSEUS: Yes. Your success would bring a double reward.
NEOPTOLEMUS: What reward? If I'm certain, I shall not refuse.
ODYSSEUS: A double title: *clever* as well as *brave*.
NEOPTOLEMUS: Right! I will do it — and goodbye to honour! 120
ODYSSEUS: You remember, then, the scheme I recommended?
NEOPTOLEMUS: Of course, now that I have agreed, once and for all.
ODYSSEUS: Very well, then.
> You stay here and wait for him.
> I shall go off: he must not see me with you.
> I shall send your man on guard back to the ship.
> But if I think too long a time has passed,
> I'll send him back again to you,
> — The same man, but disguised, dressed as a merchant captain,
> So that he can't be recognized.
> He'll tell a complicated tale, 130
> From which you'll gather hints that will help you.
> Now I'll leave you in charge,
> And go back to the ship.

I wish you luck
From Hermes, god of cunning;
And from Athene
Queen of Success, my guardian deity.

(*Exit* ODYSSEUS *Right.*)
(*Enter Right, a band of Neoptolemus's* SAILORS, *headed by
the* MATE. *The original number was fourteen, but six is probably sufficient on a modern stage. The* SAILORS *are rough
men with rough voices: they can even speak in dialect, for instance, Devonshire. The* MATE *is a young man, with an ordinary voice.*)

MATE (*going up to* NEOPTOLEMUS): Sir, what are your commands?
   I do not know this country.
   What do you wish concealed from Philoctetes?
   What may I tell him?
   He will be suspicious, won't he?
   Give me your orders.
SAILOR 1: Ay, ay, a prince knows better than other men.
SAILOR 2: He rules by the will of God.   140
SAILOR 3: And our young Leader can say he gets his throne from an-
   cient kings.
MATE: Your instructions, please, sir. I am at your service.
NEOPTOLEMUS: For the moment, probably, you want to see where
   Philoctetes lives, on the edge of the cliff.
   Take a good look, then.
   Don't be afraid.
   But when this cave-dweller comes back from his excursion,
   Fear returns with him.
   Therefore be ready, at a gesture from me,
   To be useful, as the occasion calls for it.
MATE: Your highness knows how I have always studied and   150
   watched to serve you, at the critical moment.
   And now, — where does he live, this Philoctetes?
   In what part of the island?
   In what dwelling?
SAILORS (*together*): Ay, ay, now's the time to tell us.
SAILOR 4: 'Twouldn't do if he jumped out from ambush somewhere
   on us.
SAILOR 5: Ay, ay, where has he settled?
SAILOR 6: In what parts?
MATE: Where are his tracks? Is he inside, or away?
NEOPTOLEMUS (*pointing*): You see that lair in the rock-face — a cave-
   dwelling with double entrance, running through the cliff?   160

MATE (*looking*): Poor devil! And where can he himself have got to?

NEOPTOLEMUS: To me it's obvious:

> The need for food has made him trail his damaged foot some-
> where near by.
>
> It stands to reason:
>
> He must live by hunting, with his bow and arrows.
>
> Life must be unbearable, without a friend, even to tend his
> wound.

MATE: I'm sorry for him, too.   170

> It's as you say, sir:
>
> He has no friend to nurse him, not a man.
>
> He sees no other face,
>
> He must be wretched, always alone, sick and in pain.
>
> He must go nearly mad,
>
> Wondering how to cater for his daily needs.
>
> How does a man endure such hardships?

SAILOR 1: Men can find ways of dealing with most things,

> But there's some get more than their share of misery in life.

SAILORS (*together*): Ay, ay, that's sure.

MATE (*to the others, while* NEOPTOLEMUS *walks off and looks up at the cave*): This Philoctetes — he may have been a man of noble
birth, second to none.   180

> And now, he's stripped of everything, alone, cut off,
>
> Seeing no one but the beasts — leopards and bears —
>
> Suffering from hunger, pain, anxiety.
>
> No one answers his groans,
>
> Except the echoes, over and over again,
>
> Coming back from the hills.   190

NEOPTOLEMUS (*returning, and speaking with pious earnestness*):

> I understand it all.
>
> It was a judgement from Heaven, take it from me.
>
> His trials were sent upon him by a savage goddess, Chrysê,
>
> And his present sufferings, too — his loneliness — are meant,
> without a doubt, by Providence,
>
> Who has decreed that he shall never bend his bow —
>
> Which *must* give victory —
>
> Upon the town of Troy
>
> Until the day its fall is fated.

SAILOR 1: Hush, lad! Quietly!   200

> (*He is listening Left.*)

NEOPTOLEMUS: What is it?

SAILOR 1: I heard a cry,

> The sort of sound a man will make when he's in pain.

SAILOR 2 (*who has followed him*): It came from here.

SAILOR 3: No, here!

SAILOR 4: Ay, ay, I hear it! There's no doubt —

SAILOR 5: The voice of someone limping painfully —

SAILOR 6: A long way off, and yet — I catch it!
Ay, a man in pain!
Clear as a bell it sounds!

SAILOR 2: Look out, lad! 210

NEOPTOLEMUS: Where?

SAILOR 2: Quick! Think of something new!
The man's come back: he's here, quite close at hand!

SAILOR 3: And he's no shepherd, playing on his pipe,
But he's a man who's forced to yell with pain
Each time he stumbles.

SAILOR 4: Maybe it's when he reaches the place where he can see the
empty harbour:
No ship in sight.

MATE: His cries are something awful.

(*The* SAILORS *all withdraw Right. The* MATE *also, but he stands
a little in front of them. Only* NEOPTOLEMUS *stands his ground,
as*

(PHILOCETETES *enters Left.*)

(PHILOCTETES *is a fearsome sight, with long beard, long hair,
ragged clothes. He groans as he drags his lame foot behind him,
sometimes falling on to his hands. But there are the relics of
a fine-looking man in him, and this can be seen when he sometimes draws himself up to his full height. He carries an enormous bow ornamented with gold — a quite spectacular and
extraordinary bow, in strange contrast to his own ragged appearance; and in an ornamented quiver on his back, corre-
spondingly long and handsome feathered arrows.*)

PHILOCTETES (*amazed*): Strangers, who are you?
What has brought you here from your homeland, 220
To this place that has no harbour, and no inhabitants?
If I should guess your nationality —
Should I be right?
You are dressed like Greeks —
The sight that I love best —
But I want to hear your voices.
(*Then, as they do not answer:*)
Oh, don't shrink away in terror from me, though I look a savage!
You must pity me:
I am alone, deserted, without a friend, ill, miserable.
Say something to me, if you've come as friends.

(*They are still silent. He shouts:*)
For God's sake, answer!
   (*Then remembering that he is a prince, and controlling himself.*)
It would not be right that we should part   230
Without exchanging courtesies.
NEOPTOLEMUS (*much moved, steps forward. He speaks somewhat nervously at first*):
   Well, sir, I can assure you, first of all,
   We are Greeks, if that is what you wish to hear.
PHILOCTETES: God, what a welcome sound!
   To think that I should hear a greeting, after all these years,
   From such a man!
      (*In expansive friendliness: he at once takes a fancy to NEOPTOLEMUS.*)
   Who are you, lad? What brought you?
   What need, what purpose?
   It was a lucky wind — lucky for me!
   Tell me about it all.
   I want to know: who are you?
NEOPTOLEMUS:
   My family lives on the Isle of Scyros.
   I am sailing homeward.
   My name is Neoptolemus, Achilles' son.   240
   And now you know it all.
PHILOCTETES (*beside himself with joy*):
   Son of Achilles!
   Lad, I loved your father,
   I love the land you come from.
   I remember:
   You were brought up by that old man, your grandfather.
   Where are you sailing from?
   What brings you here?
NEOPTOLEMUS (*reluctantly*):
   At the moment — well — I'm on my way from Troy.
PHILOCTETES:
   What, Troy?
   You were not with the fleet, that's certain,
   When first we started out to capture Troy.
NEOPTOLEMUS (*pretending surprise*):
   Did *you* take part in that expedition, too?
PHILOCTETES (*hurt*):
   My boy, do you mean to say you do not know me?
NEOPTOLEMUS: How could I know a man I've never seen?   250

PHILOCTETES: You never heard my name, even?
— The story of my unhappy life,
A living death?
NEOPTOLEMUS:
I assure you, I know nothing of what you tell me.
PHILOCTETES (*outraged*):
My God, how cruel, how bitter!
Not a word, even, of how I live, has reached my home,
Or trickled through to any part of Greece!
And so, while they who cast me out so wickedly laugh, and pre-
serve their secret,
My disease flourishes and increases every day!

My boy — son of Achilles — look at me: 260
I am the man you may have heard of,
He who holds the famous bow of Heracles,
Philoctetes, son of Poeas.
I am the man whom these two brother-generals,
And that prince from the western isles,
Cast out, to their dishonour,
In utter solitude, in agony,
To die of a wound inflicted by a poisonous snake.
And with that wound for company they left me upon this island,
And they sailed away —
Yes, the whole fleet.   270
How they rejoiced to see me,
After the stormy voyage across the straits,
Sleeping upon the shore, inside a cave!
And there they left me,
Yes, they went away,
When they had issued from their stores a beggarly ration of mis-
erable rags,
And food, to help me for a while:
God curse them with it!

And you, my son —
Can you imagine what my wakening was like,
To find them gone?
Can you imagine how I wept,
What anguish I felt,
To see those ships, my own contingent,
All gone?
And not an islander, no man to help me,   280
Not a man to give me aid in fighting this disease?
I gazed around,

And could see nothing else but suffering in store for me.
But of *that*, my son, good measure!

And so time passed for me, day after day,
And I was forced to think of household tasks,
Here in my narrow home, alone.
My stomach I managed to provide for, with this bow,
Shooting the doves in flight.
Anything else my arrows could shoot down,
I had to fetch, crawling along,   290
Dragging my wretched foot, until I reached it.
Then, when I needed water,
And when in frosty weather I was forced to chop some wood,
I used to drag myself painfully out to fetch these things.
Then, fire was never there.
Patiently I would rub stone on stone,
Until I made the spark, hidden within, come forth —
My constant saviour.
Such is my home:
A roof, a fire.
Together, they give me all,
Except release from pain.
Now, my son,
Let me tell you of this island.   300
No captain ever comes here willingly.
There is no port,
No place where he can trade,
No lodging.
It is a place which no sane man would choose as destination.
Sometimes, though,
Ships have been forced to call —
It is bound to happen a number of times
In the course of many years —
These men, when they arrive, my son, give pity,
And sometimes add a little food —
They are so sorry for me! —
Or a garment,
But when I mention one thing, all refuse it: 310
Rescue, a passage home.
And so I pine for the tenth year,
Miserable, starving, sick,
Working to feed my insatiable disease.
This is what Atreus' sons, and cruel Odysseus, my boy, have done to
   me

And may the Gods above inflict on them tortures as great as mine!
MATE (*stepping forward, while* NEOPTOLEMUS *broods apart*):
    Sir, son of Poeas: you have our sympathy,
    No less than that of former visitors.
NEOPTOLEMUS (*having decided, comes forward again*):
    I too can vouch for it, your tale is true,
    I know it.
       (*Loudly.*)
    I have met with the same treatment from cruel Odysseus and the
      two commanders.   320
PHILOCTETES: What! You too?
    You have a grievance?
    You are angry with those damned sons of Atreus, for some injury?
NEOPTOLEMUS: Angry!
    Give me the chance to prove it, some day, with this right hand,
    And I will show Mycenae, and Sparta too,
    Scyros can breed a man.
PHILOCTETES: Fine, my boy, fine!
    Now tell me, what's the grievance that has roused in you this furious
      hate against them?
NEOPTOLEMUS: I shall speak out, sir,
    Hard though it is to speak of the outrage that they did me   330
      when I came.
    Listen:
    When Fate decreed my father's death ——
PHILOCTETES: What! Dead? Achilles?
    Tell me no more,
    Until I hear the truth of that.
NEOPTOLEMUS: Yes, he is dead:
    Killed, but by no man's hand.
    It was an arrow shot by a god, they tell me, brought him low.
PHILOCTETES: Ah well! A noble foe for a noble victim!
    I scarcely know, my son, which to do first:
    Inquire your story, or lament your father.
NEOPTOLEMUS: I think your own misfortunes are enough, sir,
    To excuse you from lamenting those of others.   340
PHILOCTETES: You are right.
    Then tell your story.
    Start again,
    And tell me how those men offended you.
NEOPTOLEMUS: They came to seek me in a ship with prow cunningly
      carved ——
    Odysseus, and another,

My father's tutor.
And they told a tale,
— Truly or falsely —
That my father's death made *me* the man destined to capture Troy.
Their words, sir, made me eager to set sail,
Chiefly because I longed to see my father before they buried him,
For I had not seen him; *   351
And also for the glory I would win,
If I could go and end the siege of Troy.
We sailed.
And the day after,
— For the wind was fair and helped our rowing —
We touched shore near Troy:
A bitter landing!
All the men clustered around me as I stepped ashore,
Welcoming me,
Swearing they saw in me the dead Achilles come to life again.

And there he lay,
My father.
First I mourned him a little while.   360
Then I went straight to ask the generals —
Friends, naturally, I thought them —
For his belongings,
And above all, his armour.
But they — damn them! — gave a most insolent answer:
"Son of Achilles,
You may take the rest of your father's property,
Except his armour.
That now belongs to another man:
Odysseus."

The tears rushed to my eyes,
I sprang to my feet in furious anger.
Bitterly I answered:
"You scoundrels!
Have you dared to give my weapons to another man,
Without a word from me?"   370

Odysseus, who was standing near, spoke up then:

---

* Achilles left Scyros soon after Neoptolemus' birth, so that Neoptolemus could say he had never really seen his father.

"Yes, my lad:
They have given them me, and rightly:
I was the man who saved both them and him."

At that, my anger fell on *him*.
I hurled every vile name I could think of in his teeth,
If he meant to take these arms that were really mine.

This stung him,
— Though he is not easily roused —
To answer my reproaches:

"You were not here," he said, "with us:
You were absent from your duty.
In return for all your impudence,   380
You shall never carry back those arms to Scyros."

When I heard this final insult,
I took ship, and sailed for home,
Robbed of my property
By that worst scoundrel of a line of scoundrels,
Odysseus.

Oh, it is not he I blame so much, as the commanders.
Every state and army is just what its rulers make it.
Lawlessness comes from heeding bad advisers.

Well, that's my story.
I bless the man who hates those generals,
And may Heaven bless him too!   390

SAILORS (*grouped Right, stand looking across Left as if at a distant
   mountain, and sing or chant the following prayer, with arms raised*):
   Mother of gods, all-fostering Earth,
   Queen of the hills, and of those sands
   Gold-laden, borne by thy great river,
   To thee we raise our hands!

   As when the cruel sons of Atreus
   Turned on our prince their full disdain
   And gave away his father's armour,
   So now we pray again.

   They gave his armour to Odysseus.
   Oh, hear us, thou, who hast as steed

The lion that slays the bull! Give vengeance,   **400**
Most Holy, for that deed!

PHILOCTETES: Well, friends,
  It seems you have brought with you a token of grief that matches mine,
  And all your story chimes in with what I know,
  Both of these generals,
  And of Odysseus.
  It is their work, that's sure.
  How well I know that man!
  He sticks at nothing, action or word,
  By which he can achieve his ends, always dishonest.
  It is not *that* surprises me,   **410**
  But how a man like Ajax the Elder could stand by and let it happen.
NEOPTOLEMUS: Sir, he was there no longer.
  They would never have seized my arms if he had been alive.
PHILOCTETES: What, he too — gone?
NEOPTOLEMUS: Yes, gone.
PHILOCTETES: And men like him must die —
  But never scoundrels like Odysseus and Diomēdēs
  Who could well be spared!
NEOPTOLEMUS: You're right.
  I can assure you
  They are happy and flourishing in the army of the Greeks.   **420**
PHILOCTETES:
  And how's my dear old friend, Nestor of Pylos?
  A fine old man!
  Is he alive?
  His counsels often put *their* base schemes right out of action.
NEOPTOLEMUS: Yes, he is alive.
  But he has troubles now.
  He has lost his son,
  The one who was with the army.
PHILOCTETES: Another gone!
  Antilochus!
  He and Ajax are two whose deaths I least can bear to hear of.
  Ah well!
  Is life worth living, when these men are gone,
  And there's a man still here — Odysseus —
  Who should be numbered with the lost instead?   **430**
NEOPTOLEMUS: Ah, he's a clever wrestler!
  But the clever are often tripped, Philoctetes, in their schemes.

PHILOCTETES (*still running over the names of the men he knew*):
    Now, for God's sake, tell me:
    Where in all this business was your father's friend,
    Patroclus, his best friend?
NEOPTOLEMUS: He too was dead.
    I tell you, in a word:
    War never takes a bad man willingly:
    Always the best.
PHILOCTETES: That's my experience, too.
    And that reminds me:
    I must next inquire about a man —
    Worthless, but smart of speech, and clever:
    How is he getting on at present?
NEOPTOLEMUS: Surely you mean no other than Odysseus?   440
PHILOCTETES: No, no, not him.
    There was a man,
    Thersites,
    Who never was content with brevity,
    Though no one wished to hear.
    Is he alive?
NEOPTOLEMUS: I did not see him, but I heard he was.
PHILOCTETES: He would be!
    Nothing evil ever dies!
    The gods protect such things so carefully!
    They seem to take delight in turning back the wicked and
        deceitful from the tomb,
    And sending there all that is good and honest.   450
    What can I think, how praise the ways of God,
    When I find evil in the gods themselves?
NEOPTOLEMUS: I, noble sir, shall take good care to keep my distance
    Both from Troy and from the generals.
    Wherever the inferior holds the power,
    Where honesty is crushed, and smartness wins,
    — To such men I shall never give my friendship.
    No,
    My own rocky island shall content me henceforward,
    And I'll seek my joys at home.   46c

    Now I must go aboard.
    Good-bye, good-bye, sir!
    I wish you luck, most cordially, and health restored,
    As you desire.

    Come on, my men!
    We must be ready,

The moment we are granted a favourable wind,
To put to sea.

PHILOCTETES: Going?
So soon?

NEOPTOLEMUS: Yes, it is time to go where we can see the ship, and
watch the weather.

PHILOCTETES (*casting himself at* NEOPTOLEMUS' *feet*):
Now by your father and your mother,
By whatever else at home you love, my son,
I beg you on my knees,
Oh, do not leave me alone, cut off,   470
Among these miseries, so great, so many,
As you see and hear!
Give me a place somewhere!
I know too well the tiresomeness, for you, of such a cargo.
Yet undertake it!
To the generous-minded, meanness is hateful,
But a kind deed is glorious.
If you decline this charge, you earn dishonour.
If you accept it, great is your reward:
In fame, my son,
When I reach home alive.

Do it!
Your trouble will not last a day!   480
Dare it!
Throw me wherever you like, but take me!
— In the hold, in the bows, in the stern,
Anywhere, where I shall least annoy my shipmates.
Oh, consent, my son,
By the God that favours suppliants!
Oh, be persuaded!
On my knees I fall,
Weak as I am, lame, wretched!
Do not leave me thus lonely,
Far from the steps of other men!
Save me from here!
Take me no further than your *own* home,
Or the place where I can cross the straits to my own country —
That dear mountain,
Those hills,
The lovely waters of my native river!   490

And there you'll show me to my father,
Unless indeed he's gone.

As I have feared so long,
For I have sent him messages,
Often,
By those who called here,
Begging him to come for me and save me,
Fetch me home.
Yes, either he is dead,
Or else, my messengers —
Naturally, as I see it —
Thinking little of my concerns,
Sailed, with all speed straight home.

But now,
I come to you as messenger and rescuer in one; 500
Pity me, save me!
Think how, in life, all is uncertain,
Full of risks that lead to good or evil fortune.
He who stands clear of sorrow should beware.
And when one's life is smooth,
Then above all
One must keep watch against insidious ruin!

SAILORS (*turn with one accord to* NEOPTOLEMUS, *and sing, or chant in a low harmonious murmur*):
Show pity, Prince! The grievous pains,
The toils, the struggles manifold,
May never friend of mine encounter,
Such as this man has told!

You hate them, Prince, those sons of Atreus 510
So harsh! Then be advised of me:
Turning their crime to this man's profit,
Take him across the sea.

Take him, on board our own stout vessel,
Swiftly to where he longs to fly —
His home — that so the dreaded vengeance
Of Heaven may pass us by.

NEOPTOLEMUS (*to the* MATE):
Yes, *now* you are all for kindness, looking on.
But when his sickness tries you, near at hand, 520
Take care your actions suit your present words!
MATE: Of course, sir!
You shall never have to say such a thing of me truly!

NEOPTOLEMUS: Well then,

> I would be ashamed to show myself less willing than you to do a
> service for a stranger.
> Right!
> Then we sail.
> We start without delay.
> The ship will take him: *she* will not refuse.
> Only I pray:
> God bring us safely from this island
> To — the place where we are bound for.

PHILOCTETES: Oh, happiest of days!   530

> Kindest of men!
> Good sailors!
> How can I ever hope to prove by actions what a friend you've
> made in me!
> Let us go, my son,
> When we have said goodbye to my poor home in here.
> Oh, you shall see how much I've lived on
> And how brave I've been!
> I fancy, just to catch a glimpse of it would have proved too much
> for any man but me!

> (NEOPTOLEMUS *and* PHILOCTETES *turn away, to go up to the
> cave.* SAILOR 1, *who has been watching Right, stops them.*)

SAILOR 1: Wait!

> Let's find out, sir!
> Here are two men coming,
> One from our crew;
> The other man's a stranger.   540
> Find out their news, before you go inside.

> (*Enter Right, the Sailor disguised as a* MERCHANT CAPTAIN.)

MERCHANT: Sir — you are Achilles' son?

> I asked this sailor
> Who with two other men was keeping watch
> On board your ship,
> To tell me where I'd find you,
> Since unexpectedly our ways have met,
> I happened to have anchored here beside you.
> I am sailing as a trader back from Troy,
> With a small crew,
> To where I live,
> The island famous for vines, Peparethus.

And I heard that all the sailors here are of your crew.   550
So I resolved not to sail on in silence
But first to warn you, and receive my due.

Sir, you know nothing of your own affairs:
The newly-formed designs the Greeks have on you;
And not designs alone:
They are in action, without a pause.

NEOPTOLEMUS: I thank you for your kindness.
  I should be base, if I did not repay it with lasting gratitude.
  Now tell me all:
  What is this plan you know of, that the Greeks have now devised
      against me?   560

MERCHANT: They have left already in pursuit, with several ships:
  The aged tutor and the Athenian princes.

NEOPTOLEMUS: They want me back?
  By force, or by persuasion?

MERCHANT: I do not know.
  I tell you what I hear.

NEOPTOLEMUS: Are they so eager, then, to carry out the wishes of the
      generals?

MERCHANT: I assure you,
  These things are happening,
  And without delay.

NEOPTOLEMUS: Why was Odysseus not prepared to sail himself, and
      bring the message?
  Was it fear restrained him?

MERCHANT: No.
  He and his friend were starting after another man, when I set
      sail.   570

NEOPTOLEMUS: Who was the object, then, of his own voyage?

MERCHANT: It was a man ——
      (*Lowering his voice, and glancing towards* PHILOCTETES.)
  But tell me first of all:
  Who is this here?
  And do not speak too loudly.

NEOPTOLEMUS: This is the famous Philoctetes, stranger.

MERCHANT: Then ask no further questions!
  Get yourself away from here,
  As fast as ever you can!

PHILOCTETES: What is he saying, son?
  Why does he bargain, this captain, over me
  In these dark whispers?

NEOPTOLEMUS: I have not grasped his meaning yet.   580

He must speak openly,
To you and me and the men here.

MERCHANT: Oh, please, sir,
Do not get me into trouble with the army, for repeating what I
should not!
Poor as I am, I give the best I can,
And they repay me well.

NEOPTOLEMUS: I hate the generals!
This man's my dearest friend, because he hates them.
Therefore,
If you have come here to befriend me,
You must hide nothing from us, of your news.

MERCHANT: Watch what you're doing, son.

NEOPTOLEMUS: I know quite well.

MERCHANT: I shall hold *you* responsible.

NEOPTOLEMUS: Do so — but speak.   590

MERCHANT: I will.
The men I told you of,
Odysseus and his friend,
Are under oath to bring back this man *here*,
    (*Pointing to* PHILOCTETES.)
Either by pressure of words,
Or if they cannot, then by force.
That's why they sailed;
The oath Odysseus swore was heard by the whole army,
— Though his friend was not so confident of their success.

NEOPTOLEMUS: But what do the commanders want with this man,
After so long?
They cast him out, and kept him in exile many years.   600
Why this desire to get him back?
Is it some driving-force from Heaven,
Threatening vengeance for their crime?

MERCHANT: I can explain all that.
You have not heard it, perhaps.
There was a seer of noble birth, called Helenus,
Whom once Odysseus,
· – That crafty scoundrel, loathed by all the army —
Sallying forth, at night, alone,
Had captured.
He showed his prize in chains to the Greek army,
And then the seer foretold them all they asked.   610
He said, among the rest, that they could never sack Troy,
Unless they won this man (*nodding at* PHILOCTETES) by words,
And brought him from the island where he lives now.

Odysseus, when he heard the prophet's words,
Promised forthwith he would produce the man.
The prisoner would come willingly, he thought;
But otherwise, force would be used.
He offered to let the Greeks behead him, if he failed.

That's the whole story.
My advice is: Hurry!   620
Both you, and anyone who matters to you.
PHILOCTETES: Oh God!
    Can it be he,
    That utter curse,
    Who has sworn to win me back to the Greek army?
    I could as soon be won back from the grave!
MERCHANT (*staring*): I couldn't say, I'm sure,
    I must be going back to the ship.
    Good luck go with you both!
        (*Exit Sailor disguised as* MERCHANT, *Right.*)
PHILOCTETES: Is it not scandalous, my boy,
    That he, Odysseus, should expect to capture *me* with honeyed
        words,
    And hand me to the army?   630
    No!
    I would listen sooner to the viper,
    My deadliest foe,
    That made me thus a cripple!
    But he ——
    He stops at nothing, word or deed.
    And now, I am forewarned that he is coming.
    Quick, let us start, lad!
    Let us put many miles of sea between ourselves and that man's
        ship!
    Let's go!
    This is the time for working fast,
    And that brings sleep and rest another day.
NEOPTOLEMUS (*showing a strange reluctance*): Yes, we will sail,
    But we must wait until this head-wind falls.
    The weather is against us.   640
PHILOCTETES: The weather's always right for escaping trouble!
NEOPTOLEMUS: Ah, but it's blowing hard against *them* as well.
PHILOCTETES: No wind is adverse to a pirate,
    When there's plundering afoot, and violence.
NEOPTOLEMUS: All right, then:
    Let us go,

When you have fetched what most you need or want, out of your
    cave.

PHILOCTETES: Yes, there are some things,
    Though the choice is small.

NEOPTOLEMUS: What could there be, that we have not on board?

PHILOCTETES: There is a herb I keep by me,
    With which I best can soothe this sore and dull the pain.   650

NEOPTOLEMUS: Fetch it, then.
    Is there something else you want?

PHILOCTETES: One of these arrows may have slipped away;
    I must not leave it for some other man to take.

NEOPTOLEMUS: Is that the famous bow you're holding?

PHILOCTETES: It is — this bow I carry;
    This and no other.

NEOPTOLEMUS: May one come near and take a look at it,
    And hold it,
    And salute it as divine?

PHILOCTETES: *You* may, my son,
    You are allowed to handle this,
    And whatever else of mine can profit you.

NEOPTOLEMUS: (*forgetting everything in his youthful eagerness*):
    Oh, I would love to!   660
    (*Recalling himself.*)
    — That is, if my "love" is lawful.
    But if not, then let it go.

PHILOCTETES: You have said nothing wrong, my lad,
    Nothing unlawful,
    You are the one man who has given me back this sunshine — my
        own land — my aged father ——
    My friends.
    You have raised me,
    Set me out of reach of my enemies, who had me on the ground.
    Don't be afraid!
    You are allowed to touch it,
    And hand it back,
    And boast that you alone have earned this right,
    By doing a good turn,
    Just as I won it by an act of kindness.   670

    (PHILOCTETES *holds out the bow to* NEOPTOLEMUS, *and allows
    him to touch it, but without himself letting it go.*)

NEOPTOLEMUS (*thrown off his balance by this experience, speaks some-
    what awkwardly*): I am glad I found you,
    Glad you are my friend.

A man who knows how to reward a service is bound to prove a
friend above all price.

(*Indicating the cave.*)

Will you go in?

PHILOCTETES: Yes, and I'll take you with me.

My sickness needs your help and your support.

(*Exeunt* NEOPTOLEMUS *and* PHILOCTETES *into the cave. The*
SAILORS, *now that they are left alone, come forward and sing.*)

SAILOR 1:

I've heard it told in story,
— Though I have never seen —
How once a foolish mortal
Laid hands on Heaven's Queen.

SAILOR 2:

The mighty King of Heaven   680
Then hurled him to the ground,
And on the running wheel-rim
His helpless limbs he bound.

SAILOR 3:

But suffering more cruel
I never heard or saw
Than this man's, though he injured
No man, but kept the law.

SAILOR 4:

Oh, how did he endure it
There on the lonely shore,
Mourning a fate so undeserved,
Hearing the breakers roar?   690

SAILOR 5:

I marvel at his courage!
There was no neighbour near
To help him in his lameness,
His bitter cries to hear.

SAILOR 6:

No one to soothe the fever
Of his envenomed sore,
No one to bring the healing herb
And staunch the oozing gore.

SAILOR 1:

Painfully, like a baby
Without its nurse, he crept   700
This way and that, to get his food,
When the raging anguish slept.

SAILOR 2:
> He had no corn to feed him,
>> No fruits a man can grow,
> His only food was the birds brought down
>> By his far-shooting bow.   710

SAILOR 3:
> For ten long years he tasted
>> No wine to cheer his soul,
> But crawling, he would seek for
>> A stagnant water-hole.

(PHILOCTETES *and* NEOPTOLEMUS *are seen leaving the cave. The* SAILORS *take up the deception again.*)

SAILOR 4:
> But now he's met our Leader
>> And won a noble friend,
> He shall be great and happy,
>> His woes are at an end.   720

SAILOR 5:
> Our Leader, in the fulness
>> Of many months, has come,
> And on his ship, sea-cleaving,
>> Will take the exile home.

SAILOR 6:
> Home to the hills nymph-haunted,
>> Home to his native stream,
> Where Heracles went up to Heaven
>> Amid the lightning's gleam.

(*As* PHILOCTETES *and* NEOPTOLEMUS *come down from the cave, the* SAILORS *sing, all together.*)

SAILORS:
> When Heracles, the brazen-shielded,
> Climbed to the mountain-top, and yielded
> His soul, while Zeus the Father wielded
> The lightning's glorious gleam.

(NEOPTOLEMUS *leads the way slowly Right,* PHILOCTETES *stands still.*)

NEOPTOLEMUS: Come, please.   730
> (*Turns.*)
> Why do you stop without a reason,
> And stand in silence,
> As if struck dumb with fear?

PHILOCTETES (*groans*).

NEOPTOLEMUS: What's the matter?

PHILOCTETES: Nothing much. Go on, my boy.

> (*His face is contorted with pain.*)

NEOPTOLEMUS: It's not the pain from that old wound of yours?

PHILOCTETES: No, no, of course not — I shall be better soon.
Oh God!

NEOPTOLEMUS (*more and more concerned*):
Why do you groan and call on God?

PHILOCTETES: That he may visit us with saving mercy.

> (*He groans again, more deeply.*)

NEOPTOLEMUS (*going to him in great concern*): What's wrong?
Please tell me — don't stand silent there. 740
You have some dreadful pain, that's obvious.

PHILOCTETES (*breaking down*): I'm lost, my boy.
I cannot hope to hide my suffering from you.

> (*He gives a cry of pain.*)

Ah, it's going through me,
It's going through me!
Oh, what misery!
Yes, lost, my boy — this pain's devouring me.

> (*He gives three cries, each sharper and longer than the one before it.*)

For God's sake,
If you have a sword to hand, lad,
Strike my foot — here on the heel!
Mow it off, quickly!
Never mind my life!
Quick, quick, my boy! 750

NEOPTOLEMUS: What can it be, that comes so suddenly,
And makes you cry and groan with such despair?

PHILOCTETES: You know, my boy.

NEOPTOLEMUS: What is it?

PHILOCTETES: You know, my son.

NEOPTOLEMUS: What — what? I do not know.

PHILOCTETES: You *must*.

> (*He gives another sharp, long-drawn-out cry.*)

NEOPTOLEMUS: What a terrible affliction, this disease!

PHILOCTETES: Terrible beyond words.
Have pity on me!

NEOPTOLEMUS: What must I do?

PHILOCTETES: Don't give me up in terror,

This visitor comes only now and then:
Perhaps she's tired of wandering ——·

NEOPTOLEMUS: Poor man,
Worn out with every kind of suffering! 760
Would you like me to take hold of you and help you?

(*Goes to take hold of him.*)

PHILOCTETES (*shrinking back*): No, no, not that!
But my bow — here, take it,
As you asked to do just now,
And keep it safely
Until the agony of my disease abates.
As soon as it is over,
Sleep will seize me.
It will not cease till then.
And you must let me sleep peacefully.
And if, during that time, my enemies arrive,
I beg of you, in God's name, 770
Do not let them have my weapon,
Neither with nor against your will, by any means.
For if you do,
You will bring death upon yourself,
And me, who am your suppliant.

NEOPTOLEMUS (*with false heartiness*): Don't worry.
I'll be careful.
No one shall touch it but you and me.
Give it,
And luck go with it!

PHILOCTETES (*hands him the bow. At this solemn moment, there
should be a distant roll of thunder*): There, my boy!
Take it!
And pray the jealous gods
That it may not bring on you such sorrows as it brought on me
And on its former owner.

NEOPTOLEMUS: Amen, for both of us!

(*Another rumble of thunder, very faint this time.*)

And may our voyage be swift and fair, 780
To whatsoever goal God has decreed,
And our good ship is tending!

(*A last faint roll of thunder.*)

PHILOCTETES (*feels a second attack of pain beginning, and groans*): I
fear, my son, your prayers are doomed to failure.

Again the dark blood oozes forth in drops from the deep wound:
I dread a new attack.

(*He gives a cry.*)

Ah!
Heavens — this pain — (*he grasps his foot in torture*) — what
will it do to me?
It comes!
It's coming nearer! Oh, what agony!

(*He gazes round at the* SAILORS, *who are watching with great
concern.*)

You see it all!
Don't leave me, I implore you!

(*He gives another cry.*)

Oh, Prince Odysseus,   790
If this agony could stab *you* through the breast!
Oh God, oh God!
I cannot help these cries!
— And you two generals,
Agamemnon, Menelaus,
If only *you* could cherish this disease as long as I have!

(*He moans.*)

Oh Death, oh Death!
Why is it, though I call upon you daily,
You can never come?

(*To* NEOPTOLEMUS.)

My son, you are generous,
— Take me to that mountain,
The island fire, they call it,   800
That volcano,
And throw me in the flames!
Once, long ago
I earned these weapons, which you're guarding for me,
By such a service to the god-like Heracles.
What do you say, my lad?
What do you say?
Why are you silent?
What are you thinking? — say!
NEOPTOLEMUS (*evasively*): I have been grieving at your load of sorrows.
PHILOCTETES (*trying to cheer him*): Come, come, my boy!

There's room for cheerfulness!
This visitor — she's fierce, but quick to go.
Only, I beg you,
Don't abandon me.

NEOPTOLEMUS: Don't worry, we will stay.

PHILOCTETES: You'll stay?

NEOPTOLEMUS: Be sure of it!   810

PHILOCTETES: I would scorn to put you on your oath, my son.

NEOPTOLEMUS (*nods, and adds enigmatically*):
Yes. It's not lawful I should leave without you.

PHILOCTETES: Give me your hand on it.

NEOPTOLEMUS (*gives his hand*): I swear to stay.

PHILOCTETES (*as the third attack begins, points wildly to the cave*):
Take me there — there!

NEOPTOLEMUS: Where do you mean?

PHILOCTETES (*gesticulating upwards*): Up there!

NEOPTOLEMUS: Why do you rave, and gaze up at the sky?

(*He tries to take hold of* PHILOCTETES.)

PHILOCTETES (*shrinking back as before*): Let me go, let me go!

NEOPTOLEMUS: Where?

PHILOCTETES: Let me go, I tell you!

NEOPTOLEMUS (*barring his way*): I will not!

(*Goes to take hold of him again.*)

PHILOCTETES: You will kill me, if you touch me!

NEOPTOLEMUS (*gives way*): There, see!
I have let you go,
— If you are saner.

PHILOCTETES (*struggles up the path to the cave, and sinks down at the entrance*): Oh Earth, receive me,
Dying as I am!
This agony will let me stand no longer.   820

(*He lies down.*)

NEOPTOLEMUS (*carrying the great bow, goes and looks down at* PHILOCTETES. *The* MATE *follows*):
He'll be asleep, I think, before much longer.
Look how his head is sinking back,
And sweat — you see? — is breaking out all over him.
A stream of blood — how dark it is! — has gushed out of his heel.
Come, sailors, we will leave him in peace,
So that he'll fall asleep more quickly.

(NEOPTOLEMUS *comes down from the cave entrance, and*

*stands at one side, Left, looking at the bow and arrows.
Meanwhile the* SAILORS *and the* MATE *group themselves in the
centre and sing quietly.*)

SAILORS: Sleep, that knowest not grief or pain,
  Come with gentle breath, O King!
 Soothe him, spread before his eyes
  The radiance thou dost bring,   830
   O come,
  And heal his suffering!

(*Then, with a complete change of tone and attitude, they turn
to* NEOPTOLEMUS *and address him one by one, in urgent
whispers:*)

SAILOR 1: Think, son! What's your next move?
SAILOR 2: What's the next step to be?
SAILOR 3 (*nods at the sleeping* PHILOCTETES): You see how things are
 now!
SAILOR 4: What reason can there be for waiting?
SAILOR 5: Let's do it!
SAILOR 6: Now's the time!
MATE: If one is wise,
  And takes the chance that's offered,
  A swift stroke wins the Prize.
NEOPTOLEMUS (*speaks with exaltation*):
  True, he lies there hearing nothing;
  But I see we have no gain,
  For if we sail without him, we have stolen his bow in vain.   840
  His is the victory garland,
  Him the god has bade us bring,
  And to boast of failure won by lies would be a shameful thing.

(*The* SAILORS *continue to urge him, in whispers*):

SAILOR 1: God will take care of that.
SAILOR 2: But when you answer me,
  Speak softly, softly, lad!
SAILOR 3: For quick to wake is he
  Whose sleep is vexed with pain.
SAILOR 4: One thing, only one,
  Think with all your might
  How it can be done!
SAILOR 5: Take the prize by stealth!   850
SAILOR 6: You know what we mean!
MATE: In your present purpose
  Troubles can be foreseen.

SAILOR 1: Now the time is right!

SAILOR 2: Now, bereft of sight,
Helpless there he lies.

SAILOR 3: He has no command
Over foot or hand. 860

SAILOR 4: He might as well be dead.

SAILOR 5: Think if what you've said
Is sound.

MATE: So far as I
Can see, we should rely
On silent work;

SAILOR 6 (*nods*): A plan
That will not wake the man.

NEOPTOLEMUS (*has gone up to* PHILOCTETES: *bends over him*) ·
Be quiet, men!
And do not lose your wits:
His eyes are opening.
He lifts his head.

PHILOCTETES (*waking and looking round*): Sunlight,
Following sleep!
And oh, unhoped for,
Here are my guardians still,
These kindly strangers!
My son,
Never would I have dreamed
You would have shown such pity for my sufferings 870
As to stay beside me here and lend your aid.
The sons of Atreus did not bear this burden so easily,
Those valiant commanders!
But you are noble and of noble birth,
So you, my boy, made light of all of it;
My shouting,
And the loathsome smell that vexed you.
And now, I think,
For a little while there'll be forgetfulness
And rest from this affliction.
So lift me, lad, yourself,
And set me upright,
And then, when I have shaken off this weakness, 880
We can start for the ship,
And not delay our voyage.

NEOPTOLEMUS (*with restraint*): I am glad to see you living still and
breathing,
Released from pain.

I had almost given up hope:
Your symptoms seemed to augur instant death,
Regarded in the light of your disease.
But now — lift yourself up;
Or if you'd rather,
My men will carry you.
We'll spare no trouble,
Since we have both decided what to do.

PHILOCTETES: Good, my boy!
Lift me up, as you suggest.
Let your men be.
I do not want them troubled, more than is needful, by   890
the unpleasant smell.
My presence will be trial enough on board.

NEOPTOLEMUS: Very well.
Hold on to me and try to rise.

PHILOCTETES: Don't worry.
Habit will set me on my feet.

NEOPTOLEMUS (*suddenly, with a groan*): Oh God!
What am I to do next?

PHILOCTETES (*amazed*): What is it, lad?
Why this aberration in your speech?

NEOPTOLEMUS (*in great distress*): I don't know how to put it.
I am at an end ——

PHILOCTETES: An end of what?
Don't say such things, my boy!

NEOPTOLEMUS: Here I am, faced with it at last!

PHILOCTETES: Don't tell me the loathsomeness of my disease per-
suades you to refuse to take me as your passenger!   900

NEOPTOLEMUS: Everything's loathsome
When a man forsakes his nature,
And does things that do not fit him.

PHILOCTETES: You do and say nothing against the nature your father
gave you, when you help the deserving.

NEOPTOLEMUS: I shall be shown up as vile.
It tortures me!

PHILOCTETES: Not by your actions.
But your words — they daunt me.

NEOPTOLEMUS: Oh God, what shall I do?
Caught, twice a villain,
Hiding what I should tell,
Shamefully lying!   909

PHILOCTETES (*gazing at him sternly*): This man, unless I am no judge,
intends to betray me — leave me here and sail without me.

NEOPTOLEMUS: No, no, not leave you!
   But my taking you may be more bitter:
   That's what tortures me.
PHILOCTETES: What do you mean, lad?
   I don't understand.
NEOPTOLEMUS: I will tell you all.
   You are to sail to Troy,
   To the Greek army led by Atreus' sons.   920
PHILOCTETES: God, what have you said?
NEOPTOLEMUS: Do not groan, until you hear ——
PHILOCTETES: Hear what?
   What do you plan to do with me?
NEOPTOLEMUS (*desperately*): Rescue you from this misery!
   And then,
   Side by side with you,
   Sack the plains of Troy!
PHILOCTETES: This is really what you plan?
NEOPTOLEMUS: A stronger force compels me.
   Don't be angry at the hearing!
PHILOCTETES: I am lost, betrayed!
   What have you done to me, stranger?
   Oh, give it back at once,
   My bow!

   (*He goes to take it.*)

NEOPTOLEMUS (*withdraws*): No, no, I cannot!
   I am forced to obey those in command,
   By duty and expedience.
PHILOCTETES (*recoils*): You fire,
   You utter monster,
   Hateful tool of direst villainy,
   How you have worked,
   How you have cheated me!
   Have you no shame, you scoundrel, when you look at me, your
      suppliant?   930
   You took my bow — and robbed me of my life!
   Give it back, I beg you,
   Give it, I pray, my son!
   By the gods of your fathers, do not take my bow!

   (*He groans.*)

He does not even answer any more!
He looks away:
He does not mean to yield it!

(*He turns to the rocks and speaks to them.*)

Oh shores,
Oh headlands,
Oh you company of mountain animals,
Oh cliffs so sheer,
To you I cry,
For I have no one else,
And you are always there to hear my sorrows!
See what Achilles' son has done to me!   940
He swore to take me home,
And yet he takes me
To Troy!
He gave me his right hand,
Yet stole my bow,
The sacred bow of Heracles.

He wants to offer me to the Greek army.
He drags me off by force,
As though I were strong.
He does not see he kills a corpse, a shadow, a phantom!
For if I had my strength,
He never would have taken me —
Would not now, weak as I am, except by treachery.

But now, I am cheated vilely.
What shall I do?
Oh, give it back!
Repent even now,
And be your true self!
Won't you answer?   950

You are silent.
Then I am lost,
And all is misery!

(*He toils up the slope to the cave.*)

My cave, familiar shape with double entrance,
See, I return, disarmed, robbed of my living,
To waste away alone beneath your roof.

I shall no longer shoot the flying bird,
The beast that walks the mountain:
I shall be the food of those whom formerly I fed on,

And those I hunted once will now hunt me.
My blood shall pay for *their* blood —
And my end is brought about by one who seemed all innocence.
I curse you —   961
No, not yet,
Until I see if you repent.
If not — may you die wretched!

MATE (*to* NEOPTOLEMUS): What should we do?
It rests with you, sir, now,
Either to sail, or listen to his pleading.

NEOPTOLEMUS: Me?
I am filled with pity,
Searing pity for this man,
As I have been all along.

PHILOCTETES: In God's name, lad, show pity!
Do not stand convicted of this crime of robbing me!

NEOPTOLEMUS: Ah, what am I to do?
Why did I ever leave Scyros?
I am tortured by this choice!   970

PHILOCTETES: You are no villain.
But you are sent by villains,
Who have primed you with a shameful part.
Leave it to those it suits,
Give me my bow,
And sail!

NEOPTOLEMUS (*wavering*): What shall we do, men?

(ODYSSEUS *steps suddenly in Right, and checks* NEOPTOLEMUS.)

ODYSSEUS: Scoundrel, what are you doing?
Stand back, and hand this bow over to me!

PHILOCTETES: God, who is this?
Do I hear Odysseus' voice?

ODYSSEUS: Odysseus, be assured:
I whom you see.

PHILOCTETES: O, I am lost, betrayed!
So it was he,
The hand behind this capture and this robbery!

ODYSSEUS: Yes, it was I, no other,
I confess it.   980

PHILOCTETES: Give it back, lad!
Let me have my bow!

ODYSSEUS: No, that he never shall, even if he wishes.
But you must come along with it,
Or these will drag you.

PHILOCTETES: *These* will drag *me,*
    You shameless, filthy villain!
ODYSSEUS: Yes, if you won't go of your own accord.
PHILOCTETES: Oh, land of Lemnos,
    And all-conquering flame of the volcanic fire,
    Is this endurable,
    If this man drags me off from you by force?
ODYSSEUS: God, let me tell you,
    God, who rules this island,
    God has decreed it.
    I am but His servant.   9
PHILOCTETES: You wretch,
    What lies you find to utter!
    Making the gods your pretext,
    So you make them liars.
ODYSSEUS: No, they are true.
    And you must make this journey.
PHILOCTETES: I will not.
ODYSSEUS: I insist.
    You must obey.

    (*He moves towards* PHILOCTETES.)

PHILOCTETES: It was as a slave, then, after all, not a free man, my father
    gave me life!
ODYSSEUS: No: as a hero, equal to the bravest,
    With whom it is ordained
    You shall capture Troy.
PHILOCTETES: Never!
    Rather the worst that can befall me,
    So long as there is this steep drop below!   1000

    (*He crawls along as if making for the edge of the cliff.*)

ODYSSEUS: What are you trying to do?
PHILOCTETES (*standing up: wildly*): I'll dash my skull in bleeding frag-
    ments on the rocks below!
ODYSSEUS (*to the* SAILORS): Stop him!
    Don't let him have the chance of that!

    (*Two of the* SAILORS *dash up the path and seize* PHILOCTETES
    as he tries to throw himself over. There is a brief struggle.)

PHILOCTETES (*overpowered*): Oh, my poor hands,
    See how you suffer, lacking the string of that dear bow!
    This man has seized you,
    This man who knows no true or generous thought!

(*To* ODYSSEUS.)

How have you crept upon me,
Tracked me down,
Using as screen this boy I did not know,
— Too good for you — but good enough for me —
Who had no thought except to do his duty,   1010
And now displays the sorrow that he feels for his own error and
  my sufferings!
But your base soul,
For ever peeping from its ambush,
Taught him well,
Against his nature, against his will,
To be adept in evil.
And now, you beast, you have bound me,
And you plan to take me from this shore,
On which you cast me friendless,
Abandoned,
Homeless,
Dead in life.

Curse you!
How often have I cursed you so!
But the gods never grant me any pleasure: 1020
You enjoy life;
I am tormented by this very living among miseries,
Mocked at by you and by the sons of Atreus,
The two commanders, whom you serve in this.

And yet it was by trickery and compulsion you were made to join
  their fleet.
But I, poor fool,
Who freely sailed, with seven ships,
Was scorned, and dropped,
By them, or you:
Each blames the other.
And now — why do you take me?
For what purpose?
To you I have long been dead:
As good as nothing,   1030
How is it, cursed wretch, I am not *now* lame, evil-smelling?
How can you say your prayers if I sail with you?
How perform libations,
Sacrifices:
Your excuse for dropping me?

May you die miserably!
And die you will, for your crime against me,
If the gods love justice;
And that I know they do,
For you would never have sailed to fetch me from my misery
Unless a god-sent need of me had spurred you.

But oh, my country,
And ye watching gods,   1040
Bring vengeance, vengeance,
Some day, however late,
On all their heads,
If you have pity on me!
My life is wretched;
But if I could see them dead,
It would be to me like health restored!

SAILOR 1 (*murmuring*): He's bitter.

SAILOR 2: Ay, his words are bitter, Prince.

SAILOR 3: He does not bow the neck before his troubles.

ODYSSEUS: I could say much in answer to his speech,
If I had time.
But now, I have one theme:
I shape myself to suit the moment's needs.
When there's a competition in the virtues,   1050
You will find none more holy than myself.
It is my nature to desire success,
— Except with you
     (*To* PHILOCTETES, *contemptuously.*)
To you I gladly yield.
     (*To the* SAILORS.)
    Yes, let him go.
Don't touch him any more.
He can stay here.
We have no need of *you*
Now that we have this bow.
We have a man in the army, Teucros, skilled in archery,
And there's myself, as fit as you, I fancy,
To handle this and take as true an aim.
Why should we want you?
You can pace your Lemnos with pleasure!   1060
Let us go.
Perhaps your prize will bring *me* fame that should have gone to
     you.

PHILOCTETES (*groans*): Ah, God, what shall I do?

Will you display yourself before the Greeks,
Decked with my weapon?

ODYSSEUS: Argue no more with me.
I am going now.

PHILOCTETES (*to* NEOPTOLEMUS): Son of Achilles,
And will you, too, leave me,
Without a farewell word?

ODYSSEUS (*to* NEOPTOLEMUS): Come on!
Don't cast a glance at him,
For generous as you are,
You still may wreck the whole of our success.

PHILOCTETES (*to the* SAILORS):
And am I to be thus abandoned, strangers, by you too?   1070
Have you lost all pity for me?

MATE (*awkwardly*): This young man here's our captain.
Anything he says to you,
Well, that's what we say, too.

NEOPTOLEMUS: I shall be told that I am too soft-hearted,
  ~ By *him*.
      (*Nodding towards* ODYSSEUS, *who has gone on Right.*)
Still, you can stay,
If he (*indicating* PHILOCTETES) would like it,
But only till the crew has made all ready,
And we have said a prayer.
Meanwhile,
Maybe he'll think this matter over,
And conceive some better mind towards us.
— We will go, then;
And you — (*to the* SAILORS) — come quickly, when I give the
  word.   1080

      (*Exeunt* ODYSSEUS *and* NEOPTOLEMUS *Right.*)
      (*In the following scene,* PHILOCTETES *stays by the mouth of the
      cave, and absorbed in his misery, talks almost to himself. The
      SAILORS group themselves below, and watch him, interspersing
      their arguments.*)

PHILOCTETES: My cave within the hollow rock,
Now hot, now bitter cold;
Then I am doomed to leave you never more,
And you will witness when I die!

Oh dwelling filled with my despair,
How shall I live from day to day?
Where shall I find a hope of food?   1090

The timid doves will wing their way through the shrill breeze,
For I can stay their flight no more.
SAILORS (*in a murmur*): It was your doing, unhappy man.
    You are not held by chance or force.
    You could have shown your common sense.
    Instead, you chose the foolish course.   1100
PHILOCTETES: Ah, I am crushed, by suffering!
    For now at last, for evermore,
    I shall live wretched and abandoned,
    And die alone upon this shore.

    No longer can I find my nurture,
    No more the feathered shafts shall fly from my strong hands.
    A treacherous soul cheated me with its cunning lie.   1111
    Would he could suffer even as I,
    And for so long!
SAILORS: It was your fate, decreed by God,
    No trick of mine;
    So do not bend your bitter curse at me: 1120
    Remember,
    And do not scorn it,
    I'm your friend.
PHILOCTETES (*unheeding*): Ah God!
    Somewhere he sits and laughs,
    By the grey sea, upon the shore,
    Wielding my bow, my hope of life,
    That no man ever held before.

    Ah, my beloved bow,
    Thus wrenched from hands that loved you!
    Do you sorrow,
    If you have sense,   1130
    To know the friend of Heracles has lost you?
    Morrow will never dawn when he will bend you once again,
    But one will borrow your might,
    A hateful man and vile,
    Treacherous, wicked, full of guile,
    Worker of troubles without end,
    — Odysseus —
    Against *me*.
SAILORS: It's human to proclaim the right,   1140
    But spiteful words should be restrained.
    He was the one they chose,
    To do this deed by which his friends have gained.

PHILOCTETES: Oh feathered prey,

And tribes of beasts with glowing eyes, who roam this land and
walk the hills,

You need not leap back from my cave in flight;

My hand is empty of its former strength,   1150
My bow and arrows.
Do not fear,
But roam at large,
And in revenge, fall on my quivering flesh and tear your food
apart,
For I am near to death.
I cannot anywhere find food,
And who can live on air?   1160
I cannot till the bounteous earth.
Helpless I die, in utter dearth.

(PHILOCTETES *sinks down in despair.*)
(*The* MATE *approaches him.* PHILOCTETES *repudiates him
violently.*)

MATE: In God's name,

Do not scorn a friend who comes to you in all good will,
Believe, believe it rests with you to seek release from this great ill.
A curse she is to feed,
And woes, countless, she brings with her,
Yet knows no patience to instil.

PHILOCTETES (*half-rising painfully*):

Again, again you have reminded me,   1170
You, kinder than all earlier visitors,
Of my old grief,
Why do you kill me?
Why have you done it?

MATE: What do you mean?

PHILOCTETES: You want to take me to the land of Troy,
The place that I hate most.

MATE: Ay, for I think it best.

PHILOCTETES (*violently*): Then leave me — leave me!

(*The* MATE *rejoins the* SAILORS, *and all make as if to go.*)

SAILORS (*chant or sing as they go, Right*): Your command is welcome;
Gladly, gladly we obey.
Each man to his place aboard!   1180
Come, men, let's get away.

PHILOCTETES: No, no, in God's name, do not go!

MATE: Keep calm!

PHILOCTETES: Oh stay, friends, I implore you!

MATE: Why do you call us?

PHILOCTETES: Oh God!

Condemned to death!

Oh crippled foot, what shall I do with you, in this existence that
lies before me?

Oh my friends, come back! 1190

MATE: What can we do that's different from before? — from what
you told us?

PHILOCTETES: Don't be angry with me,

If in my madness, buffeted with pain, I speak unreasonably.

MATE (*returns impulsively*): Come with us, then!

Do as we tell you, poor unhappy man!

PHILOCTETES: No, never, never!

Know that, once for all!

Not if the god who wields the lightning-flash burn me to ashes
with his blazing stroke!

To hell with Troy! 1200

And all before her walls who had the heart to cast this crippled
body away!

But grant me, friends, one thing I beg for!

MATE: What do you want?

PHILOCTETES (*wildly*): A sword, if you can get one,

Or a hatchet,

— any tool,

But give it me!

MATE: What feat do you want to try now?

PHILOCTETES: I will hew my flesh in pieces,

Hack away my limbs!

Blood, blood is all my thought!

(*He staggers to his feet and looks round wildly.*)

MATE: What is it?

PHILOCTETES: I seek — my father. 1210

MATE: Where is he?

PHILOCTETES: In the grave.

He cannot be alive.

My country, oh my country!

Oh that I could behold thee!

Fool that I was to leave thy sacred stream,

And go to help the cause of the Greeks,

My enemies!

And now I am nothing.

(PHILOCTETES *crawls to the cave, and then into it, out of sight.*)

MATE (*goes Right and looks out*): I should have left you long before,
 and gone back to the ship;   1219
 But I can see, quite near, Odysseus and our chief coming this way

(*Enter* NEOPTOLEMUS *carrying the bow, and* ODYSSEUS *hurrying
after, Right.*)

ODYSSEUS (*to* NEOPTOLEMUS): Will you explain why you are hurrying
 all the way back at this tremendous speed?
NEOPTOLEMUS (*curtly*): To undo the mistake I made a while ago.
ODYSSEUS: You talk in riddles.
 What was the mistake?
NEOPTOLEMUS: In doing what you said, and the whole army.
ODYSSEUS (*contemptuously*): What have you done, that was not proper
 for you?
NEOPTOLEMUS (*fiercely*): I caught a man with filthy lies and trickery!
ODYSSEUS: What man?
 (*Glancing at the cave.*)
 No, no!
 You can't intend to alter ——
NEOPTOLEMUS: I alter nothing; but to Philoctetes ——   1230
ODYSSEUS: What will you do?
 A fear comes over me ——
NEOPTOLEMUS: — From whom I took this bow, I shall once more ——
ODYSSEUS: God, what comes next?
 You cannot mean to give it ——
NEOPTOLEMUS: Yes! — for I got it basely and dishonestly.
ODYSSEUS: In heaven's name!
 Is this some joke of yours?
NEOPTOLEMUS: If truth is funny, then it is a joke.
ODYSSEUS: What are you saying, man?
 What is this story?
NEOPTOLEMUS: Must I repeat the same thing twice or thrice?
ODYSSEUS: I wish I had not heard it even once.
NEOPTOLEMUS: Well, now you know.
 That's all I have to say.   1240
ODYSSEUS: And yet — you can be stopped:
 I know by whom!
NEOPTOLEMUS: What?
 Where's the man who'll stop me doing this?
ODYSSEUS: The army of the Greeks, of whom I am one.
NEOPTOLEMUS: *You* may be clever — but your words are stupid.
ODYSSEUS: *You* show stupidity in word and deed!
NEOPTOLEMUS: If it is right, it overrides what's clever.

ODYSSEUS: How can it be right, to give back what you won by my devices?

NEOPTOLEMUS: It was a crime, and shameful.
Now I shall try to put it right again.

ODYSSEUS: Have you no fear of the army, if you do this?   1250

NEOPTOLEMUS: Right is with me:
I do not feel your fear.
Even to your force, I would not give obedience.

ODYSSEUS: I see it is not Troy we must fight, but you.

NEOPTOLEMUS: Let come what may.

(*He goes towards the cave.*)

ODYSSEUS: Look!
Do you see my hand upon my sword-hilt?

NEOPTOLEMUS (*turns threateningly*): Look yourself, and see how I
am doing the the same, and just as quickly!

ODYSSEUS (*retreats*): Well, I will leave you.
But the assembled army shall hear of this,
And they will punish you.

NEOPTOLEMUS: You're wise!
And if you show such common-sense in future,
You'll avoid troubles, perhaps.   1260

(*Exit* ODYSSEUS, *Right.*)
(NEOPTOLEMUS *shouts cheerfully up to the cave.*)

NEOPTOLEMUS: Now, Philoctetes!
Philoctetes, I say!
Come out, and leave that rocky home of yours!

PHILOCTETES (*appears at the mouth of the cave, dazedly*):
What is this noise of shouting, near my cave again?
Why do you call me, sailors?
What do you want?
(*He sees* NEOPTOLEMUS.)
Ah!
This means trouble!
Have you come to add to the harm you've done to me already?

NEOPTOLEMUS: Don't be alarmed!
Hear what I've come to tell you.

PHILOCTETES: Ah, but I am afraid!
I came to grief before, through listening to fine speeches — yours!

NEOPTOLEMUS: Can a man not be allowed to change his mind?   1270

PHILOCTETES: That's how you sounded when you stole my bow:
Trustworthy,
But in secret, my destroyer.

NEOPTOLEMUS: Ah, but not now!
  Tell me — I want to hear —
  Are you resolved to stay here and endure,
  Or sail with us?
PHILOCTETES: Stop!
  You need go no further!
  What you can say will all be said in vain.
NEOPTOLEMUS: You are resolved?
PHILOCTETES: More than I say, believe me.
NEOPTOLEMUS: I would have liked to get you to accept my reasoning;
  But if the time is wrong to speak,
  I am silent.
PHILOCTETES: All you could say is useless.   1280
  You never could recover my good will,
  You, who by trickery have robbed me of my means of life,
  And then come back to preach me a sermon,
  Hateful son of a hero-father!
  Curse you!
  — The generals above all,
  And then Odysseus,
  And you!
NEOPTOLEMUS: Curse me no further,
  But take your bow — here — back from my hand.

  (*He holds out the bow.*)

PHILOCTETES: What's this?
  Is this some second trick you're playing me?
NEOPTOLEMUS: No, by the sacred glory of God most high!
PHILOCTETES: Oh, joyful words,
  — If it's genuine, what you say!   1290
NEOPTOLEMUS: The deed will show it clearly.
  Here, stretch out your hand,
  And take possession of your weapons!

  (*Distant roll of thunder.*)
  (PHILOCTETES *advances to take the bow. He has almost
  reached* NEOPTOLEMUS *when* ODYSSEUS *enters, Right.*)

ODYSSEUS: No, I forbid it! —
  Be the Gods my witness! —
  In the name of the army of Greece and its commanders!

  (*But* ODYSSEUS *is too late to step between them.* PHILOCTETES
  takes the bow from NEOPTOLEMUS' *hands. Roll of thunder.*)

PHILOCTETES: My son, whose voice is that?
  Was it Odysseus I heard?

ODYSSEUS (*stepping forward*): You heard aright,
 And now you see me:
 The man who will drag you back to the plains of Troy.
 With or without the wish of Neoptolemus.
PHILOCTETES (*aiming the bow*): It will cost you dear,
 If this can hit the mark!
NEOPTOLEMUS (*seizing his arm*): No, no, for God's sake!
 Do not shoot that arrow!   1300
PHILOCTETES (*struggling*): Let me go, for the love of God!
 Let go my arm, dear boy!
NEOPTOLEMUS: I will not.

 (ODYSSEUS *slips out Right.*)

PHILOCTETES: Ah!
 Why have you robbed me of the chance to shoot my greatest
  enemy?
NEOPTOLEMUS (*gently*): That would not bring honour to you, or me.
PHILOCTETES: Well, you can see one thing:
 The army leaders, the lying emissaries of the Greeks, are cowards
  when faced with steel,
 Though bold in words.
NEOPTOLEMUS (*changing the subject*): Good: now you have your bow,
 And you've no cause for further anger or complaint against me.
PHILOCTETES: I grant it.
 You have proved the stock, my son, from which you sprang. 1310
 No Sisyphus, *your* father,
 But Achilles, greatest name among the living,
 While he still lived,
 And now, among the dead.
NEOPTOLEMUS: It gives me joy to hear you praise my father,
 And myself also.
 But I want one thing from you.
 Listen:
 There are misfortunes sent from above which men are forced to
  bear.
 But when they cleave to self-inflicted sufferings,
 As you do,
 Then one cannot pardon them in justice, or be sorry for them
  either.   1320
 You have grown savage:
 You will not accept advice,
 And if one offers it in kindness,
 You hate him, and consider him your enemy.
 Still I will speak.

God knows my words are true!
And you must heed, and write them in your soul.

The wound you suffer from was heaven-sent,
For you disturbed the goddess Chrysê's guardian,
The hidden snake who keeps her roofless shrine.
And you are doomed never to find release from this affliction,
While the sun rises *there* in the east, 1330
And sinks *here* in the west again,
Until you go yourself to the plains of Troy,
And see Asclepius' sons, our army doctors.
There you'll be cured;
And with your bow,
And me to help you,
You will achieve the fall of Troy.

I know it is so.
I will tell you how.

We have a man captured from Troy,
A prophet unrivalled, Helenus,
Who states quite clearly that this must happen,
And moreover, that it is inevitable Troy shall fall during the
present summer. 1340
Otherwise he says, they can kill him — if it does not come true.

There now,
You know the facts.

Agree to come!
Think what a glorious prize,
To be the one chosen as bravest of the Greeks,
To win, first healing,
And then everlasting fame
As the man who caused the fall of suffering Troy!

PHILOCTETES: Oh hateful Time,
Why do you keep me here alive?
Why have you not sent me to my grave?
What shall I do? 1350
How can I disregard his words, spoken out of good will towards
me?
Am I to yield?
But then, how could I bear to show my wretched self?
Who'd speak to me?

How could these eyes of mine,
That have seen all my story,
Bear to see me mixing with those two commanders, who were
my destroyers,
And with Odysseus, that accursed pest!

It is not pain over the past that stings me,
But what I still would suffer at their hands I can imagine.
Once a mind conceives evil designs, its fruits are always
evil.   1360

And that is what amazes me in you:
You should have stayed away from Troy yourself, and held me
back.
They have insulted you,
Stolen your father's treasure,
Adjudged his arms to Odysseus,
And you still intend to fight with them,
And you would have me do the same!

Don't do it, lad!
But as you swore to me,
Carry me home!
And stay yourself in Scyros,
And let these scoundrels perish miserably.
Thus you will win from me a double thanks, as from my father,
and avoid the name of being like the villains you are
helping.   1370
NEOPTOLEMUS: There's sense in what you say.
But still, I wish you would have faith in God, and in my words,
And sail away from here with me — your friend.
PHILOCTETES: You mean, to Troy,
And to that man I hate,
— Agamemnon —
With this crippled foot of mine?
NEOPTOLEMUS: I mean, to those who can relieve the pain of your
ulcered foot,
— Cure you of your disease.
PHILOCTETES: You give me cruel advice.
What are you saying?   1380
NEOPTOLEMUS: What I see will work out best, for both of us.
PHILOCTETES: Aren't you ashamed, before God, to say such things?
NEOPTOLEMUS: What shame is there in trying to help your friends?
PHILOCTETES: This help — is it meant for me,
Or for your generals?

NEOPTOLEMUS: For you.

    I am your friend, and speak as such.

PHILOCTETES: What, when you want to hand me to my enemies?

NEOPTOLEMUS (*sighs*): Man, man!

    Learn to be less stiff-necked in trouble!

PHILOCTETES (*torn*): You'll kill me,

    — Yes, I know you —

    With your talk!

NEOPTOLEMUS: No, no, not I!

    You don't understand, I say!

PHILOCTETES: And don't I know those generals cast me out?   1390

NEOPTOLEMUS: Yes.

    But consider if they now can save you.

PHILOCTETES: Never — if I must agree to go to Troy!

NEOPTOLEMUS (*exasperated*): What can I do, if with my arguments

    I cannot get you to agree at all?

    The easiest thing for me is to stop talking,

    And you — to live on as before, unrescued.

PHILOCTETES (*gently*): Leave me to follow out my destiny.

    And as you promised, giving me your hand,

    Carry me home!

    Do *this* for me, my son,

    Do not delay it!

    Make no further mention of Troy,   1400

    For it has cost me tears enough.

NEOPTOLEMUS: Very well, then.

    Let us go.

PHILOCTETES: Oh, generous word!

NEOPTOLEMUS: Lean on me as you walk.

PHILOCTETES: With all my strength.

NEOPTOLEMUS: How can I escape the blame of the Greeks?

PHILOCTETES: Don't think of it!

NEOPTOLEMUS: What if they ravage Scyros?

PHILOCTETES: I'll be there.

NEOPTOLEMUS: What can you do to help?

PHILOCTETES: The bow of Heracles ——

NEOPTOLEMUS: You mean? ——

PHILOCTETES: — Will fend them off.

NEOPTOLEMUS: Now say good-bye to the soil of Lemnos,

    And set forth with me.

        (*The stage goes dark, as* NEOPTOLEMUS *helps* PHILOCTETES,
        painfully past the group of SAILORS *to the exit Right.*)
        (*Suddenly there is a roll of thunder, and several flashes of*

*(ightning. In front of the cave above, HERACLES appears. He
is a huge golden-haired bearded man, wearing a lionskin and
carrying a great club. He stands in a golden radiance. The
SAILORS fall on their knees. NEOPTOLEMUS and PHILOCTETES
halt before him, facing him. After another roll of thunder he
speaks.)*

HERACLES: Not yet, my Philoctetes.
   First listen to me.   1410
   You hear the voice,
   You see the face, of Heracles.
   My care for you has brought me down from Heaven,
   To reveal the will of God to you.
   And stay you from your present journey,
   Now,
   Pay heed to what I say.
   First I will tell you of my own good fortune:
   How after many toilsome labours ended,
   I won immortal fame, as you can see.   1420

   Now learn:
   For you, too, such a fate is fixed:
   From your present toils to build a life of fame.
   You are to go, with this man here, to Troy,
   Where first, you shall be cured of this disease,
   And then, the chosen champion of the army, shall fight the cause
      of all this misery — Paris —
   And with this bow of mine, rob him of life.
   You shall sack Troy, and take your booty home,
   — The prize of valour given by the army —
   To your father, and to your own native hills.   1430
   Do not forget to take a part of all they give you to my pyre,
   In gratitude for this my bow.
   You too, Achilles' son,
   Heed my advice.
   You are not strong enough without him, to take Troy.
   Nor he without you.
   But like two lions roving side by side,
   Guard each the other.

   I will send Asclepius to Troy,
   To be the healer of your sore.
   For Troy must fall again,
   — The second time —
   Before my bow.   1440

One thing remember:
When you sack the land,
Respect whatever's sacred.
For Zeus, our father, holds of less account all else.
Piety does not die with mortals:
In life, in death, it never is destroyed.

PHILOCTETES: Ah, voice I longed to hear!
Ah, vision long delayed!
Thy words shall be obeyed.

NEOPTOLEMUS: I too shall not fail.

HERACLES: Do not delay,
The time has come. 1450
The wind is in the sail.

> (*Roll of thunder.* HERACLES *fades. More thunder. Darkness.
> Then the stage grows light again.*)
> (*They all prepare to go out Right.*)

PHILOCTETES: As I go, I'll bid this land good-bye.
Farewell, my cave, my home,
And ye,
Nymphs of the meadows and the stream,
And deep-voiced roaring of the sea.
Often the south wind sought me in my cave,
And drenched my head with spray,
Often the mountain echoed back my raging cries, from far
away! 1460

And now I leave you, fount and spring,
Leave you at last!
To think that I should rise so far above my hope!
Goodbye, O Lemnian Land, goodbye!

Grant me a voyage safe and sure,
To where great Destiny shall lead,
And my friends' purpose,
And that God Almighty, who has thus decreed.

> (*They go out Right,* NEOPTOLEMUS *helping* PHILOCTETES.)
> (*The* SAILORS *follow, singing:*)

SAILORS: Come, all together, comrades!
When we have said a prayer
To the Sea-Nymphs: 1470
May they grant us
A voyage safe and fair!

EURIPIDES

ALCESTIS

□

Translated by Richard Aldington

INTRODUCTION

THE *Alcestis* is probably the most touching of all the Greek dramas to a modern audience; whether it was equally compelling to the Greeks when it was presented in 438 B.C. has not been disclosed; it was the fourth play in a tetralogy, not a distinguished position, and Sophocles won first prize on the same occasion. Its theme of self-sacrifice by a noble and all-too-loving wife, who is nevertheless represented as a quite human person with a natural fear of death, is unique in ancient tragedy. Homer (*Iliad* II. 715) called her the "loveliest of all the daughters of Pelias" and mentioned her in the catalogue of Greek ships; her son Eumelos sailed eleven ships to Troy.

The plot of the *Alcestis* is simple. It is based upon a somewhat complicated legend that has been reconstructed by Wilamowitz-Moellendorff from the fragments of a lost poem of Hesiod (see his *Isyllos von Epidauros*, p. 57: Isyllos wrote five brief hymns in the third century B.C., two of them chiefly in praise of Apollo and Asclepius, the patron god of medicine; these were discovered at Epidaurus in the temple of Asclepius toward the end of the nineteenth century). Asclepius, the son of Apollo and the nymph Coronis, became a great physician. He presumed even to bring the dead to life. For this subversion of the natural course of things, Zeus killed him with the thunderbolt at Delphi, his father's sanctuary. Apollo in anger slew the Cyclopes who had forged the thunderbolt. Zeus was persuaded by Leto to save Apollo from Tartarus, but he was forced to serve a mortal for one year on earth. King Admetus of Pherae in Thessaly was that mortal; Apollo tended his flocks for him near Lake Boebeis. Admetus treated his illustrious shepherd kindly. In return Apollo caused him to prosper and aided him to win Alcestis for his queen by yoking a lion and a boar to a chariot as the suitors of Alcestis were commanded to do by her father Pelias. Admetus brought her home in triumph but offended Apollo's sister Artemis Brimo of Pherae by forgetting to make a sacrifice to her. She showed her displeasure for this affront by placing a nest of snakes in his wedding chamber. Apollo interpreted this sinister omen to Admetus, saying that his sister sought the life of Admetus but would be pacified by a proper sacrifice on condition that some other life should be offered in place of Admetus' own. In due time Admetus fell ill and lay close to death. None of his friends and relations, not even his aged father and mother, would consent to die in his place. At last Alcestis agreed to do so. As Admetus revived, Alcestis sickened and died. Persephone, however, who is Artemis Brimo in the underworld, took pity on Alcestis and restored her to life.

The story as told by Euripides employs a different and more exciting means to achieve the same happy ending. No sooner has Alcestis been buried than Hercules, an old friend of Admetus, comes visiting to Pherae. Half-tipsy and in a great good humor, he questions the gate-keeper and the rest of the staff for the cause of the gloom which grips the household. Upon learning the truth, he makes light of the situation in his hearty, kind, and vulgar manner and declares that he will wrestle Death for Alcestis and bring her back to Admetus. He sets out on one of his greatest labors. In the last scenes of the play he leads a veiled woman back to Admetus, pretending at first that he is bringing him a second wife (whom he has won at an athletic contest) to console his sorrow for the first one. Since Alcestis, if it is really she, cannot speak for three days after her return from Hades, as Hercules explains, we are not certain as the play closes who the third figure on the stage may be: a gruesome ambiguity.

D. L. Drew has, in fact, put forward the well-argued, if repulsive, theory that the woman whom Hercules holds in his arms and offers to Admetus is really the corpse of Alcestis, not a living woman (*Am. Jour. of Phil.* 52, 295–319). The cowardice and abject poltroonery of Admetus, upon whose elaboration Euripides has lavished so much space, has led him to break in quick succession after her death the oaths he had sworn to Alcestis: that he would mourn her forever and remain celibate; that he would entertain no more friends with wine and song in his house, and that he would have a statue of her made to be placed permanently in his bed. The drunken and somewhat simple-minded Hercules, whom Admetus had deceived upon his arrival as to the true nature of the situation in the palace, whom Admetus had entertained at almost the very moment of his wife's burial, even shutting the doors of the banquet-hall against the sound of wailing, now, whether through a ghoulish taste for humor or a malevolent wish to return the deception, plays his own outrageous joke. He brings on stage a dead woman whom he first urges Admetus to accept and keep for him until he returns from his ninth labor; if he does not return Admetus may keep her as a concubine. At last, after ineffectual protests which one feels are not sincere, Admetus accepts her. Thus in a blood-curdling one hundred and fifty lines at the end of the play the dead wife of Admetus returns — to take him with her to the grave: a fit repayment for his treacherous and abominable behavior.

No other theory so conveniently explains her silence throughout this scene. She is not a live body which was dead nor is she in a trance, as Verrall believed: she is dead and therefore cannot speak. The two-actor convention Euripides follows is made absurd by Admetus' question (1143), "Why does she stand here without speaking?" if indeed the playwright did not intend to imply by the scene that Alcestis is dead.

In his early career, to which the *Alcestis* belongs, Euripides tried to amuse the Athenians with unusual, less often treated, subjects: hence his choice of a tale from the royal house of Iolcus, a comparatively obscure source of dramatic legend. The play has been variously interpreted. K. O. Mueller regarded it as a chthonic myth, that is, an identification of underground divinities with human beings. Admetus was originally Pluto, god of the underworld, and Alcestis his wife Persephone. After slaying the Python, Apollo was forced to serve Pluto in Hades for a time. This tale became localized in Thessaly, where the name of Admetus was frequent in occurrence; thus Pluto was transformed into a Greek king. Euripides seems to have followed Hesiod closely, laying emphasis upon the hospitality of Admetus and doubtless exaggerating the conjugal loyalty of Alcestis. He was forty-two when the play appeared; his interest seems to have already turned toward the north where he was to end his days and to present his last play, the *Bacchae*, at the court of Archelaus in Macedonia.

The *Alcestis* has definite comic elements; in fact, those who used the theme after Euripides turned it into comedy. It was presented actually in the chronological position of a satyr-play in a tetralogy which included the *Cretan Women*, *Alcmeon in Psophis*, and *Telephus*: a strange combination of subjects. But it is not a true comedy or even a burlesque in either the Greek sense or in ours. Hercules provides most of the comedy, and he appears in only the last third of the play, although it is true that the treatment of Death and the absurd quarrel between Admetus and Pheres have a strongly comic flavor. The plot is very well made and moves swiftly. Next to the *Heracleidae* and *Cyclops* it is the shortest play of Euripides. The best American edition of the Greek text is by H. W. Hayley (1898); he lists and discusses many representations of the story in ancient sculptural art and in painting, especially upon sarcophagi, where it was a favorite with artists. The Etruscans as well as the Greeks and Romans used it often. Browning's *Balaustion's Adventure* is an adaptation of Euripides worth reading as a modern use of the story by a poet who knew his Greek dramatists well even if he could not translate them into English with any real success. Another modern version is the one by Dudley Fitts and Robert Fitzgerald.

The problem of the stage-setting indicates that both players and chorus are on the same level; the palace front has two doors in it. Mr. Aldington prefers two stage levels. The chorus withdraws once from the stage, as it does in Aeschylus' *Eumenides*, Sophocles' *Ajax*, and Euripides' *Helen* and *Rhesus*. Apollo speaks the prologue and fixes the locality of the play. The use of masks for Death and Alcestis can be made most effective along the lines suggested by Fitts and Fitzgerald.

L. R. LIND

ALCESTIS

□

CHARACTERS

APOLLO, *the god of sunlight*
DEATH
CHORUS *of Old Men*
A WOMAN SERVANT
ALCESTIS, *the queen, wife of Admetus*
ADMETUS, *king of Thessalia*
EUMELUS, *their child*
HERACLES, *the heroic saviour*
PHERES, *father of Admetus*
A MAN SERVANT

The Prologue

SCENE. *At Pherae, outside the Palace of Admetus, king of Thessalia. The centre of the scene represents a portico with columns and a large double-door. To the left are the women's quarters, to the right the guest rooms; each with a separate entrance. In front and on a slightly lower level is the circular Orchestra for the Chorus.*

The Stage is empty. Then the centre doors slowly open inwards. A pause. From the Palace comes PHOEBUS APOLLO, god of sunlight, healing and song. In his left hand he carries a large unstrung golden bow. He moves slowly and majestically, turns, and raises his right hand in salutation to the Palace.

APOLLO: Dwelling of Admetus, wherein I, a God, deigned to accept the food of serfs! (*He turns, and faces the audience.*)

The cause was Zeus. He struck Asclepius, my son, full in the breast with a bolt of thunder, and laid him dead. Then in wild rage

216

I slew the Cyclopes who forge the fire of Zeus. To atone for this my
Father forced me to labour as a hireling for a mortal man; and I
came to this country, and tended oxen for my host. To this hour I
have protected him and his. I, who am just, chanced on the son   10
of Pheres, a just man, whom I have saved from Death by tricking the
Fates. The Goddesses pledged me their faith Admetus should escape
immediate death if, in exchange, another corpse were given to the
Under-Gods.

One by one he tested all his friends, and even his father and the
old mother who brought him forth — and found none that would
die for him and never more behold the light of day, save only his
wife. Now, her spirit waiting to break loose, she droops upon his
arm within the house; this is the day when she must die and render
up her life.   20

But I must leave this Palace's dear roof, for fear pollution soil me
in the house. (*He pauses, and looks to the right.*)

See! Death, Lord of All the Dead, now comes to lead her to the
house of Hades! Most punctually he comes! How well he marked
the day she had to die!

(*From the right comes* DEATH, *with a drawn sword in his hand.
He is like one of the grim figures on Etruscan tombs, horrible of
aspect, bearded, huge-winged, dressed in black. This is Death
the Destroyer, not Death the Healer. He moves stealthily
towards the Palace; then sees* APOLLO *and halts abruptly. The
two Deities confront each other.*)

DEATH: Ha! Phoebus! You! In this city! Before this Palace! Law-
lessly would you grasp, abolish the rights of the Lower Gods!   30
Did you not beguile the Fates and snatch Admetus from the grave?
Does not that suffice? Now, once again, you have armed your hand
with the bow, to guard the daughter of Pelias who must die in her
husband's stead!

(*Now begins the swift dispute of the Gods in rapid interchange
of speech. Death speaks sharply and querulously;* APOLLO *more
gently, restraining himself, pleading with the implacable
Enemy.*)

APOLLO (*conciliatory*): Fear not! I hold for right, and proffer you just
words.

DEATH (*suspiciously*): If you hold for right, why then your bow?

APOLLO: My custom is ever to carry it.   40

DEATH (*querulously*): Yes! And you use it unjustly to aid this house!

APOLLO: I grieve for a friend's woe.

DEATH: So you would rob me of a second body?

APOLLO: Not by force I won the other.

DEATH: Why, then, is he in the world and not below the ground?

APOLLO: In his stead he gives his wife — whom you have come to take.

DEATH: And shall take — to the Underworld below the earth!

APOLLO (*angrily*): Take her, and go! (*Restraining himself*) I know not if I can persuade you. . . .

DEATH: Not to kill her I must kill? I am appointed to that task.

APOLLO (*pleading*): No, no! But to delay death for those about to die.

DEATH (*sneering*): I hear your words and guess your wish!   51

APOLLO: May not Alcestis live to old age?

DEATH: No! I also prize my rights!

APOLLO: Yet at most you win one life.

DEATH: They who die young yield me a greater prize.

APOLLO: If she dies old, the burial will be richer.

DEATH: Phoebus, that argument favours the rich.

APOLLO (*surprised*): What! Are you witty unawares?

DEATH: The rich would gladly pay to die old.

APOLLO: So you will not grant me this favour?   60

DEATH: Not I! You know my nature.

APOLLO: Yes! Hateful to men and a horror to the gods!

DEATH: You cannot always have more than your due.

APOLLO (*suddenly changing his tone. He becomes both threatening and prophetic*): Yet you shall change, most cruel though you are! For a man comes to the dwelling of Pheres, sent by Eurystheus to fetch a horse-drawn chariot from the harsh-wintered lands of Thracia; and he shall be a guest in the house of Admetus, and by force shall he tear this woman from you. Thus shall you gain no thanks from us, and yet you shall do this thing — and my hatred be   70 upon you!

(APOLLO *goes out.* DEATH *gazes after him derisively.*)

DEATH: Talk all you will, you get no more of me! The woman shall go down to the dwelling of Hades.

(*He turns to the Palace*) Now must I go to consecrate her for the sacrifice with this sword; for when once this blade has shorn the victim's hair, then he is sacred to the Lower Gods!

(DEATH *enters the Palace by the open main door, and the Stage is left silent and empty.*)

[END OF THE PROLOGUE]

The Parodos:

or Entry of the Chorus

(The Stage is empty. The chorus, *led by the flute-player, enters the Orchestra from the right. The Chorus, as usual, numbers fifteen; one of whom is the* chorus-leader. *They enter three abreast in five files, in silence, and take up their position in the centre of the Orchestra. They are the Elders or Notables of the city, and therefore move slowly, leaning upon their staffs. Their dance is far more dramatic gesture and movement of the hands than actual dancing. The whole of the Parodos, like other Stasima, is accompanied by music. The passages in italics were sung; the others declaimed to a musical accompaniment. The object of this opening Chorus is, naturally, to show the city's anxiety as to the fate of Alcestis, and to create a dramatic suspense.)*

chorus-leader (*gazing towards the Palace*): Why is there no sound outside the Palace? Why is the dwelling of Admetus silent? (*A pause, as they look and listen.*)

Not a friend here to tell me if I must weep for a dead Queen   80
or whether she lives and looks upon the light, Alcestis, the daughter
of Pelias, whom among all women I hold the best wife to her spouse!

chorus: *Is a sob to be heard?*
            Or the beating of hands
            In the house?
            The lament for her end?

            Not one,
            Not one of her servants
            Stands at the gate!   90

            Ah! to roll back the wave of our woe,
            O Healer,
            Appear!

first semi-chorus:
            Were she dead
            They had not been silent.

second semi-chorus:
            She is but a dead body!

first semi-chorus:
            Yet she has not departed the house.

SECOND SEMI-CHORUS:

> *Ah! Let me not boast!*
> *Why do you cling to hope?*

FIRST SEMI-CHORUS:

> *Would Admetus bury her solitary,*
> *Make a grave alone for a wife so dear?*

CHORUS: *At the gate I see not*
> *The lustral water from the spring*
> *Which stands at the gates of the dead!*   100
> *No shorn tress in the portal*
> *Laid in lament for the dead!*
> *The young women beat not their hands!*

SECOND SEMI-CHORUS:

> *Yet to-day is the day appointed. . . .*

FIRST SEMI-CHORUS:

> *Ah! What have you said?*

SECOND SEMI-CHORUS:

> *When she must descend under earth!*

FIRST SEMI-CHORUS:

> *You have pierced my soul!*
> *You have pierced my mind!*

SECOND SEMI-CHORUS:

> *He that for long*
> *Has been held in esteem*   110
> *Must weep when the good are destroyed.*

CHORUS: *No!*
> *There is no place on earth*
> *To send forth a suppliant ship —*
> *Not to Lycia,*
> *Not to Ammon's waterless shrine —*
> *To save her from death!*
> *The dreadful doom is at hand.*
> *To what laden altar of what God*
> *Shall I turn my steps?*   120

> *He alone —*
> *If the light yet shone for his eye —*

> *Asclepius, Phoebus's son,*
> *Could have led her back*
> *From the land of shadows,*
> *From the gates of Hades.*
> *For he raised the dead*
> *Ere the Zeus-driven shaft*
> *Slew him with thunder fire. . . .*
> *But now*
> *What hope can I hold for her life?*　　　130

CHORUS-LEADER:

> *The King has fulfilled*
> *Every rite;*
> *The altars of all the Gods*
> *Drip with the blood of slain beasts:*
> *Nothing, nothing avails.*

[END OF THE PARODOS]

The First Episode

(*The Stage is still empty. The* CHORUS *range themselves in two Semi-Choruses on either side of the Orchestra. The* CHORUS-LEADER *stands apart, half-facing the Stage. From the women's quarters in the left wing of the Palace comes a woman in tears. She is not a slave, but one of the personal attendants on the Queen.*

The limitations of the Greek stage made it impossible for Euripides to present this expository scene directly, even if he had wished to do so. His stage is set once for all outside the Palace; therefore he can only relate indirectly what is going on inside. It must be imagined that the SERVANT *mimes the actions of Alcestis as she describes them and repeats the Queen's words.*)

CHORUS-LEADER (*to the* CHORUS. *These words are accompanied by the flute-player*): But now from the house comes one of her women servants, all in tears. What now shall I learn? (*To the weeping Servant, after a pause*) It is well to weep when our lords are in sorrow — but tell us, we would know, is she alive, is she 140 dead? (*The flute accompaniment ceases.*)

SERVANT: You may say she is both alive and dead.

CHORUS-LEADER: How can the same man be dead and yet behold the light?

SERVANT: She gasps, she is on the verge of death.

CHORUS-LEADER (*Thinking of Admetus*): Ah, unhappy man! For such
a husband what loss is such a wife!

SERVANT: The King will not know his loss until he suffers it.

CHORUS-LEADER: Then there is no hope that her life may be saved?

SERVANT: The fated day constrains her.

CHORUS-LEADER: Are all things befitting prepared for her?

SERVANT: The robes in which her lord will bury her are ready.

CHORUS-LEADER: Then let her know that she dies gloriously, the best
of women beneath the sun by far!   150

SERVANT (*indignantly*): How should she not be the best! Who shall
deny it? What should the best among women be? How better
might a woman hold faith to her lord than gladly to die for him?

(*More calmly*) This the whole city knows, but you will marvel
when you hear what she has done within the house.

(*Emphatically*) When she knew that the last of her days was
come she bathed her white body in river water, she took garments
and gems from her rooms of cedar wood, and clad herself   160
nobly; then, standing before the hearth-shrine, she uttered this
prayer:

"O Goddess, since now I must descend beneath the earth, for the
last time I make supplication to you: and entreat you to protect
my motherless children. Wed my son to a fair bride, and my daughter to a noble husband. Let not my children die untimely, as I
their mother am destroyed, but grant that they live out happy lives
with good fortune in their own land!"

To every altar in Admetus's house she went, hung them   170
with garlands, offered prayer, cut myrtle boughs — unweeping, un-
lamenting; nor did the coming doom change the bright colour of
her face.

Then to her marriage-room she went, flung herself down upon
her bed, and wept, and said:

"O my marriage-bed, wherein I loosed my virgin girdle to him
for whom I die! Farewell! I have no hatred for you. Only me you
lose. Because I held my faith to you and to my lord — I   180
must die. Another woman shall possess you, not more chaste indeed than I, more fortunate perhaps."

She fell upon her knees and kissed it, and all the bed was damp
with the tide of tears which flooded to her eyes. And when she
was fulfilled of many tears, drooping she rose from her bed and made
as if to go, and many times she turned to go and many times turned
back, and flung herself once more upon the bed.

Her children clung to their mother's dress, and wept; and she
clasped them in her arms and kissed them turn by turn, as   190
a dying woman.

All the servants in the house wept with compassion for their Queen. But she held out her hand to each, and there was none so base to whom she did not speak, and who did not reply again.

(*A pause.*) Such is the misery in Admetus's house. If he had died, he would be nothing now; and, having escaped, he suffers an agony he will never forget.

CHORUS-LEADER: And does Admetus lament this woe — since he must be robbed of so noble a woman?   200

SERVANT: He weeps, and clasps in his arms his dear bedfellow, and cries to her not to abandon him, asking impossible things. For she pines, and is wasted by sickness. She falls away, a frail burden on his arm; and yet, though faintly, she still breathes, still strives to look upon the sunlight, which she shall never see hereafter — since now for the last time she looks upon the orb and splendour of the sun!

(*She turns towards the Palace.*) I go, and shall announce that you are here; for all men are not so well-minded to their lords   210
as loyally to stand near them in misfortunes, but you for long have been a friend to both my lords.

(*She goes back into the women's quarters of the Palace, and the Stage is again left empty.*)

[END OF THE FIRST EPISODE]

Stasimon I:
or Second Chant of the Chorus

FIRST SEMI-CHORUS:
> *O Zeus,*
> *What end to these woes?*
> *What escape from the Fate*
> *Which oppresses our lords?*

SECOND SEMI-CHORUS:
> *Will none come forth?*
> *Must I shear my hair?*
> *Must we wrap ourselves*
> *In black mourning folds?*

FIRST SEMI-CHORUS:
> *It is certain, O friends, it is certain!*
> *But still let us cry to the Gods;*
> *Very great is the power of the Gods.*

CHORUS: *O King, O Healer,*   220
      Seek out appeasement!
      To Admetus's agony!
      Grant this, Oh, grant it!
      Once before did you find it;
      Now once more
      Be the Releaser from death.
      The Restrainer of blood-drenched Hades!

SECOND SEMI-CHORUS:
      Alas!
      O Son of Pheres.
      What ills shall you suffer
      Being robbed of your spouse!

FIRST SEMI-CHORUS:
      At sight of such woes
      Shall we cut our throats?
      Shall we slip
      A dangling noose round our necks?   230

CHORUS: *See! See!*
      She comes
      From the house with her lord!
      Cry out, Oh, lament.
      O land of Pherae,
      For the best of women
      Fades away in her doom
      Under the earth,
      To dark Hades!

[END OF STASIMON I]

The Second Episode

(*From the central door of the Palace comes a splendid but tragical procession. Preceded by the royal guards,* ADMETUS *enters, supporting* ALCESTIS. *The two children, a boy and a girl, cling to their mother's dress. There is a train of attendants and waiting women. Admetus and Alcestis are both in royal dress. Admetus wears a long embroidered tunic with a royal-purple mantle, but does not carry the sceptre. Alcestis is dressed in a purple tunic with a long train — probably held by attendants — and a white cloak edged with purple; she wears many jewels. The attendants bring a low throne for the fainting Alcestis. Admetus, Alcestis, and the children are grouped by this throne in the centre of the Stage, with the attendants and guards on either side, and the Chorus facing them from the Orchestra. Other guards remain standing in the raised portico.*

The technical inconvenience of the Greek stage is revealed in this important scene — why should Alcestis die outside the Palace except to suit the convenience of the dramatist? At best he manages to suggest a reason in Alcestis's opening words, i.e., that in her delirium she had insisted upon seeing the sun and sky once more before she died.)

CHORUS-LEADER (*declaimed to flute accompaniment*): Never shall I say that we ought to rejoice in marriage, but rather weep; this have I seen from of old and now I look upon the fate of the King,   240 who loses the best of wives, and henceforth until the end his life shall be intolerable. (*Flute-player ceases.*)

ALCESTIS (*in delirium*):

> Sun, and you, light of day,
> Vast whirlings of swift cloud!

ADMETUS: The sun looks upon you and me, both of us miserable, who have wrought nothing against the Gods to deserve death.

ALCESTIS:

> O Earth, O roof-tree of my home,
> Bridal-bed of my country, Iolcus!

ADMETUS: Rouse up, O unhappy one, and do not leave me!   250 Call upon the mighty Gods to pity!

ALCESTIS (*starting up and gazing wildly in terror*):

> I see the two-oared boat,
> I see the boat on the lake!
> And Charon,
> Ferryman of the Dead,
> Calls to me, his hand on the oar:
> "Why linger? Hasten! You delay me!"
> Angrily he urges me.

ADMETUS: Alas! How bitter to me is that ferrying of which you speak! O my unhappy one, how we suffer!

ALCESTIS (*shrieking in terror, and clinging to* ADMETUS):

> He drags me, he drags me away —
> Do you not see? —

> *To the House of the Dead,* 260
> *The Winged One*
> *Glaring under dark brows,*
> *Hades! —*
> *What is it you do?*
> *Set me free! —*
> *What a path must I travel,*
> *O most hapless of women!*

ADMETUS: O piteous to those that love you, above all to me and to these children who sorrow in this common grief!

ALCESTIS:

> *Loose me, Oh, loose me now;*
> *Lay me down;*
> *All strength is gone from my feet.*

(*She falls back in the throne.*)

> *Hades draws near!*
> *Dark night falls on my eyes,*
> *My children, my children,*
> *Never more, Oh never more* 270
> *Shall your mother be yours!*
> *O children, farewell,*
> *Live happy in the light of day!*

ADMETUS (*declaimed to the flute*): Alas! I hear this unhappy speech, and for me it is worse than all death. Ah! By the Gods do not abandon me! Ah! By our children, whom you leave motherless, take heart! If you die, I become as nothing; in you we have our life and death; we revere your love. (*Flute-player ceases.*)

ALCESTIS (*recovering herself and sitting upright*): Admetus, you see the things I suffer; and now before I die I mean to tell you what I wish. 280

To show you honour and — at the cost of my life — that you may still behold the light, I die; and yet I might have lived and wedded any in Thessalia I chose, and dwelt with happiness in a royal home. But, torn from you, I would not live with fatherless children, nor have I hoarded up those gifts of youth in which I found delight. Yet he who begot you, she who brought you forth, abandoned you when it had been beautiful in them to die, beautiful to die with dignity to save their son! They had no child but you, no hope if you were dead that other children might be born to them. Thus I should have lived my life out, and you too, and you would not lament as now, made solitary from your wife, that you must rear our children motherless! 290

(*With a gesture of resignation*) But these things are a God's doing and are thus.

(*With solemn adjuration*) Well! Do not forget this gift, for I shall ask — not a recompense, since nothing is more precious   300 than life, but — only what is just, as you yourself will say, since if you have not lost your senses you must love these children no less than I.

(*Appealingly*) Let them be masters in my house; marry not again, and set a stepmother over them, a woman harsher than I, who in her jealousy will lift her hand against my children and yours. Ah! not this, let not this be, I entreat you! The new stepmother hates the first wife's children, the viper itself is not more cruel.   310 The son indeed finds a strong rampart in his father — but you, my daughter, how shall you live your virgin life out in happiness? How will you fare with your father's new wife? Ah! Let her not cast evil report upon you and thus wreck your marriage in the height of your youth! You will have no mother, O my child, to give you in marriage, to comfort you in childbed when none is tenderer than a mother!

And I must die. Not to-morrow, nor to-morrow's morrow comes this misfortune on me, but even now I shall be named with   320 those that are no more. Farewell! Live happy! You, my husband, may boast you had the best of wives; and you, my children, that you lost the best of mothers! (*She falls back.*)

CHORUS-LEADER: Take heart! I do not hesitate to speak for him. This he will do, unless he has lost his senses.

ADMETUS (*speaking with deep emotion, although his egotism makes him think more of himself than her*): It shall be so, it shall be! Have no fear! And since I held you living as my wife, so, when dead, you only shall be called my wife, and in your place no   330 bride of Thessalia shall salute me hers; no other woman is noble enough for that, no other indeed so beautiful of face. My children shall suffice me; I pray the Gods I may enjoy them, since you we have not enjoyed.

(*Passionately*) I shall wear mourning for you, O my wife, not for one year but all my days, abhorring the woman who bore me, hating my father — for they loved me in words, not deeds. But you — to save my life you give the dearest thing you have! Should I   340 not weep then, losing such a wife as you?

(*Thinking piteously and selfishly of his own future life*) I shall make an end of merry drinking parties, and of flower-crowned feasts and of the music which possessed my house. Never again shall I touch the lyre, never again shall I raise my spirits to sing to the Libyan flute — for you have taken from me all my joy. Your image,

carven by the skilled hands of artists, shall be laid in our marriage-
bed; I shall clasp it, and my hands shall cling to it and I shall   350
speak your name and so, not having you, shall think I have my dear
wife in my arms — a cold delight, I know, but it will lighten the burden of my days. Often you will gladden me appearing in my dreams;
for sweet it is to look on those we love in dreams, however brief the
night.

(*Wildly*) Ah! If I had the tongue and song of Orpheus so that
I might charm Demeter's Daughter or her Lord, and snatch you
back from Hades, I would go down to hell; and neither   360
Pluto's dog nor Charon, Leader of the Dead, should hinder me
until I had brought your life back to the light!

(*More calmly*) At least await me there whenever I shall die, and
prepare the house where you will dwell with me. I shall lay a solemn
charge upon these children to stretch me in the same cedar shroud
with you, and lay my side against your side; for even in death let
me not be separate from you, you who alone were faithful to me!

CHORUS-LEADER (*to* ADMETUS): And I also will keep this sad mourning
with you, as a friend with a friend; for she is worthy of it.   370

ALCESTIS (*kissing her children*): O my children, you have heard your
father say that never will he set another wife over you and never
thus insult me.

ADMETUS (*emphatically*): Again I say it, and will perform it too!

ALCESTIS (*placing the children's hands in his*): Then take these children from my hand.

ADMETUS (*drawing them to him*): I take them — dear gifts from a
dear hand.

ALCESTIS: Now you must be the mother for me to my children.

ADMETUS: It must be so, since they are robbed of you.

ALCESTIS (*looking yearningly at her children*): O children, I should
have lived my life out — and I go to the Underworld.

ADMETUS: Alas! What shall *I* do, left alone by you?   380

ALCESTIS (*quietly*): Time will console you. The dead are nothing.

ADMETUS (*stung by her irony*): Take me with you, by the Gods!
Take me to the Underworld!

ALCESTIS: It is enough that I should die — for you.

ADMETUS: O Fate, what a wife you steal from me!

ALCESTIS (*growing faint*): My dimmed eyes are heavily oppressed.

ADMETUS: O woman, I am lost if you leave me!

ALCESTIS (*more faintly*): You may say of me that I am nothing.

ADMETUS (*desperately*): Lift up your head! Do not abandon your
children!

ALCESTIS (*piteously*): Ah! Indeed it is unwillingly — but, farewell,
my children!

ADMETUS (*wildly*): Look at them, look. . . .

ALCESTIS (*very faintly*): I am nothing.   390

ADMETUS (*clutching her*): What are you doing? Are you leaving me?

ALCESTIS (*falling back dead*): Farewell.

ADMETUS (*clasping his head, and staring at the body*): Wretch that
  I am, I am lost!

CHORUS-LEADER: She is gone! The wife of Admetus is no more.

EUMELUS:

> *Ah! Misery!*
> *Mother has gone,*
> *Gone to the Underworld!*
> *She lives no more,*
> *O my Father,*
> *In the sunlight.*
> *O sad one,*
> *You have left us*
> *To live motherless!*
>
> *See, Oh, see her eyelids*
> *And her drooping hands!*
> *Mother, Mother,*
> *Hearken to me, listen,*
> *I beseech you!* (Sobbing.)   400
> *I — I — Mother! —*
> *I am calling to you,*
> *Your little bird fallen upon your face!*

(*Throws himself on her body.*)

ADMETUS: She hears not, she sees not. You and I are smitten by a
  dread calamity.

EUMELUS (*leaping up, and runing to his father*):

> *Father, I am a child,*
> *And I am left*
> *Like a lonely ship*
> *By the mother I loved.*
> *Oh! The cruel things I suffer!*
> *And you, little sister,*   410
> *Suffer with me.*
>
> *O my Father,*
> *Vain, vain was your wedding,*
> *You did not walk with her*

> To the end of old age.
> She died first;
>
> And your death, O Mother,
> Destroys our house.

(A *pause*.)

CHORUS-LEADER: Admetus, you must endure this calamity. You are not the first and will not be the last to lose a noble wife. We all are doomed to die.

ADMETUS (*royally*): I know it.

Not unawares did this woe swoop down on me; for long it   420
has gnawed at me.

But, since I shall ordain the funeral rites for this dead body, you must be there, and meanwhile let a threnody re-echo to the implacable God of the Underworld. And all you men of Thessalia whom I rule — I order you to share the mourning for this woman with severed hair and black-robed garb. You who yoke the four-horsed chariot and the swift single horse, cut the mane from their necks with your steel.

Let there be no noise of flutes or lyre within the city until   430
twelve moons are fulfilled. Never shall I bury another body so dear to me, never one that has loved me better. From me she deserves all honour, since she alone would die for me!

(*The body of Alcestis is carried solemnly into the Palace, followed by* ADMETUS, *with bowed head, holding one of his children by each hand. When all have entered, the great doors are quietly shut, and the Stage is left empty.*)

[END OF SECOND EPISODE]

Stasimon II:

or Third Chant of the Chorus

CHORUS: *O Daughter of Pelias,*
Hail to you in the house of Hades,
In the sunless home where you shall dwell!
Let Hades, the dark-haired God,
Let the old man, Leader of the Dead,   440
Who sits at the oar and helm,
Know you:
Far, far off is the best of women
Borne beyond the flood of Acheron
In the two-oared boat!

Often shall the Muses' servants
Sing of you to the seven-toned
Lyre-shell of the mountain-tortoise,
And praise you with mourning songs at Sparta

When the circling season
Brings back the month Carneius   450
Under the nightlong upraised moon,
And in bright glad Athens.
Such a theme do you leave by your death
For the music of singers!

Ah! That I had the power
To bring you back to the light
From the dark halls of Hades,
And from the waves of Cocytus
With the oar of the river of hell!
Oh, you only,
O dearest of women,   460
You only dared give your life
For the life of your lord in Hades!
Light rest the earth above you,
O woman.

   If your lord choose another bridal-bed
He shall be hateful to me
As to your own children.

When his mother
And the old father that begot him
Would not give their bodies to the earth
For their son's sake,
They dared not deliver him — O cruel!
Though their heads were grey.   470
But you,
In your lively youth,
Died for him, and are gone from the light!
Ah! might I be joined
With a wife so dear!
But in life such fortune is rare.
How happy were my days with her!

[END OF STASIMON II]

The Third Episode
Scene I

(*The Stage is again empty. The* chorus *is ranged on either side of the Orchestra in two Semi-Choruses, with the* leader *apart. From the left enter* heracles. *He is black-bearded and of great physical strength; he wears a lion-skin over his shoulders and carries a large club. He moves to the centre of the Stage, opposite the main entrance to the Palace, and addresses the* chorus.)

heracles (*with a gesture of salutation*): Friends, dwellers in the lands of Pherae, do I find Admetus in his home?

chorus-leader (*returning the salutation*): The son of Pheres is in his home, O Heracles. (*Inquisitively*) But, tell us, what brings you to the land of Thessalia and to the city of Pherae?   480

heracles: I have a task I must achieve for Eurystheus of Tiryns.

chorus-leader: Where do you go? To what quest are you yoked?

heracles: The quest of the four-horsed chariot of Diomedes, the Thracian.

chorus-leader: But how will you achieve it? Do you know this stranger?

heracles: No, I have never been to the land of the Bistones.

chorus-leader (*with friendly discouragement*): You cannot obtain the horses without a struggle.

heracles (*calmly*): I cannot renounce my labours.

chorus-leader: You must kill to return, or you will remain there dead.

heracles: It will not be the first contest I have risked.

chorus-leader (*sarcastically*): And if you conquer the King   490
will you gain anything?

heracles: I shall bring back his foals to the lord of Tiryns.

chorus-leader: It is not easy to thrust the bit into their jaws.

heracles (*sarcastic in his turn*): Only if they breathe fire from their nostrils!

chorus-leader: But they tear men with their swift jaws.

heracles: You speak of the food of wild mountain beasts, not of horses.

chorus-leader: You may see their mangers foul with blood.

heracles: Of what father does the breeder boast himself the son?

chorus-leader: Of Ares, the lord of the gold-rich shield of Thracia!

heracles (*at last somewhat moved*): In this task once more you remind me of my fate, which is ever upon harsh steep ways,   500
since I must join battle with the sons of Ares — first with Lycaon, then with Cycnus, and now in this third contest I am come to match myself with these steeds and their master!

chorus-leader (*pointing to the Palace door behind Heracles*): But see, the lord of this land, Admetus himself, comes from the house!

[END OF EPISODE III, SCENE I]

The Third Episode
Scene II

(The central doors of the Palace have opened, and ADMETUS *comes slowly on the Stage, preceded and followed by guards and attendants. The King has put off all symbols of royalty, and is dressed in black. His long hair is clipped close to his head.* ADMETUS *dissembles his grief throughout this scene, in obedience to the laws of hospitality, which were particularly reverenced in Thessalia. The behaviour of* HERACLES *compels us to assume a certain worthy obtuseness in him.)*

ADMETUS *(with a gesture of greeting)*: Hail! Son of Zeus and of the blood of Perseus!

HERACLES *(returning the greeting)*: And hail to you, Admetus, 510 lord of the Thessalians!

ADMETUS: May it be so! I know your friendship well.

HERACLES: What means this shorn hair, this mourning robe?

ADMETUS *(sadly)*: To-day I must bury a dead body.

HERACLES: May a God avert harm from your children!

ADMETUS: The children I have begotten are alive in the house.

HERACLES: Your father was ripe for death — if it is he has gone?

ADMETUS *(grimly)*: He lives — and she who brought me forth, O Heracles.

HERACLES *(suddenly remembering, anxiously)*: Your wife — Alcestis — she is not dead?

ADMETUS *(evasively)*: Of her I might make a double answer.

HERACLES: Do you mean that she is dead or alive? 520

ADMETUS *(ambiguously)*: She is and is not — and for this I grieve.

HERACLES *(perplexed)*: I am no wiser — you speak obscurely.

ADMETUS: Did you not know the fate which must befall her?

HERACLES: I know she submitted to die for you.

ADMETUS *(prolonging the ambiguity)*: How then can she be alive, having consented to this?

HERACLES *(mistaking his meaning)*: Ah! Do not weep for your wife till that time comes.

ADMETUS *(gloomily)*: Those who are about to die are dead, and the dead are nothing.

HERACLES: Men hold that to be and not to be are different things.

ADMETUS: You hold for one, Heracles, and I for the other.

HERACLES *(weary of quibbling)*: Whom, then, do you mourn? Which of your friends is dead? 530

ADMETUS: A woman. We spoke of her just now.

HERACLES *(again mistaking his meaning)*: A stranger? Or one born of your kin?

ADMETUS: A stranger, but one related to this house.

HERACLES: But how, then, did she chance to die in your house?

ADMETUS: When her father died she was sheltered here.

HERACLES (*turning away*): Alas! Would I had not found you in this grief, Admetus!

ADMETUS: What plan are you weaving with those words?

HERACLES (*going*): I shall go to the hearth of another friend.

ADMETUS (*stopping him*): Not so, O King! This wrong must not be.

HERACLES (*hesitating*): The coming of a guest is troublesome to those who mourn. 540

ADMETUS (*decisively*): The dead are dead. Enter my house.

HERACLES (*uneasily*): But it is shameful to feast among weeping friends.

ADMETUS: We shall put you in the guest-rooms, which are far apart.

HERACLES (*making a last appeal*): Let me go, and I will give you a thousand thanks.

ADMETUS (*obstinately*): No, you shall not go to another man's hearth. (*To a servant*) Guide him, and open for him the guest-rooms apart from the house. (HERACLES *enters the Palace by the guests' door; when he has gone in,* ADMETUS *turns to the other servants.*) Close the inner door of the courtyard; it is unseemly that guests rejoicing at table should hear lamentations, and be saddened. (*The attendants go into the Palace.*) 550

CHORUS-LEADER (*in amazement*): What are you about? When such a calamity has fallen upon you, Admetus, have you the heart to entertain a guest? Are you mad?

ADMETUS (*calmly*): And if I had driven away a guest who came to my house and city, would you have praised me more? No, indeed! My misfortune would have been no less, and I inhospitable. One more ill would have been added to those I have if my house were called inhospitable. I myself find him the best of hosts when I enter the thirsty land of Argos. 560

CHORUS-LEADER: But why did you hide from him the fate that has befallen, if the man came as a friend, as you say?

ADMETUS: Never would he have entered my house if he had guessed my misfortune.

To some, I know, I shall appear senseless in doing this, and they will blame me; but my roof knows not to reject or insult a guest. (*He goes into the Palace.*)

[END OF THIRD EPISODE]

Stasimon III:
or Fourth Chant of the Chorus

O house of a bountiful lord,
Ever open to many guests,
The God of Pytho,
Apollo of the beautiful lyre,   570
Deigned to dwell in you
And to live a shepherd in your lands!
On the slope of the hillsides
He played melodies of mating
On the Pipes of Pan to his herds.

And the dappled lynxes fed with them
In joy at your singing;
From the wooded vale of Orthrys
Came a yellow troop of lions;   580
To the sound of your lyre, O Phoebus,
Danced the dappled fawn
Moving on light feet
Beyond the high-crested pines,
Charmed by your sweet singing.

He dwells in a home most rich in flocks
By the lovely moving Boebian lake.   590
At the dark stabling-place of the Sun
He takes the sky of the Molossians
As a bourne to his ploughing of fields,
To the soils of his plains;
He bears sway
As far as the harbourless
Coast of the Aegaean Sea,
As far as Pelion.

Even to-day he opened his house
And received a guest,
Though his eyelids were wet
With tears wept by the corpse
Of a dear bedfellow dead in the house.
For the noble spirit is proclaimed by honour;   600
All wisdom lies with the good.
I admire him:
And in my soul I know
The devout man shall have joy.

[END OF STASIMON III]

The Fourth Episode
Scene I

(The Stage is empty. The funeral procession of ALCESTIS *enters from the door of the women's quarters. The body, carried on a bier by men servants, is followed by* ADMETUS *and his two children. Behind them comes a train of attendants and servants carrying the funeral offerings. All are in mourning.* AD-METUS *addresses the* CHORUS.)

ADMETUS: O friendly presence of you men of Pherae! Now that the body is prepared, and the servants bear it on high to the tomb and the fire, do you, as is fitting, salute the dead as she goes forth on her last journey. 610

(Enter, to them, PHERES, *the father of Admetus, followed by attendants bearing funeral offerings.* PHERES *is dressed in royal garments, but wears the white-haired mask of old age, and totters along, leaning on a staff.)*

CHORUS-LEADER: But I see your father, tottering with an old man's walk, and his followers bearing in their hands for your wife garments as an offering to the dead.

PHERES (*speaking in an old man's trembling voice*): My son, I have come to share your sorrow, for the wife you have lost was indeed noble and virtuous — none can deny it. But these things must be endured, however intolerable they may be.

Take these garments, and let her descend under the earth. Her body must be honoured, for she died to save your life, my son; she has not made me childless, nor left me to be destroyed with- 620 out you in my hapless old age; and she has given glorious fame to all women by daring so noble a deed! (*He lifts his hand in salutation to the body of* ALCESTIS.) O woman, who saved my son, who raised me up when I had fallen, hail! Be happy in the halls of Hades! I de-clare it — such marriages are profitable to mankind; otherwise, it is foolish to marry.

(After listening to this unctuous speech with extreme impatience, ADMETUS *turns furiously upon his father.)*

ADMETUS: It was not my wish that you should come to this burial, and I deny that your presence is that of a friend! She shall never 630 wear these garments of yours; she needs not your gifts for her burial. You should have grieved when I was about to die; but you stood aside, and now do you come to wail over a corpse when you, an old man, allowed a young woman to die?

(*Striking his chest*) Were you in very truth father of this body of mine? Did she, who claims to be and is called my mother, bring me forth? Or was I bred of a slave's seed and secretly brought to your wife's breast? You have proved what you are when it comes   640 to the test, and therefore I am not your begotten son; or you surpass all men in cowardice, for, being at the very verge and end of life, you had neither courage nor will to die for your son. But this you left to a woman, a stranger, whom alone I hold as my father and my mother!

Yet it had been a beautiful deed in you to die for your son, and short indeed was the time left you to live. She and I would   650 have lived out our lives, and I should not now be here alone lamenting my misery.

You enjoyed all that a happy man can enjoy — you passed the flower of your age as a King, and in me your son you had an heir to your dominion; you would not have died childless, leaving an orphaned house to be plundered by strangers. You will not say that you abandoned me to death because I dishonoured your old age, for above all I was respectful to you — and this is the gratitude I have from you and my mother!   660

(*Furiously*) Beget more sons, and quickly, to cherish your old age and wrap you in a shroud when dead and lay your body out in state! This hand of mine shall not inter you. I am dead to you. I look upon the light of day because another saved me — I say I am her son, and will cherish her old age!

(*More calmly, but bitterly*) Vainly do old men pray for death, regretting their age and the long span of life. If death draws   670 near, none wants to die, and age is no more a burden to him!

CHORUS-LEADER (*vulgarly shocked*): Admetus! The present misfortune is enough. Do not provoke your father's spirit.

(ADMETUS *turns angrily to depart, but* PHERES *prevents him.*)

PHERES: My son, do you think you are pursuing some hireling Lydian or Phrygian with your taunts? Do you know I am a Thessalian, a free man lawfully begotten by a Thessalian father? You are over-insolent, and you shall not leave thus, after wounding me with your boyish insults. I indeed begot you, and bred you up to be Lord   680 of this land, but I am not bound to die for you. It is not a law of our ancestors or of Hellas that the fathers should die for the children! You were born to live your own life, whether miserable or fortunate; and what is due to you from me you have. You rule over many men, and I shall leave you many wide fields even as I received them from my own father. How, then, have I wronged you? Of what have I robbed you? Do not die for me, any more than I die for you.   69c You love to look upon the light of day — do you think your father hates it? I tell myself that we are a long time underground and that life is short, but sweet.

But you — you strove shamelessly not to die, and you are alive, you shirked your fate by killing her! (*points to* ALCESTIS) And you call me a coward, you, the worst of cowards, surpassed by a woman who died for you, pretty boy? And now you insult those who   700 should be dear to you, when they refuse to die for a coward like you!

Be silent! Learn that if you love your life, so do others. If you utter insults, you shall hear many, and true ones too!

CHORUS-LEADER (*pacific*): These insults and those that went before suffice. Old man, cease to revile your son.

ADMETUS (*to* PHERES): Speak on! I shall refute you. If the truth wounds you when you hear it you should not have wronged me.

PHERES (*contemptuously*): I should have wronged you far   710 more if I had died for you.

ADMETUS (*sarcastically*): It is the same then to die an old man and in the flower of life?

PHERES: We should live one life, not two.

ADMETUS (*ironically*): May you live longer than God!

PHERES: Do you curse your parents when they have done you no wrong?

ADMETUS: I see you are in love with long life.

PHERES (*pointedly*): But you are not carrying her dead body in place of your own?

ADMETUS (*furiously*): It is the proof of your cowardice, O worst of men.

PHERES (*coolly*): You cannot say she died for me!

ADMETUS: Alas! May you one day need my help.

PHERES (*taunting him*): Woo many women, so that more may die for you.   720

ADMETUS: To your shame be it — you who dared not die.

PHERES: Sweet is the daylight of the Gods, very sweet.

ADMETUS: Your spirit is mean, not a man's.

PHERES: Would you laugh to carry an old man's body to the grave?

ADMETUS: You will die infamous, whenever you die.

PHERES: It will matter little enough to me to hear ill of myself when I am dead!

ADMETUS: Alas! Alas! How full of impudence is old age!

PHERES (*pointing to* ALCESTIS): She was not impudent, but foolish.

ADMETUS (*losing his temper again*): Go! Leave me to bury her body.

PHERES (*turning away*): I go. You, her murderer, will bury her   730 — but soon you must render an account to her relatives. Acastus is not a man if he fails to avenge his sister's blood on you!

(PHERES *goes out by the way he entered, followed by his attend-ants.* ADMETUS *gazes angrily after him.*)

ADMETUS: Go with a curse, you, and she who dwells with you! Grow old, as you ought, childless though you have a child. You shall never return to this house. And if I could renounce your hearth as my father's by heralds, I would do it. (*He turns to the funeral procession.*) But we — since this sorrow must be endured — let us go, and set her body on the funeral pyre. 740

(*The Procession moves slowly along the Stage, and is joined by the* CHORUS. *As they pass, the* CHORUS-LEADER *salutes the body of* ALCESTIS.)

CHORUS-LEADER (*to flute accompaniment*): Alas! Alas! You who suffer for your courage, O noblest and best of women, hail! May Hermes of the Dead, may Hades, greet you kindly. If there are rewards for the dead, may you share them as you sit by the bride of the Lord of the Dead!

[END OF EPISODE IV, SCENE I]

The Fourth Episode

SCENE II

(*The Stage is empty.* A SERVANT *in mourning hurries out from the guests' quarters, and faces the audience.*)

SERVANT: Many guests from every land, I know, have come to the Palace of Admetus, and I have set food before them, but (*pointing behind him to the Palace*) never one worse than this guest have I welcomed to the hearth. 750

First, though he saw our Lord was in mourning, he entered, and dared to pass through the gates. Then, knowing our misfortune, he did not soberly accept what was offered him, but if anything was not served to him he ordered us to bring it. In both hands he took a cup of ivy-wood, and drank the unmixed wine of the dark grape-mother, until he was encompassed and heated with the flame of wine. He crowned his head with myrtle sprays, howling discordant songs. There was he caring nothing for Admetus's misery, and we 760 servants weeping for our Queen; and yet we hid our tear-laden eyes from the guest, for so Admetus had commanded.

And now in the Palace I must entertain this stranger, some villainous thief and brigand, while she, the Queen I mourn, has gone from the house unfollowed, unsaluted, she who was as a mother to me and all us servants, for she sheltered us from a myriad troubles by softening her husband's wrath. 770

Am I not right, then, to hate this stranger, who came to us in the midst of sorrow?

(HERACLES *comes from the Palace. He is drunkenly merry, with a myrtle wreath on his head, and a large cup and wine-skin in his hands. He staggers a little.*)

HERACLES (*sees the* SERVANT): Hey, you! Why so solemn and anxious? A servant should not be sullen with guests, but greet them with a cheerful heart.

You see before you a man who is your Lord's friend, and you greet him with a gloomy, frowning face, because of your zeal about a strange woman's death. (*Drinks*) Come here, and let me make you a little wiser!

(*With drunken gravity*) Know the nature of human life? Don't think you do. You couldn't. Listen to me. (*Swaying to   780 and fro*) All mortals must die. Isn't one who knows if he'll be alive to-morrow morning. Who knows where Fortune will lead? Nobody can teach it. Nobody learn it by rules. (*With drunken cheeriness*) So, rejoice in what you hear, and learn from me! Drink! Count each day as it comes as Life — and leave the rest to Fortune. (*Expansively*) Above all, honour the Love Goddess, sweetest of all the Gods to mortal men, a kindly goddess! Put all the rest   790 aside. Trust in what I say, if you think I speak truth — as I believe. Get rid of this gloom, rise superior to Fortune. Crown yourself with flowers and drink with me, won't you? I know the regular clink of the wine-cup will row you from darkness and gloom to another haven.

(*Drinks*) Mortals should think mortal thoughts. To all solemn and frowning men, life I say is not life, but a disaster.   800

SERVANT (*contemptuously*): We know all that, but what we endure here to-day is far indeed from gladness and laughter.

HERACLES (*more soberly*): But the dead woman was a stranger. Lament not overmuch, then, for the Lords of this Palace are still alive.

SERVANT: How, alive? Do you not know the misery of this house?

HERACLES (*at last becoming uneasy*): Your Lord did not lie to me?

SERVANT (*indignantly*): He goes too far in hospitality!

HERACLES (*bewildered*): But why should I suffer for a stranger's   810 death?

SERVANT: It touches this house only too nearly.

HERACLES: Did he hide some misfortune from me?

SERVANT (*sarcastically*): Go in peace! The miseries of our Lords concern us.

HERACLES (*still uncertain*): That speech does not imply mourning for a stranger!

SERVANT: No, or I should not have been disgusted to see you drinking.

HERACLES: Have I then been basely treated by my host?

SERVANT: You did not come to this house at a welcome hour. We

are in mourning. You see my head is shaved and the black garments
I wear.

HERACLES (*angrily*): But who, then, is dead? One of the children?
The old father? 820

SERVANT (*mournfully*): O stranger, Admetus no longer has a wife.

HERACLES (*amazed*): What! And yet I was received in this way?

SERVANT: He was ashamed to send you away from his house.

HERACLES (*thinking of* ADMETUS): O hapless one! What a wife you
have lost!

SERVANT: Not she alone, but all of us are lost.

HERACLES (*now completely sobered*): I felt there was something when
I saw his tear-wet eyes, his shaven head, his distracted look. But he
persuaded me he was taking the body of a stranger to the grave.
Against my will I entered these gates, and drank in the home of
this generous man — and he in such grief! (*Throws down* 830
the cup and wine-skin, and tears off the wreath) And shall I drink
at such a time with garlands of flowers on my head? (*Indignantly*)
You, why did you not tell me that such misery had come upon this
house? Where is he burying her? Where shall I find him?

SERVANT: Beside the straight road which leads to Larissa you will see
a tomb of polished stone outside the walls. (*Returns to the servants'
quarters.*)

HERACLES (*with deep emotion*): O heart of me, much-enduring heart,
O right arm, now indeed must you show what son was born to
Zeus by Alcmene, the Tirynthian, daughter of Electryon! For I must
save this dead woman, and bring back Alcestis to this house 840
as a grace to Admetus.

(*Energetically*) I shall watch for Death, the black-robed Lord
of the Dead, and I know I shall find him near the tomb, drinking
the blood of the sacrifices. If I can leap upon him from an ambush,
seize him, grasp him in my arms, no power in the world shall tear
his bruised sides from me until he has yielded up this woman. If I
miss my prey, if he does not come near the bleeding sacrifice, 850
I will go down to Kore and her Lord in their sunless dwelling, and I
will make my entreaty to them, and I know they will give me Alcestis
to bring back to the hands of the host who welcomed me, who did
not repulse me from his house, though he was smitten with a heavy
woe which most nobly he hid from me! Where would be a warmer
welcome in Thessalia or in all the dwellings of Hellas?

He shall not say he was generous to an ingrate! (*Goes.*) 86c

[END OF EPISODE IV, SCENE II]

The Fourth Episode
SCENE III

(The Stage is left empty. ADMETUS *and his attendants, followed by the* CHORUS, *return from the burial of* ALCESTIS.*)*

ADMETUS *(accompanied by the flute-player)*: Alas!
   Hateful approach, hateful sight of my widowed house! Oh me!
   Oh me! Alas! Whither shall I go? Where rest? What can I say?
   What refrain from saying? Why can I not die? Indeed my mother
   bore me for a hapless fate. I envy the dead, I long to be with them,
   theirs are the dwellings where I would be. Without pleasure I look
   upon the light of day and set my feet upon the earth — so precious
   a hostage has Death taken from me to deliver unto Hades!   870

CHORUS: *Go forward,*
             Enter your house.

ADMETUS: *Alas!*

CHORUS: *Your grief deserves our tears.*

ADMETUS: *O Gods!*

CHORUS: *I know you have entered into sorrow.*

ADMETUS: *Woe! Woe!*

CHORUS: *Yet you bring no aid to the dead.*

ADMETUS: *Oh me! Oh me!*

CHORUS: *Heavy shall it be for you*
             Never to look again
             On the face of the woman you love.

ADMETUS *(accompanied by the flute-player)*: You bring to my mind
   the grief that breaks my heart. What sorrow is worse for a man
   than the loss of such a woman? I would I had never married, never
   shared my house with her. I envy the wifeless and the child-   880
   less. They lived but one life — what is suffering to them? But the
   sickness of children, bridal-beds ravished by Death — dreadful!
   when we might be wifeless and childless to the end.

CHORUS: *Chance, dreadful Chance, has stricken you.*

ADMETUS: *Alas!*

CHORUS: *But you set no limit to your grief.*   890

ADMETUS: *Ah! Gods!*

CHORUS: *A heavy burden to bear, and yet. . . .*

ADMETUS: *Woe! Woe!*

CHORUS: *Courage! You are not the first to lose. . . .*

ADMETUS: *Oh me! Oh me!*

CHORUS: *A wife.*
             Different men
             Fate crushes with different blows.

ADMETUS (*accompanied by the flute-player*): O long grief and mourning for those beloved under the earth!
   Why did you stay me from casting myself into the hollow grave to lie down for ever in death by the best of women? Two lives, not one, had then been seized by Hades, most faithful one to the   900
other; and together we should have crossed the lake of the Underworld.

CHORUS: *A son most worthy of tears*
             Was lost to one of my house,
             Yet, childless, he suffered with courage,
             Though the white was thick in his hair
             And his days were far-spent!   910

ADMETUS (*stands before his Palace door. Accompanied by the flute-player*): O visage of my house! How shall I enter you? How shall I dwell in you, now that Fate has turned its face from me? How great is the change! Once, of old, I entered my house with marriage-songs and the torches of Pelias, holding a loved woman by the hand, followed by a merry crowd shouting good wishes to her who is dead and to me, because we had joined our lives, being both noble and born of noble lines. To-day, in place of marriage-songs are   920
lamentations; instead of white garments I am clad in mourning, to return to my house and a solitary bed.

CHORUS: *Grief has fallen upon you*
             In the midst of a happy life

Untouched by misfortune.
But your life and your spirit are safe.
She is dead,
She has left your love.   930
Is this so new?
Ere now many men
Death has severed from wives.

ADMETUS (*turns from the Palace and faces the* CHORUS): O friends,
whatsoever may be thought by others, to me it seems that my wife's
fate is happier than mine. Now, no pain ever shall touch her again;
she has reached the noble end of all her sufferings. But I, I who
should have died, I have escaped my fate, only to drag out a   940
wretched life. Only now do I perceive it.

How shall I summon strength to enter this house? Whom shall
I greet? Who will greet me in joy at my coming? Whither shall I
turn my steps? I shall be driven forth by solitude when I see my bed
widowed of my wife, empty the chairs on which she sat, a dusty floor
beneath my roof, my children falling at my knees and calling for
their mother, and the servants lamenting for the noble lady lost
from the house!

Such will be my life within the house. Without, I shall be   950
driven from marriage-feasts and gatherings of the women of Thessalia. I shall not endure to look upon my wife's friends Those who
hate me will say: "See how he lives in shame, the man who dared
not die, the coward who gave his wife to Hades in his stead! Is that
a man? He hates his parents, yet he himself refused to die!"

This evil fame I have added to my other sorrows. O my friends,
what then avails it that I live, if I must live in misery and   960
shame?

(*He covers his head with his robe, and crouches in abject misery
on the steps of his Palace.*)

[END OF FOURTH EPISODE]

Stasimon IV:

or Fifth Chant of the Chorus

I have lived with the Muses
And on lofty heights:
Many doctrines have I learned;
But Fate is above us all.
Nothing avails against Fate —

Neither the Thracian tablets
Marked with Orphic symbols,
Nor the herbs given by Phoebus
To the children of Asclepius 970
To heal men of their sickness.

None can come near to her altars,
None worship her statues;
She regards not our sacrifice.
O sacred goddess,
Bear no more hardly upon me
Than in days overpast!
With a gesture Zeus judges,
But the sentence is yours.
Hard iron yields to your strength; 980
Your fierce will knows not gentleness.

And the Goddess has bound you
Ineluctably in the gyves of her hands.
Yield.
Can your tears give life to the dead?
For the sons of the Gods
Swoon in the shadow of Death. 990
Dear was she in our midst,
Dear still among the dead,
For the noblest of women was she
Who lay in your bed.

Ah!
Let the grave of your spouse
Be no more counted as a tomb,
But revered as the Gods,
And greeted by all who pass by!
The wanderer shall turn from his path, 1000
Saying: 'She died for her lord;
A blessed spirit she is now.
Hail, O sacred lady, be our friend!'
Thus shall men speak of her.

[END OF STASIMON IV]

Exodos:

or Finale of the Play

(ADMETUS *is still crouched on the Palace steps, when* HERACLES *enters from the side, leading a veiled woman.*)

LEADER OF THE CHORUS: But see! The son of Alcmene, as I think, comes to your house.

(ADMETUS *uncovers his head, and faces the new-comer.*)

HERACLES: Admetus, a man should speak freely to his friends, and not keep reproaches silent in his heart. Since I was near you in your misfortune, I should have wished to show myself your friend. 1010 But you did not tell me the dead body was your wife's, and you took me into your house as if you were in mourning only for a stranger. And I put a garland of flowers upon my head, and poured wine-offerings to the Gods, when your house was filled with lamentation. I blame you, yes, I blame you for this — but I will not upbraid you in your misfortune.

Why I turned back and am here, I shall tell you. Take and keep this woman for me until I have slain the King of the Bis- 1020 tones and return here with the horses of Thracia. If ill happens to me — may I return safely! — I give her to you to serve in your house.

With much striving I won her to my hands. On my way I found public games, worthy of athletes, and I have brought back this woman whom I won as the prize of victory. The winners of the easy tests had horses; heads of cattle were given to those who won in 1030 boxing and wrestling. Then came a woman as a prize. Since I was present, it would have been shameful for me to miss this glorious gain. Therefore, as I said, you must take care of this woman, whom I bring to you, not as one stolen but as the prize of my efforts. Perhaps in time you will approve of what I do.

ADMETUS (*He has listened to this long and surprising speech with amazement, annoyance and embarrassment, especially since the woman reminds him poignantly of Alcestis. But, true to his tradition of hospitality, he answers politely at first, though the emotion of his grief soon overcomes him.*)

Not from disdain, nor to treat you as a foe, did I conceal my wife's fate from you. But if you had turned aside to another man's hearth, one more grief had been added to my sorrow. It was enough 1040 that I should weep my woe.

(*Hesitantly*) This woman — O King, I beg it may be thus — enjoin some other Thessalian, one who is not in sorrow, to guard her. In Pherae there are many to welcome you. (*Losing his self-control*)

Do not remind me of my grief. Seeing her in my house, I could not restrain my tears. Add not a further anguish to my pain, for what I suffer is too great. And then — where could I harbour a young woman in my house?

For she is young — I see by her clothes and jewels. Could 1050 she live with the men under my roof? How, then, could she remain chaste, if she moved to and fro among the young men? (*Persuasively*) Heracles, it is not easy to restrain the young. . . . I am thinking of your interests. . . . (*Breaking down again*) Must I take her to my dead wife's room? How could I endure her to enter that bed? I fear a double reproach — from my people, who would accuse me of betraying my saviour to slip into another woman's bed, and from my dead wife, who deserves my respect, for which 1060 I must take care.

(*Turning to the veiled woman*) O woman, whosoever you may be, you have the form of Alcestis, and your body is like hers.

(*Violently to* HERACLES) Ah! By all the Gods, take her from my sight! Do not insult a broken man. (*With tears*) When I look upon her — she seems my wife — my heart is torn asunder — tears flow from my eyes. Miserable creature that I am, now I taste the bitterness of my sorrow. (*He turns aside to conceal his weeping.*)

CHORUS-LEADER: I do not praise this meeting; but, whatever happens, we must accept the gifts of the Gods. 1070

HERACLES (*putting his hand on* ADMETUS's *shoulder*): Oh, that I might bring your wife back into the light of day from the dwelling of the Under-Gods, as a gift of grace to you!

ADMETUS (*touched*): I know you would wish this — but to what end? The dead cannot return to the light of day.

HERACLES: Do not exaggerate, but bear this with decorum.

ADMETUS (*bitterly*): Easier to advise than bear the test.

HERACLES: How will it aid you to lament for ever?

ADMETUS: I know — but my love whirls me away. 1080

HERACLES: Love for the dead leads us to tears.

ADMETUS: I am overwhelmed beyond words.

HERACLES: You have lost a good wife — who denies it?

ADMETUS: So that for me there is no more pleasure in life.

HERACLES: Time will heal this open wound.

ADMETUS: You might say Time, if Time were death!

HERACLES: Another woman, a new marriage, shall console you.

ADMETUS: Oh, hush! What have you said? A thing unbelievable!

HERACLES: What! You will not marry? Your bed will remain widowed?

ADMETUS: No other woman shall ever lie at my side. 1090

HERACLES: Do you think that avails the dead?

ADMETUS: Wherever she may be, I must do her honour.

HERACLES: I praise you — but men will call you mad.

ADMETUS: Yet never more shall I be called a bridegroom.

HERACLES: I praise your faithful love to your wife.

ADMETUS (*fervently*): May I die if I betray her even when dead!

HERACLES (*offering him the veiled woman's hand*): Receive her then into your noble house.

ADMETUS (*fiercely*): No, by Zeus who begot you, no!

HERACLES (*meaningly*): Yet you will do wrong if you do not take her.

ADMETUS: If I do it, remorse will tear my heart.   1100

HERACLES: Yield — perhaps it will be a good thing for you.

ADMETUS: Ah! If only you had not won her in the contest!

HERACLES: But I conquered — and you conquered with me.

ADMETUS: It is true — but let the woman go hence.

HERACLES: She shall go, if she must. But first — ought she to go?

ADMETUS: She must — unless it would anger you.

HERACLES: There is good reason for my zeal.

ADMETUS (*very reluctantly*): You have conquered then — but not for my pleasure.

HERACLES: One day you will praise me for it — be persuaded.

ADMETUS (*to his attendants*): Lead her in, since she must be received in this house.   1110

HERACLES (*intervening*): No, I cannot leave such a woman to servants.

ADMETUS (*impatiently*): Then lead her in yourself, if you wish.

HERACLES (*insistently*): I must leave her in your hands.

ADMETUS: I must not touch her — let her go into the house.

HERACLES: I trust only in your right hand.

ADMETUS (*protesting*): O King, you force me to this against my will.

HERACLES (*firmly*): Put forth your hand and take this woman.

ADMETUS (*turning aside his head*): It is held out.

HERACLES: As if you were cutting off a Gorgon's head! Do you hold her?

ADMETUS: Yes.

HERACLES: Then keep her. You shall not deny that the son of Zeus is a graceful guest. (*Takes off the veil and shows* ALCESTIS.)   1120
Look at her, and see if she is not like your wife. And may joy put an end to all your sorrow!

ADMETUS (*drops her hand and starts back*): O Gods! What am I to say? Unhoped-for wonder! Do I really look upon my wife? Or I am snared in the mockery of a God?

HERACLES: No, you look upon your wife indeed.

ADMETUS: Beware! May it not be some phantom from the Underworld?

HERACLES: Do not think your guest a sorcerer.

ADMETUS: But do I indeed look upon the wife I buried?

HERACLES: Yes — but I do not wonder at your mistrust.　　1130

ADMETUS: Can I touch, speak to her, as my living wife?

HERACLES: Speak to her — you have all you desired.

ADMETUS (*taking* ALCESTIS *in his arms*): O face and body of the dearest of women! I have you once more, when I thought I should never see you again!

HERACLES: You have her — may the envy of the Gods be averted from you!

ADMETUS: O noble son of greatest Zeus, fortune be yours, and may your Father guard you! But how did you bring her back from the Underworld to the light of day?

HERACLES: By fighting with the spirit who was her master.　　1140

ADMETUS: Then did you contend with Death?

HERACLES: I hid by the tomb and leaped upon him.

ADMETUS: But why is she speechless?

HERACLES: You may not hear her voice until she is purified from her consecration to the Lower Gods, and until the third dawn has risen. Lead her in.

And you, Admetus, show as ever a good man's welcome to your guests.

Farewell! I go to fulfil the task set me by the King, the　　1150 son of Sthenelus.

ADMETUS: Stay with us, and share our hearth.

HERACLES: That may be hereafter, but now I must be gone in haste. (*Goes.*)

ADMETUS (*gazing after him*): Good fortune to you, and come back here!

(*to the* CHORUS) In all the city and in the four quarters of Thessalia let there be choruses to rejoice at this good fortune, and let the altars smoke with the flesh of oxen in sacrifice! To-day we have changed the past for a better life. I am happy. (*He leads* ALCESTIS *into the Palace.*)

CHORUS-LEADER:

> *Spirits have many shapes,*
> *Many strange things are performed by the Gods.*　　1160
> *The expected does not always happen,*
> *And God makes a way for the unexpected.*
> *So ends this action.*

EURIPIDES

SUPPLIANTS

Translated by L. R. Lind

INTRODUCTION

THE *Suppliants* is a war play and therefore always a timely one. Ir it Euripides has shown us how war makes its most tragic impact upor those who have lost a loved one in the fighting; and he has shown us in a play unique in dramatic literature, the remorse and degradatior of those who start wars they cannot win. To those for whom war i largely a violent interruption of their peaceful activities, to those who have lost no one in it, he has brought home nevertheless its patho and desolation. For the spectator of this play, death remains no longer something private in whose presence he need look merely gravt and sympathetic; Euripides makes him a participant in the commor suffering of the Argive women who form the chorus. They are the mothers of the dead, theirs are the cries of an unassuageable grief, grief without hope.

What Euripides says about war has been said before and after hi time; his pacifism is echoed frequently in Greek history after his death. His logic, the logic of all decent, sensitive men who are outraged by the injustice of war, seems to make no difference to those who begin the wars. We may not be moved, therefore, by the remorse of Adrastus, the war-lord who has failed; even Evadne's heartbroken suicide may appear to us superfluous melodrama. But we cannot forget the sorrow of the Argive women; we have seen that sorrow before, in our town, in our street.

Euripides also speaks of politics; and grief can come from bad politics. Nowhere else in Greek drama is the problem of military aggression and its consequences presented so dramatically. The suppliant women, the weeping children, Adrastus in his utter disgrace, the pathetic death of Evadne, her father's anguish, all heighten the tragic effect of political misjudgment and underline the moral that emerges from inexorable events set in motion by rash and dogmatic spirits. Adrastus grovels before Theseus in the hope that the Athenian king will negotiate a peace for him, a peace as much for his guilty conscience as one through which the Argive women may recover their dead. Theseus, the high-minded administrator, hopes in his turn to arbitrate the question, but he too is forced to fight; against relentless and determined aggression no other argument save force can prevail. His fight, however, is a carefully contained operation; he defines his objective and remains faithful to it. The orderly use of force in the cause of justice wins more than a moral victory in the end.

The ancient scholiast wrote of this play, "It is a praise of Athens";

and most of the later critics have taken their cue from him. It is rather a praise of Theseus, who clearly represents for Euripides the truly enlightened ruler, astute and humane beyond the customs of Greek warfare. Having won the fight, he could have massacred the Thebans; no higher law except his given word prevented him from doing so. Not only, in the light of what we know about Greek treachery from the pages of Thucydides, does he show unusual self-control and pity; his original decision to aid the Argives is, at his insistence, ratified by democratic vote at Athens so that his act of mercy becomes not personal but social, the mercy of one city-state toward another in an age when the practice was to wipe out the conquered at once. The logical conclusion of this kind of elevated diplomacy appears when Athena requests Theseus to exact a mutual defense pact from the Argives as the price for his intervention. But it cannot be said that the play ends on such a lofty note. Athena turns to the children of the seven dead heroes — the Epigoni of later legend — and preaches war against Thebes when they are grown. Thus high-minded diplomacy remained an illusion as far as permanent peace in Greece was concerned. It was the historical fate of the Greeks that they did not learn from Euripides nor follow Theseus in curbing the deadly antagonisms of their cities; they did not solve their international problems in such a simple and civilized manner.

The *Suppliants* is full of typically Euripidean ideas, well-turned phrases, brilliant argument, and skillful characterization. The situation is one of deep pathos, far transcending the specific circumstances. Its pacifism is stated on that level which places Euripides among the greatest of anti-war playwrights. The hamartia of Adrastus lay in an aggression which was not justified by Polynices' exile from Thebes, for he too had tried wrongfully to possess sole power there by refusing to give up the rule by alternate years which had been agreed upon by Eteocles and Creon. No play of Euripides except perhaps the *Trojan Women* and *Hecuba* shows more plainly the wanton waste of all wars. In it the particular situation of Adrastus and the suppliant women and children is merged with the universal aspects of that sorrow which all who attack society in warfare must suffer sooner or later.

The faults of Euripides as a dramatist have recently been pointed out once again by Gilbert Norwood in an essay somewhat ironically entitled "Toward Understanding Euripides" (in *Essays on Euripidean Drama*, 1954). These faults include his sometimes tedious prologues, the awkward "god from the machine," his sardonic piquancy that often reveals the absurdity in human affairs but sometimes leads to an impairment of consistent tone, and his fondness for melodrama. He is, for Norwood, "not a classical writer at all, but a romantic, who entered the theatre still groping." Yet he is immensely stimulating and readable. More than this, he chooses the greatest of themes and places them under the concentrated light of rational inquiry upon the stage; as in the plays of Ibsen, the basic social problems and ideas are never lost to view. He forces us to think about the very bases of political and social existence.

The latest study of the *Suppliants* is also by Norwood, in the volume just mentioned. He tries to show, with much convincing evidence, that this play is really made up from two plays, one by Euripides, the other by a fourth century B.C. poet named Moschion, put together by some unknown person. Whether Norwood can establish this view or not, he has made many searching comments on the constitution of the chorus, the technique and language of the play, the political sentiments expressed by Theseus, and on certain passages he considers un-Euripidean. Why anyone should have gone to the trouble of mutilating a genuine play by Euripides and contaminating it (according to the practice of the Latin comedy writers, Plautus and Terence) with parts from a second and inferior play is still not made clear; one may still believe that the *Suppliants* is fundamentally by Euripides.

The translation of this play and of the *Andromache* imitates as far as is possible in a non-quantitative language the meters of the original Greek text, although the lines of the chorus can establish only a visible, not audible, approximation of length, without any pretense of suggesting the complex rhythms of Euripides. The six-beat iambic of the dialogue is, on the other hand, an easy rhythm to reproduce; its sole difficulty is that the reader, and particularly the actor, who has never seen it before in English may find it strange to discipline himself to what is, after all, nothing but an English blank verse line plus two more syllables and one beat. It is the neatest and most natural of rhythms in speech and can become so to us as it was to the Greeks.

The style of these translations is as close to the Greek as I can make it. The style of Euripides sometimes lacks elevation. Like Ibsen, he was not interested in a fine style for its own sake, although he often achieves it, but in a style adapted for conveying his ideas simply and forcefully. His defects in structure and his neglect of the chorus show that certain parts of the dialogue held his chief interest.

The Greek text of both plays is Gilbert Murray's, in the Oxford Classical series; in the *Suppliants* I have bracketed the lines he brackets for omission, but I think the brackets are unnecessary in this play, and the reader may ignore them if he wishes. I have found no verse translations of either play and suspect that none exists which could be read with pleasure. I have made no unnecessary omissions or rearrangements and have experimented with the transliteration of certain

Greek interjections with the hope that they may provide something of an authentic flavor; every translator of Greek drama is hard pressed to find synonyms expressing sorrow. At least I can say that I have not used the word "Alas!" even once in what are two very sad plays.

The traditional date given for the presentation of the *Suppliants* is around 421 B.C., on the evidence of the sharp criticism of Thebes and of Argos in the play, at a time when both cities were planning an alliance which would have been against the interest of Athens. The scene is at Eleusis; there is a cliff behind the temple front from which Evadne throws herself. The chorus is formed of the Argive women, mothers of the dead heroes who attacked Thebes, and their attendants.

L. R. LIND

SUPPLIANTS

◧

CHARACTERS

AITHRA, *mother of Theseus of Athens*
CHORUS *of Argive women, mothers of the dead*
THESEUS
ADRASTUS *of Argos*
THEBAN HERALD
MESSENGER *from Thebes*
EVADNE, *wife of Capaneus*
IPHIS, *father of Evadne*
BOYS, *grandsons of the Argive women*
ATHENA

SCENE: *Before the temple of Demeter at Eleusis, near Athens. The* CHORUS *of Argive women, mothers of the slain Seven against Thebes, and the temple attendants are gazing at* AITHRA. ADRASTUS, *lone survivor of the Seven against Thebes, lies at her feet, weeping. She raises her arms, faces the statue of the goddess, and speaks the prologue.*

AITHRA: Demeter, guarding the hearth in Eleusinian land,
    And you, the priests who serve her in her dwelling place,
    I pray that you may keep my Theseus safe, my child,
    The city of the Athenians and Pittheus' land,
    In which, when he had raised me in a happy home,
    My father gives me, Aithra, to Pandion's son,
    To Aegeus as his wife, by Loxias' * command.

---

* Apollo.

    I have made my prayer with my gaze fixed on these
Old women who have left their homes in Argive land,
With suppliant bough have fallen here beside my knees;   10
A dreadful pain they suffer, since around the gates
Of Cadmus they have lost their seven noble sons,
Whom once Adrastus, ruler of the Argives, led,
Wishing to seize the heritage of Oedipus
For the exile, his son-in-law Polynices.
Their mothers yearn to bury the spear-slain bodies,
But those who rule will not allow the gathering-up
And thus dishonor all the sacred laws of heaven.
Adrastus bears his burden too with these and me;
He lies in tears, he groans because he sent the host,   20
The spear from home, the most unlucky in the world.
He urges me to win my son's consent with prayers
To take the bodies off by argument or strength
Of spear and thus to share the blame of burial,
Setting this task, and only this, upon my son
And on the town of Athens. But I happen to
Be here in sacrifice for harvest of the soil
And coming from my home, here to this sacred shrine
Where first the bearded grain shows ripe above the ground,
This chainless chain of leaves* I hold and here I stay   30
Beside the holy altars of the goddesses,
Of Cora and of Demeter, in pity for
These white-haired childless mothers mourning for their sons
And reverence for their sacred garlands; at my word
A herald went to call my Theseus from the town
So he may cast the grief of these out of the land
Or loose their suppliant bonds through holy deeds toward gods,
Since it is best for women who have common sense
To get all things of this sort done by way of men.

CHORUS: I, an old woman, beg you   40
      Here with my aged mouth, forward
        Falling beside your knee,
      Lawless . . . to free my children, you who
      Leave the members of corpses
In limb-relaxing death as food for mountain beasts.

      Seeing about my eyes
      Piteous tears on the lids
        And wrinkles on aged flesh

---

* She is bound only by religious feeling, symbolized by the garlands of the women.

Torn by my finger nails, what
Must I do who see my dead children   50
Neither laid out in my home nor hid in a tomb of heaped earth?

You too have borne a son, O queen,
    Making your bed a delight
    To your husband; share with me then
    My feelings, O share with me too
The grief which I bear for my loss,
    For the dead I have borne;
Prevail on your son, O, I beg you,
    To come to Ismenus and place
In my hands the young bodies, the lost, the untombed.

Not as the holy custom bids but forced, I come   60
    To fall in suppliant prayer
    At the altars that kindle flame.
    But I have just cause, and you
Have the power through your good son
    To take from me all my sorrow.
In pitiable suffering I ask
You to place my child in my hands,
That I may embrace his poor limbs, the corpse of my boy.

Another struggle of groans, of groans, comes on,
Following mine; the hands of the servants resound.   70
    Go, fellow-singers of sorrow,
    Go, you who suffer with me.
    Hades honors your dance!
    Scratch your white nail on your cheek,
Bloody, and bloody your skin:
    The care of the dead
    Is an honor to those alive.

Insatiate, this grace of sorrow leads me,
Full of my woe, as from a sun-burnt rock
    The water drop trickles down   80
    Unceasing ever; their sorrow
    For children of theirs who die
Nature has placed upon women,
A suffering grown out of tears. Ee, ee,
    May I forget
    My pain in death.

(*Enter* THESEUS.)

THESEUS: What are these groans I hear, these beatings of the breast,
　These dirges for the dead that echo from the temple?
　How fear has fluttered over me, a fear for mother!
　I guide my steps to her, fearing the news she brings:　　　90
　She has been gone so long from home.
　　　　　　　　　　　　　　　　Ah, what is this?
　I see a new beginning of the song of sorrow.
　My grey-haired mother is sitting on the altar step
　Among these stranger women, not all in one fashion
　Keening their woe, and from their aged eyes let fall
　The piteous tears; their locks are shorn; they do not wear
　The flowing festal robes that fit the worshipper.
　　　　What *is* this, mother? It's for you to tell me all,
　For me to listen; I suspect it's something new.
AITHRA: O son, these women are the mothers of the boys　　　100
　Who died around the gates of the Cadmeian town,
　The seven leaders; and with suppliant branches they
　Keep guard encircling me, as you can see, my son.
THESEUS: But who is this who groans so piteously at the gates?
AITHRA: Adrastus, as they say, the Argive general.
THESEUS: These children round about him: are they of these women?
AITHRA: No, they're the sons of those whose corpses you see here.
THESEUS: Why have they come to us with hands of suppliants?
AITHRA: I know; but they must speak to you, my son, henceforth.
THESEUS: You, dressed in woolen cloak, I ask you, tell me first.　110
　Take off the cover from your head; stop groaning; speak.
　You get nowhere with me unless you use your tongue.
ADRASTUS: O noble lord victorious of Athenian land,
　Theseus, I come to you and yours a suppliant.
THESEUS: Upon the hunt for what? And what is it you need?
ADRASTUS: You know the fateful expedition which I led.
THESEUS: Of course; you did not pass through Greece so silently.
ADRASTUS: Here fell the bravest fighters of the Argive men.
THESEUS: Such are the wretched sorrows caused by wretched war.
ADRASTUS: I came to this city to ask for the bodies of the dead.　120
THESEUS: You trust in Hermes' heralds? You have come to bury?
ADRASTUS: Yes, but the slayers will not let me bury them.
THESEUS: What do they tell you, since you ask a holy favor?
ADRASTUS: Yes, what! They don't know how to bear their good fortune.
THESEUS: You've come for my advice? Or is it something else?
ADRASTUS: I want you, Theseus, to carry off the Argive sons.
THESEUS: But where is Argos now? Or were her boasts in vain?
ADRASTUS: We stumbled; we are done for; we have come to you.
THESEUS: Was this your own idea or did Argos know?

ADRASTUS: All of the Danaans beg you to inter their dead.   130
THESEUS: Why did you lead your seven divisions on to Thebes?
ADRASTUS: I did it as a favor for my sons-in-law.
THESEUS: To whom among the Argives did you give your daughters?
ADRASTUS: I did not join them in alliance with my house.
THESEUS: But did you marry off the Argive girls to strangers?
ADRASTUS: To Tydeus and Polynices, born at Thebes.
THESEUS: And how was it you came to wish this marriage-bond?
ADRASTUS: The hard-to-riddle riddles of Phoebus baffled me.
THESEUS: What said Apollo to bring about the virgin marriage?
ADRASTUS: That I should give my daughters to a boar, a lion.   140
THESEUS: But how did you unravel the god's strange web of words?
ADRASTUS: There came two runaways to my gates at dead of night
THESEUS: Who and who? Tell me. You speak of two at once.
ADRASTUS: Tydeus had joined battle with Polynices.
THESEUS: And to this pair, as wild beasts, did you give your daughters?
ADRASTUS: Yes, likening their warfare unto that of beasts.
THESEUS: How did they come to you and leave their fathers' lands?
ADRASTUS: Tydeus fled the blood-curse he had raised at home.
THESEUS: The son of Oedipus, in what way did he leave Thebes?
ADRASTUS: Under his father's curses, lest he kill his brother.   150
THESEUS: You speak of flight in wisdom, flight of one's accord.
ADRASTUS: But those who stayed did wrong to those who went away.
THESEUS: How's that? His brother took away his wealth by fraud?
ADRASTUS: I went to make a judgment and I was undone.
THESEUS: And did you visit seers? See flames of sacrifice?
ADRASTUS: O woe! You're driving me to the place I stumbled.
THESEUS: It doesn't seem you went there with the gods' good will.
ADRASTUS: It's more than that! I went against Amphiareus' * will.
THESEUS: Did you so easily twist away from godly power?
ADRASTUS: The eager shouts of young men left me panic struck.   160
THESEUS: You strove for courage rather than for prudent counsel.
ADRASTUS: Yes; what I did has killed many other generals.
 But you, O bravest man in all the land of Greece,
 Ruler of Athens, it is part of my disgrace
 To fall obeisant on the ground and grasp your knee,
 A grey-haired man like me, a happy king before;
 Yet all the same force makes me yield to my misfortune.
 O save the corpses for me, pity all my woes
 And pity the mothers of the slaughtered children,
 On whom grey age has come in all their childlessness.   170
 They have endured to come here and their stranger feet

---

* His brother-in-law, who warned him not to go against Thebes.

To shuffle slowly, moving all their aged limbs,
An embassy not for Demeter's mysteries,
But to inter the corpses who have rightful cause
Beneath these women's hands to find fit burial.
For it is wise that rich men look at poverty
And for the poor to look upon the wealthy man
In yearning, so that love of wealth may grip him too,
And so the fortunate fear the pitiable.

(*Some lines are missing.*)

So too the poet may create the poems he makes,   180
Rejoicing as he does so; if he feels no joy,
He could not, being troubled in affairs at home,
Delight his hearers, for his feeling would be false.
Perhaps you might say, "Why leave out the land of Pelops
And set this task on the Athenian state alone?"
I know I'm right in giving you this explanation:
Sparta is cruel and cunning in her devious ways;
The other states are small and strengthless; but your city
Alone would be equipped to undertake the toil.
For it has looked on sorrow, it has youthfulness   190
In you, and a good shepherd, through the want of whom
Many a town has perished, lacking a general.

CHORUS: I too speak here to you the same word as this man;
Theseus, you should take pity on my evil lot.

THESEUS: With other men I've grappled in this argument.
Who was it said among us mortals all things worse
Outnumber better things, outnumber them by far?
But my opinion is the exact reverse of this.
There are more good than bad things here for mortal men,
For if there weren't we would not live and look on light.   200
I praise whichever god was first to bring our life
From its confused and beastly state to something orderly,
Giving us our intelligence and then our tongue
As messenger to thoughts, to learn to know our speech,
The nurture of the fruit and for that nurture heaven's
Sweet drops of rain so crops might spring up out of earth
And fill the stomach; in addition, winter clothes
He fashioned, clothes to keep off burning heat of summer,
And sailings over sea that we might bring exchange
To one another of the goods each land might need.   210
But things obscure and things we do not clearly know
By looking into flames and folds of inward parts
The seers foretell, and from the sweep of flying birds.

Are we not then presumptuous when a god has given
Such gear for livelihood, to be unsatisfied?
Our mortal wisdom seeks to be more than a god's;
The haughty pride we harbor in our human wits
Makes us think we are wiser than any of the gods.
  Of this division you seem to be, not being wise,
When, bound by Phoebus' oracles, you gave your daughters   **220**
To utter strangers just as if the gods existed,
And mingled your clear ancestral blood with turbid blood.
You laid a sore upon your house; wise men should not
Join bodies of the unjust to bodies of the just
But win for their descendants prosperous relatives.
The god who deems our fortunes held in common lot
By miseries of the sick man has destroyed the man
Who was not sick and had not done an injury.
In leading all the Argives on this expedition,
When seers gave forth pronouncements, you did grave dishonor
To spurn the gods, by violence to destroy the town,   **231**
Through young men led astray who like to hold command,
Rejoice in their increase of wars unjustly waged,
Destroying citizens: in order that one may
Be general of the army; that one may be wanton
With power in his hand that makes him wreak outrage;
Another, for the sake of gain, not looking out
To find how all the people suffer, suffering war.
For there are three divisions of the citizens:
The rich and useless, always craving more and more;   **240**
The ones who have not, and eke out a scanty life;
The dangerous, who give their envy greater sway,
Shooting its evil darts against the idle rich,
And cheated, deceived by tongues of crooked counsellors.
The middle one of these three parts saves every city.
Preserving whatsoever order it sets up.
And then shall I become allied to fight with you?
What fine excuse shall I give all my citizens?
Go, and farewell; if you have counselled lucklessly
Let fate press hard on you, but let my people be.   **250**
CHORUS: He sinned; yet this is of the young man's temperament,
  A fault we must forgive; so let it be with him.
  But now to you as to a doctor, lord, we come.
ADRASTUS: I chose you not as judge of my mistaken deeds,
  Nor, if I should be found to have acted with dishonor,
  To censure me and punish me for this, O lord,
  But that you might be helpful. If you do not wish

To aid me, I must acquiesce. What can I do?
    Come, grey-haired women, go your way and leave the dark
Green grass the leaves have covered as they flutter down,   **260**
Calling the gods to witness, call the earth, and her,
The goddess fire-bearing, Demeter, and the sun,
That prayers made in gods' names avail us not at all.
CHORUS: (*A line is missing here.*)
Who was the son of Pelops, we from Pelops' land
Possess the same blood on the father's side with you.
What are you doing? Will you forsake and cast them forth,
Old women who have not won what they should have won?
Not so! The beast has refuge in a rocky lair,
The slave has altars of the gods, city has city
To crouch beside when tempest-tossed; of mortal lives   **270**
There is not one that's happy to the very end.

Come down, poor soul, come down, from Persephone's sacred environs,
Come down to approach her and throw your arms round her knees
    in entreaty
To pick up the bodies, the dead, and to bury them . . . O how I
    suffer!
The strong young sons who have perished beneath the high walls of
    the Thebans!

        Ah sorrow! Take me, bear me, guide me,
          lift me by my poor old hands!

By your beard I beseech you, O friend, the most noble in Hellas,
I grasp at your knee and your hand as I fall in my grief here before
    you;
Pity me for my dead children, a suppliant wandering, wailing;   **280**
Let them not lie there, my son, a joy to the beasts in Cadmeian
Land; look not on unburied boys who were like you, so youthful.
Look at the tear on my eyelids, who fall at your feet for your favor,
Clasping your knees in my passion to win for my children a tomb.
THESEUS: Mother, why do you weep and bring your veil up to
Your eyes? Is it because you hear the desolate
Groans of these women? Something has touched me too.
Lift up your white head; do not cry again, my dear,
Sitting beside the hallowed hearth of Demeter.
AITHRA: Ai, ai!
THESEUS: You should not groan because these women sorrow.   **290**
AITHRA: O wretched women!
THESEUS: You were not born one of them.

AITHRA: May I say something fine for you and for our city?

THESEUS: Of course; from women too come words of great wisdom.

AITHRA: The word I hide brings hesitation to me now.

THESEUS: A shameful thing, to hide good words from us, your own.

AITHRA: I shall not later on be blamed for keeping still
Because I now stayed silent so dishonorably,
Nor, cowed because it is supposed to be useless
For women to speak well, yield my honor to fear.
O son, I ask you, first consider godly things, 300
Lest you be overthrown by dishonoring them;
For here alone you waver, right in all the rest.
To add to this, if it were wrong to be so bold
For those who have been wronged, I would have kept so still.
But now this brings for you as much of honor too
As it brings me no fear to urge you on, my son,
That you should lay your hand to this necessity
Against fierce men who try to keep the helpless dead
From burial and their full share of funeral gifts,
And stop them from confounding all the laws of Greece. 310
For this it is that holds men's cities firm and safe,
This: when each man upholds the laws in honor bound.
Someone will say it was in cowardice of hand,
With chance to win a crown of glory for your city,
You feared and stood apart; although you fought a boar,
Contending in an easy struggle with the beast,
When it was yours to look at spear-point and on helm
And had to fight, they found that you were cowardly.
  O don't do this, my son, since you are really mine.
You see how, ridiculed as lacking counsellors, 320
Your country lifts a Gorgon's eye at those who mock?
Amid great toils it grows and grows and wins increase.
But states that act in quiet darkness, all of them,
See everything in darkness, taking too much caution.
Will you not go to aid the women and their dead?
I do not fear for you, by justice set in motion;
And seeing the folk of Cadmus who have fared so well,
I trust that they will make another throw of dice;
For god turns all things upside down and back again.

CHORUS: O dearest one for me, you've spoken honorably 330
To this man and to me; this is a double joy.

THESEUS: The words that I have spoken, mother, rightly hold
As they concern this man, and I have brought to light
The reason why the plans he laid brought him to ruin.
I see the sense, I too, of your admonishment.

It is not fitting for a man with ways like mine
To run from danger. I've done honorable deeds;
This is the conduct I have chosen toward the Greeks:
To be the man who punishes the evil doer.
It is not possible for me to shun war's toils.   340
For what will the mortals who hate me say of me
When it's my mother, very much afraid for me,
Who is the first to urge me to take up this toil?
    I'll do it; I will go and liberate the dead,
Persuading Thebes with words; if not, by force of spears.
This shall be done if gods do not begrudge success.
But I desire that this be approved by all the city.
It will approve if I am willing, and in giving
Its own approval the folk will be more favorable.
For it was I who brought them to a monarchy   350
And set the city free for an equal suffrage.
But taking Adrastus as a proof for all my words
I'll go to the mass of citizens and win consent,
Collecting first the best young men of Athens town.
Then sitting under arms I'll send my arguments
To Creon, asking him to give the bodies up.
    Now, aged women, take away the holy garlands
From mother, as I lead her on to Aegeus' house,
Taking her dear hand; for children who do not
Serve faithfully their parents are a luckless lot —   360
The loveliest of gifts if shared, for he who gives,
Receives from his own children what he gives his parents.

CHORUS: Horse-feeding Argos, ancestral land of mine,
      You have heard, you have heard,
      The words of a king that are reverent
      Toward gods, both great through Pelasgia
        And throughout Argos.

      Now to the end of my sorrows, and even beyond,
        May he come and bear off
        The blood-stained glory of the mothers,   370
        Make the land of Inachus friendly,
          Doing this kindness.

      A marvellous glory for cities is a worshipful deed,
        It holds its graciousness ever.
      What will the city agree to? Friendship to me
        Will it pledge? Shall we bury our sons?

Aid me, a mother; O city of Pallas, be kind!
   Defile not the laws of the gods.
Surely you reverence justice, assigning the lesser
   Share to injustice, and help the bereft.   380

THESEUS (*to an Athenian herald*):
   Possessing the art of heraldry, you minister
   To me and to the city, carrying messages.
   Passing beyond Asopus and Ismenus' water,
   Speak to the haughty ruler of Thebes the words I say:
   "Theseus requests of you as favor to bury the dead;
   Dwelling as neighbor, he has a neighbor's right to this.
   You should make friends also of Erechtheus' sons."
   If they say yes, come back at once to tell me so.
   If they refuse, here is your second argument:
   "Receive my Bacchic revellers all bearing shields;   390
   The army stands full armed and goes upon parade
   Round holy Callichorus; it is well prepared.
      Yes, willingly and gladly did the city receive
   This task, when it perceived that I was willing too."
   Hold on!
            Who comes to interrupt this speech of mine?
   A Theban herald is what he looks like; I'm not sure.
   Stop, wait; he may relieve you of an envoy's task
   By coming here to parley as to my requests.

      (*Enter the* THEBAN HERALD.)

THEBAN HERALD: Who's tyrant in this land? To whom shall I report
   The words of Creon who rules the land of Cadmus now,   400
   With Eteocles dead beside the seven gates
   Under the hand of his brother Polynices?
THESEUS: First, stranger, you have started off your speech all wrong,
   Seeking a tyrant here; the city is not ruled
   By one man only; it's a city of the free.
   The people rule by class in yearly interchange;
   They do not give the bulk of power to the rich:
   The poor man also rules in turn with equal strength.
HERALD: You put us one ahead, as if you played at draughts;
   My city has a one-man rule, no mob-control.   410
   There is no one who blusters, blows it up with words,
   Or turns it this way, that way just for private gain.
   For he who now is pleasant and gives much delight,
   Next moment does an injury and covers up
   With new-made slander, slips away from punishment.

Besides, how could the folk who do not judge aright
The words of men rule rightly any town at all?
Time gives us, and not haste, a better knowledge.
But a poor man who earns his living from the soil
Even if he were not ignorant, because he toils   420
He could not oversee the common interest.
Surely this would be harmful to the better class
When crooked rascals hold official posts of power,
And upstart rich men rule the people with their tongues.

THESEUS: The herald's clever, he handles words like an expert.
But since in this talking contest you have had your say,
Listen: you've challenged me to a full-dress debate.
There's nothing more sinister for a city than tyrants,
Where first of all there are not any laws in common;
There one man, keeping laws unwritten, holds the rule   430
Himself unto himself, and power is not equal.
But where the laws are written down both weak and strong,
Both rich and poor, have equal power and equal right.
The weaker man can there talk back on even terms
To those who are more prosperous, if they use him ill.
The small can beat the great with justice on his side.
And this is the cry of liberty: "Who wants to give
Good counsel to the city, bring it to our midst?"
The man who does so wins great glory, but the man
Who does not sits in silence. What's more fair than this?   440
    And truly where the people run the government
They are rejoiced by good young citizens coming up.
The absolute king regards this as a dangerous state;
He kills the best men who he thinks have minds they use;
He is afraid his tyranny will not endure.
But how then could a city come into its strength
When some one cuts the springtime meadow flowers down,
Removing boldness, plucking out the younger men?
Why should a man earn livelihood and wealth for sons
When all his toil makes tyrants live a richer life?   450
Or raise up girls as virgins in a decent home
As dainty pleasures for the tyrant, when he chooses,
But tears for those who reared them: may I cease to live
When my dear children shall be married off by force.
    These are the words I've shot as arrows at your words.
What is it that you wish? Why do you come to us?
You would have come ill-fated had the state not sent
You, speaking past all measure: proper heralds say
Just what they're told to say and then go back again

As swiftly as they came. In future let the king   460
Of Thebes send some one less a blabber-mouth than you.
CHORUS: O grief! When god assigns success to evil men,
They run amuck in pride as though good luck would last.
HERALD: I'll speak out now. As far as this debate's concerned,
You may believe you've won; I take the other view.
    I warn you, I and all Cadmeian folk as well,
Not to allow Adrastus to stay in this land.
But since he's here, before the sunset comes again,
Breaking the mystic wreaths he wears as suppliant,
Drive him away nor try to take the dead by force,   470
Since nothing in the Argive city is your concern.
If you obey me, you will steer your city straight,
Without upsetting waves; but if you don't, a huge
Deluge of spears will fall on you and your allies.
    Think carefully, and do not grow enraged at my
Advice, because you rule a city that is free,
And in exchange of heated words flex muscles too.
The hope that springs from arms is unreliable
As many cities have learned in their excess of wrath.
For when war comes to be put to vote before the folk,   480
No one weighs carefully the thought of his own death;
He turns aside to others this calamity.
But if death stood before our eyes on voting day,
Spear-crazy Greece would never be at brink of ruin.
And yet of these two words — the good, the bad — we men,
All of us, know which is the better and how much
More good peace gives to mortal souls than bloody war.
Peace, the first and best beloved by all the Muses,
But hateful to the Avengers, loves to have good children,
Loves to have wealth; we evil fools discard them both   490
Whenever we choose war, enslaving men and cities.
    But do you benefit the dead and hostile men
Raising for burial those whom insolent pride destroyed?
Is it not just that Capaneus's body smoke,
Stricken by lightning, on the upright ladder rungs
He placed against the gates of Thebes the time he swore
To crush the city whether god willed it or not?
Did not a chasm yawn to snatch away the seer *
And fold his four-horse chariot in its awful gulf?
Don't other leaders lie in death before the gates,   500
The sutures of their bones crushed utterly with rocks?

---

* Amphiareus.

Boast now that you have better sense than Zeus himself,
Or grant that justly gods destroy the evil man.
The wise men then should love their children first of all,
Next those who bore them, next their country, if they wish
To make it great, not break it; reckless pilots are
A danger to their men; the steady sailor's wise
At the right time; foresight shows manly courage too.
CHORUS: Great Zeus has visited full punishment on these,
But you should not insult them, insolently proud.   510
ADRASTUS: You utter villain —
THESEUS: Keep quiet, Adrastus; shut your mouth.
Bring not your curses out before I give my speech:
This herald does not come to speak to you, but me;
It is my duty and not yours to make reply.
And first of all I'll answer the first words you said.
I do not think that Creon is my master yet,
Or stronger than I am, so that he can bring force
On Athens to do this; for water would flow uphill
If thus indeed he really could command my city.
I have not come to settle this warfare of yours,   520
Nor did I come with these people to Cadmus' land.
I claim the right, upholding Panhellenic law,
To bury the corpses without harming your city
Nor bringing on a conflict that will cut men down.
You tell me: which of these requests dishonors me?
For even if you've suffered under Argive swords,
They're dead, you've thrown them back in justice and in honor,
Disgrace is on their heads, their suffering is complete.
Allow the corpses now to be covered up in soil,
For whence each part came once into the light of day,   530
There it has gone, the spirit into upper air,
The body into earth; we can not call it ours
Except to use and dwell in it throughout our lives.
And then the earth that nourished it receives it back.
Do you suppose, not burying them, you harm Argos?
By no means; it's a common question for all Greece
If anyone defraud the dead of what's their right
And keep them tombless. For the bravest men will be
Called cowards all, if this law be laid down indeed.
To me you've come to utter dreadful menaces;   540
But do you fear the dead if they should hide in earth?
Lest what should happen? Lest they should dig up your land
Where they are buried? Or breed children in their hole
By whom revenge, some punishment, be laid on you?

This is indeed ill-omened, foolish waste of words
For you to stand in dread of evil, empty fears.
    But, O vain fools, learn here about the ills of men.
This life is struggle; some of us grow fortunate,
Some swiftly, others later; some are lucky now.
But god is fickle; he who is unfortunate   **550**
Honors the god so that he may be fortunate.
The prosperous who fears the breath of wealth may fly
Lifts up the god in praise. Then since we know these facts,
When injured slightly we ought not bear wrath in heart
And do such wrongs as will bring harm upon the state.
    How might this be? Give us the right to burial
For corpses and to honor those who plead with us.
Or what I do hereafter's plain; I'll go, use force.
I'll never let the word be spread among the Greeks
That ancient sacred law came to Pandion's city,   **560**
To me, and met no one who would respect it here.
CHORUS: Courage: for while you save the light of Righteousness,
    You will escape the many slanderous words of men.
HERALD: Shall I join speech with you for just a little space?
THESEUS: Speak, if you wish; you're not the one to stay close mouthed.
HERALD: You'll never take the Argive sons out of the land.
THESEUS: Now, if you please, hear what I have to say in turn.
HERALD: I'll listen; it's your privilege to speak again.
THESEUS: I'll bury the corpses, take them from Asopian land.
HERALD: Then you must run the risk of death among our shields. **570**
THESEUS: Well, I have fought before this, many other fights.
HERALD: Your father then begot you as a match for all?
THESEUS: At least for all the violent; the good I spare.
HERALD: It is your custom, and your city's, to mix and meddle.
THESEUS: It's just because we labor much that she grows strong.
HERALD: Come, so the sown spear may catch you within the city.
THESEUS: What raging Ares ever sprang from dragon blood?
HERALD: You'll learn through suffering; you are a young man still.
THESEUS: You do not rouse me to be angry in my heart
    With these loud words; despatch yourself out of this land   **580**
And take the empty boasts you brought along with you.
We do no good delaying here.
                  To arms! To arms!
Let every full-armed soldier and each charioteer
Press on, and make the war-horse shake his bridle-discs
And drop his foam, and gallop on the Cadmeian land.
I shall proceed to the seven gates of Cadmus' city,
With my sharp steel in hand, announcer of my own

Arrival. But I charge you to remain behind,
Adrastus; do not mingle your bad luck with mine.
For under my own god I lead my army on,   590
A warrior fresh and new with fresh, new spear I ride!
One wish alone I utter: may the gods give aid,
The ones who honor justice, for with their support
I'll win the fight; but courage does not signify
Unless you have a willing god to help your side.

CHORUS:
> — O miserable mothers of miserable chiefs,
>> How green fear sits and broods upon my heart —
> — What new voice do you bring me?
> — How will Athena's army settle this?
> — You mean by spears or by exchange of words?   600
> — That would be profit; but if Ares-slaying
>> Bloody battle, smiting breasts, appear throughout
>>> The wretched city,

What debt shall I, the cause of this, take on myself?

> — But on the man who shines with fortune now
>> Some fate may seize. This bold hope folds me round.
> — You speak indeed of gods as just.
> — What other creatures guide events for us?
> — I see great differences in god-given affairs.
> — You perish with your former fear.   610
>> Right calls for right and murder calls for murder,
>> But respite from our ills

The gods deal out to mortals, they who hold the ends of all.

> — How might we come to those bright-towered plains,
>> Leaving the goddess' water, Callichorus —
> — Would that a god might give me wings to fly,
>> To the two-rivered city.
> — So you would know, would know the fates of friends.
> — What lot, what chance awaits
>> The noble leader of   620
>>> This land?

> — Once more we call on gods we've called upon;
> — This our best hope in fear.
> — Ho Zeus! The husband of
>> Our ancient mother, heifer-child of Inachus.
> — Be now a helpful ally to the city;

The glorious prize, your statue
   In the square, I bear away,
   Insulted, to the pyre.

MESSENGER: Women, I come to tell you many pleasant things,   630
   Rescued myself; for I was captured in the battle
   Where fought the army of the seven dead leaders
   (The exact spot they fought at is by Dirce's stream.)
   I now report that Theseus won. A longer speech
   I'll spare you, for I was the servant of Capaneus,
   Whom Zeus destroyed by striking with his thunderbolt.
CHORUS: O dearest man, you do announce happy return
   And news of Theseus; if you add that the army
   Of Athens too is safe, all of your words are sweet.
MESSENGER: Safe; and he did what Adrastus should have done him-
      self,   640
   When, having led his Argives from the Inachus,
   He marched to set attack upon the Cadmeian city.
CHORUS: How did the son of Aegeus set his trophies up,
   Rewards for Zeus, he and his comrades of the spear?
   Tell me; since you were there, delight us absent ones.
MESSENGER: A brilliant ray of sunshine, clear and sparkling beam,
   Fell slantwise on the earth; around Electra's gates
   I stood and watched full-view upon a tower.
   I saw three tribes from out the three divisions come:
   First, weapon-bearing mass of folk that stretched up to   650
   Ismenus' banks (that's the report) and then the king
   Himself, the famous offspring of king Aegeus,
   And those who marched with him, arranged upon the right,
   The men who have their homes in old Cecropian land,
   Equal in number; and the chariots of full-armed men
   And coastal men from Paralus equipped with spears
   Close by the spring of Ares, and the cavalry
   Massed near the flanks of the encampment in their might.
   The folk of Cadmus crouched before their fort-like walls;
   They placed the dead behind, for whom the quarrel arose,   660
   Below the monuments set up for Amphion.
   And armored horsemen turned to face a horseman foe,
   While chariots turned to chariots their four-wheeled threat.
   The herald of Theseus spoke these words to all of them:
   "Keep silence, people; silence, rank and file of Cadmus,
   In silence hear us; we are come to take the dead
   We wish to bury, preserving Panhellenic law.
   We do not wish to shed your blood in battle here."

And Creon made no counter-cry to these stout words,
But sat in silence under arms; the chariot drivers   670
Began the battle in their four-wheeled vehicles.
Driving them all athwart each other in the field,
They set the men they carried down, spear against spear.
And these fought steel to steel; the drivers turned again
Their horses to stand guard and aid their fighting men.
But Phorbas, chief of cavalry, who saw the mass,
With single horses of the sons of Erechtheus
And those appointed to avert a flank attack,
Clashed with the Thebans, beat them, then was beaten too.
I saw this fight, I now repeat no hearsay — I   680
Was on the spot where chariots and their warriors fought —
I do not know, of all the wild calamities,
Which one to tell of first — the dust that reached the sky
(How much there was!), or of the horsemen borne aloft
Amid the chariot-traces, or borne down to death;
The blood that flowed in rivers, those who fell and those
Who tumbled like a diver when their chariots crashed
Headlong to earth and left their lives in the debris.
When Creon saw your horsemen winning in the fight
From where he sat, he took a shield into his hands   690
And moved before despair should strike his allied friends.
And clashing fiercely in the midst of all the foe,
Their men were killed, and they killed too, and passed the word
Of cheer to one another with a mighty shout:
"Kill! Stab the spear into the sons of Erechtheus!"
But Theseus' troops did not give way to panic fear;
They pressed straight onward, snatching up their shining arms.
The band that grew to men, sprung from the dragon's teeth,
Now wrestled fiercely, made the left wing turn and flee;
Our men gave way; but their right wing was crushed, turned
    too,   700
And fled; the contest then became an equal one.
And at this point one could approve our general;
He did not press advantage on the wing that won
But went to help the wing that wavered in defeat,
And roared so loudly that he shook the earth beneath:
"Boys, if you don't turn back their steel, the men who sprang
From seed will win, the city of Pallas will be gone."
Then courage rose through all the host of Danaans.
And he himself took up his Epidaurian mace
With frightful war-head, and he swung it like a sling,   710
Harvesting heads and necks and cutting from their stalks

The fighters' helmets where the wood crashed, sickening, home.
Yet with great effort they turned the enemy to flight.
I raised the war-cry, and I went into a dance,
And clapped my hands, but they streamed toward the Theban gates.
The wail of lamentation rose throughout the city
Of young and old; they filled the temple precincts full,
In terror. Though he could have gone right through the walls,
Theseus held off. For he had said he did not come
To sack the city but to gather up the dead.   720
      This is the kind of general that a city should choose,
One brave in danger, one who hates a violent folk
Who, faring well, still seek to climb the highest rungs
Of ladders to lose the happiness they might enjoy.
CHORUS: Now looking on this day I did not hope to see,
    In gods I do believe, and think that my bad luck
    Is less since these have paid their proper penalty.
ADRASTUS: O Zeus, why do men say poor mortal men are wise?
    We all depend on you; we do what you permit.
    Once Argos was a city irresistible   730
    With many young men, strong of arm, who formed our group.
    When Eteocles offered peace on equal footing
    And moderate terms we did not wish to deal with him.
    And then we perished. He in turn then fortunate,
    Just like a poor man coming into sudden wealth,
    Grew proudly wanton; in his pride his people fell,
    The foolish folk of Cadmus: mortal empty-heads,
    Who stretch the bow beyond the limit that is just!
    You suffer just deserts who suffer many ills;
    You heed not friends but only bitter circumstance.   740
    And, cities, when you could turn woes aside through words,
    You settle matters by the sword, not common sense.
      But why say this? I'd like to know how you yourself
    Were saved from death; and then I'll ask you all the rest.
MESSENGER: When uproar shook the city, as spears were shaken too,
    I passed the gates through which the warriors had come.
ADRASTUS: And do you bring the dead for whom the fight arose?
MESSENGER: Yes, all the seven chiefs from seven noble homes.
ADRASTUS: What's that you say? But where's the rest of those who
    died?
MESSENGER: They're given to their tombs in glens of Cithaeron.   750
ADRASTUS: On their side or near our side? Who has buried them?
MESSENGER: Theseus, where rises the shady Eleutherian rock.
ADRASTUS: Where did you leave the dead he left above the ground?
MESSENGER: Nearby. For very close is all we've struggled for.

ADRASTUS: No doubt in bitterness the servants bore them off.

MESSENGER: There was no servant there to bury any dead.

ADRASTUS: . . . .

MESSENGER: You'd call him noble if you saw his deep respect.

ADRASTUS: And did he wash the wounds of the wretched ones himself?

MESSENGER: Yes; and he spread the couches, covered up their frames.

ADRASTUS: A dreadful burden, one that might have brought him
    shame.   760

MESSENGER: What shame is there among men's troubles, each to each?

ADRASTUS: Ah, grief! I wish that I had died along with them.

MESSENGER: You mourn in vain; you draw from these a mournful tear.

ADRASTUS: I seem to do so; these women are my teachers.
    But come; I'll lift my hand and go to meet the dead.
  The song of death that flows with tears I'll sing for them.
  I'll greet my friends; bereft of them I'm miserable,
  Alone, alone. This is the only loss for men
  We can't bring back, a mortal life; wealth we can reach.

CHORUS: — Some things are well, but some unhappy;   770
        A good report to the city,
        For those who bore the spear
        A double honor now.

      For me to look on the limbs of my children,
      A bitter yet honorable sight if I shall see
        The day unhoped for,
      I who have seen the greatest grief of all.

      — Would that unmarried ever up to this time
        The ancient father of days,
        Chronus, had brought me this day!   780
        What need of children had I?
      Then I should have hope against suffering
      The wildest of woes, had I been unwed,
        But now I see clearly, too clearly,
      This evil, deprived of dear sons.

      — But now I look on the bodies
      Of children departed: poor me!
      Would I had died with my darlings,
        Gone down with them, down into Hades!

ADRASTUS: Your lament, O mothers,   790
        For corpses that go underground,
      Utter, raise up, in answer to mine,
        As you hear my lament.

CHORUS:	O children, O bitter the greeting Of mothers who love you, I speak to you, dead as you are.

ADRASTUS: Io, io!
CHORUS: I wail for my woe.
ADRASTUS: Ai, ai!
CHORUS: . . . . . .
ADRASTUS: We have suffered, oh . . .
CHORUS: Such grief as a dog should not suffer.
ADRASTUS: O city of Argos, do you behold not my plight?   800

CHORUS: They look upon me, the pitiful,
            Shorn of my sons.

ADRASTUS: Bring on the blood-dripping bodies
            Of ill-fated youths
            Cut down unworthily by an unworthy foe
            Who decided the struggle.

CHORUS: Give them to me, so enfolding
            My hands for embrace I can press
            Their dear bodies within my arms.

ADRASTUS: You have them, you have them.
CHORUS: The weight of our grief is too much.   810
ADRASTUS: Ai, ai!
CHORUS: Do you sigh as well for the mothers?
ADRASTUS: Listen to me.
CHORUS: You groan for the sorrows of both.
ADRASTUS: Would that the ranks of the Thebans had slain me amid
            the dust!

CHORUS: Would that my body had never
            Been yoked in wedlock to a man!

ADRASTUS: Look on this sea of troubles, O
            You wretched mothers of children!

CHORUS: Our faces are furrowed with nail-prints; we have
            Poured dust around our heads.

ADRASTUS: Io, io, for me! For me!   820
            Would that earth's plain would engulf me,
            A whirlwind might seize me,
        A flame of fire from Zeus fall on my head!

CHORUS: You have looked upon bitter marriage,
                   Bitter prophecy of Phoebus;
               Upon you has come the Fury of many wails;
               She has left the lone house of Oedipus for you.

           (*Enter* THESEUS.)

THESEUS: What I was about to ask you when you poured forth grief
       For the army, I'll let that pass, leave out the words
       I had in mind for you; Adrastus now I see.   830
       Whence ever were born these soldiers of spirit surpassing
       All mortals? Speak to me, since you are the wiser,
       And to the younger citizens, since you understand.
       For you* saw greater deeds of daring done by them
       Than one could tell, by which they hoped to take the city.
       One thing I shall not ask you; you would only laugh:
       Against whom each of these stood up to wage the fight
       Or which gave which the spear-wound that he bore away.
       For these are empty stories, both for those who listen
       And for the one who tells, whoever goes to fight   840
       And stands while spears are whizzing thickly past his eyes
       To give a clear report on who was brave or not.
       I could not ask this question, nor could I believe
       The man who dared to say he knew the truth of it;
       It would be hard for anyone who faced the foe
       To see the things he had to see to stay alive.
ADRASTUS: Hear me then; the opportunity you give to me
       For speaking praise of those dear friends I wish to praise
       Is one I welcome, and to say what's just and true.
             You see this delicate corpse, through which the lightning flew?
       This is Capaneus; he was a man who had great wealth,   851
       But took small pride in it; nor did his mind aspire
       Beyond the thoughts of poor men; he was not a man
       To mix with diners whose table always swelled with food,
       Disdaining moderation; for he often said
       That good lay not in gluttony but in just enough.
       He was a friend to all his friends both tried and true,
       To those at hand and those away: such friends are few.
       He never lied; his character was amiable;
       He never made a promise he did not fulfill   860
       To citizens or servants. Here lies the second man,

---

* I emend εἶδον (844) to εἶδες, (i.e., Adrastus) since Theseus did not see
the battle of the Seven against Thebes.

Eteoclus, another who practiced virtue too;
He was a youth without much means of livelihood,
But yet he had the greatest honors in the Argive land.
When many times his friends would offer to give him gold
He did not take it into his house to make his ways
Like those of slaves yoked slavishly to things alone.
He hated those who missed the mark, he did not hate
The city, because the city itself is not to blame
When a bad helmsman brings it into bad repute.   870
   The third of these, Hippomedon, was good by nature.
While yet a boy he struggled not for the delights
The Muses give, nor for the ease of leisured life;
He lived outdoors and made his mind and body strong,
Rejoiced in manliness, went on long hunting trips,
Rejoiced in horses, stretched the bow in his own hands,
Wishing to make his person useful to the city.
   This other body, son of the huntress Atalanta,
Parthenopaeus, most renowned for his good looks,
Was an Arcadian, but he came to Inachus' river   880
To spend his youth in Argos, and was reared up there.
First, as befits all guests who share another state,
He was not troublesome nor a nuisance to the city.
He did not quarrel with words (prime cause of those
Ill feelings between foreigners and citizens).
He took his place in the army like an Argive born,
Defended Argos; whenever the city was well off,
He felt great joy, but he was sad if it fared ill.
Men loved him, many, and the women not a few;
He kept his head and never once wronged any one.   890
   The great glory of Tydeus I'll sum up in brief:
[Not brilliant at a speech, he was a clever man
At fighting with a shield and wise in strategy.
His brother Meleager had a better brain,
But Tydeus was his equal in the art of war,
And made an exact science of the shield and spear.]
His character was rich in love of honor, but
His mind was fitted more for noble deeds than words.
   From all the things I've said don't be surprised, Theseus,
That these men dared to die before the Theban towers.   900
Trained to be noble from their youth, they shunned disgrace;
For every man trained to good deeds would be ashamed
To be a coward. Human courage is a thing
That must be taught to men, just as the child is taught
To say and hear the things it has no knowledge of.

And what he learns a person often keeps in mind
Until old age. So educate your children well.

CHORUS: Oh, my child, unhappy
　　　　　I bore you, under my heart
　　　　　I suffered the pains of childbirth; now　　　910
　　　　　Hades has all the labor
　　　　　I suffered for you;
　　　　　I have no child to cherish my old age,
　　　　　I who gave birth to you.

THESEUS: Truly the gods who snatched away the noble child *
Of Oicleus alive into the earth's dark depths
With chariot and all gave him clear eulogy;
Yet praising Oedipus's son, Polynices,
We should not tell a lie; he was a guest of mine
Before he left the city of Cadmus in his flight,　　　920
Self-chosen, passing over to the Argive land.
But do you know what I want done about these things?
ADRASTUS: I don't know more than one fact: to obey your words.
THESEUS: Capaneus, stricken by the thunderbolt of Zeus ...
ADRASTUS: You wish to bury him apart, an awesome corpse?
THESEUS: Yes; all the others may be burnt in one great fire.
ADRASTUS: Where will you place his monument quite separate?
THESEUS: Right here; I'll build his tomb close to this very house.
ADRASTUS: The slaves shall shortly undertake this mournful task.
THESEUS: We'll care for them; now let the load of dead approach.　930
ADRASTUS: Go, wretched mothers, now approach your lifeless sons.
THESEUS: Adrastus, most unfitting are the words you've spoken.
ADRASTUS: How so? Ought not the mothers come to touch their sons?
THESEUS: They'd die if they should see them changed so terribly.
ADRASTUS: A bitter sight are blood and scars upon the dead.
THESEUS: Why do you wish to add that grief to all they bear?
ADRASTUS: I yield: the women must wait patiently; Theseus
Speaks well; but when we place the dead upon the fire,
Take up the charred bones. O you suffering mortal men,
Why own a spear and use it to destroy, to kill　　　940
Each other? Stop: but when you've given up your war,
Guard quietly your cities in tranquillity.
A little thing is life; but we should spend it well,
As easily and free from labor as we can.

---

* Amphiareus.

CHORUS: — No longer fair children, fair
Offspring have I, nor a
Share among mothers of children in Argos,
No; Artemis, goddess of
Childbirth, says nothing to
Childless women.   950
My life is no life,
And like a driven cloud
I am harried by terrible winds.

— Seven mothers, we bore seven
Sons, we wretched ones,
The seven most famous in Argos;
Now childless, bereft of sons,
I grow old most miserably,
Unnumbered among the
Dead and the living,   960
Possessing a lot that is separate from these.

— Tears only are left me;
Sad memories at home,
The locks I cut from his hair,
The garlands I placed on his head,
[Libations poured out for the dead]
And songs which the golden-haired god
Apollo does not receive;
And awakened so early by groans,
I wet, ever damp with my tears,   970
The folds of the robe on my breast.

— And here I see the bridal chamber
Of Capaneus and his holy tomb.
Outside the house
The offerings of Theseus I see,
And the noble wife of the dead
Slain by the lightning, Evadne,
Whom king Iphis begot as his child.
Why does she stand on the rock
That towers above this house   980
Turning her steps this way?

EVADNE: What light, what brilliant beam
Did the sun then chariot
Through the sky, and the moon

Through upper air so fine?
Where the swift-footed nymphs
Carry their torches like riders
Through night, when for my marriage
The city of Argos raised
Its song of happiness high   990
As a tower for me and my husband,
Capaneus, ai ai, of bronze armor.
I have come to you from my house,
   Frantic with Bacchic desire
   To seek for myself the fire,
   The tomb that is his,
To loosen in Hades my life,
   Weary with trouble and care.
   Sweetest of deaths to die
   With dear ones who are dying,   1000
    If god might bring this to pass.

CHORUS: Indeed you see the pyre near which you took your stand,
   The treasure-chest of Zeus in which your husband lies,
   Subdued in death beneath the flaming thunderbolts.

EVADNE: I see the end at last
Where I have stood; good fortune
Joins my journey here.
But for the sake of honor
I'll rush from off this rock
And leap into the fire   1010
   Mingling my body in bright
Flame with my darling, my dear,
Joining my flesh to his flesh,
I'll come to Persephone's room.
   I'll never betray you though dead,
   Underground, by clinging to life.
    Farewell the torch, the wedding bed;
    Farewell whatever marriages
And decent nuptials may take place in Argos,
   With those who follow me.   1020
   Holy a lawful wedded husband,
   Flesh joined to flesh in guiltless breath,
   Loved by a noble wife.

CHORUS: Indeed it is your father who is stepping near,
   The aged Iphis come to hold a younger speech

Which ignorant of before he will be grieved to hear.

IPHIS: Poor woman, I'm an old man and I'm wretched too;
I come here with a double grief upon my house:
To bring by sea the body of Eteoclus,
My son who died in war at Thebes back home again;   1030
To seek my daughter too, who is Capaneus' wife;
She vanished from my home, eager to die with him.
I kept her guarded in the house before; and when
I eased my watch, in sorrow with my present ills,
She left me. But no doubt I'll find her here with you;
Please tell me if you know where I can find her now.

EVADNE: Why do you ask the women? Here; I'm on this rock;
Like some wild bird above Capaneus' funeral fire
I teeter lightly in my wretchedness, father.

IPHIS: Daughter, what wind has blown you here? What clothes are
these?   1040
Why did you run away from home and come into this land?

EVADNE: You would be angry if you heard my plots and schemes.
I do not wish that you should hear them, father dear.

IPHIS: Why not? Is it not right for your own father to know?

EVADNE: You would not be a wise judge of what I must do.

IPHIS: But why this dress? It's different from the ones you wear.

EVADNE: This dress means something famous and well-known, father.

IPHIS: It's not the proper mourning garment for a widow.

EVADNE: I've dressed myself for something new and strange to hear.

IPHIS: And then you stand beside the tomb, beside the fire?   1050

EVADNE: Yes, here indeed I come a glorious conqueror.

IPHIS: Winning what victory? I'd like to know from you.

EVADNE: I conquer all women whom the sun looks on.

IPHIS: In handwork of Athena or the mind's shrewd plan?

EVADNE: In courage; when I die I'll lie beside my man.

IPHIS: What do you say? What hollow riddle do you pose?

EVADNE: I'll leap upon this pyre of dead Capaneus.

IPHIS: O daughter, do not say these words before the crowd.

EVADNE: That's just the thing I want, that all Argives should know.

IPHIS: But I shall never let you do the deed you plan.   1060

EVADNE: It's all the same to me. You cannot catch my hand.
I've let my body go — it won't be pleasant for you,
But this is what I want, to burn with him to death.

(EVADNE *throws herself from the rock onto the pyre.*)

CHORUS: O woman, you have done a terrible thing.

IPHIS: I'm lost, I'm done for, daughters of the Argive men.

CHORUS: Ee, ee, suffering these cruelties.

You will see a deed beyond all daring deeds.

IPHIS: No one could find another that shocks me more than this.

CHORUS: Oh miserable!

You share the fate of Oedipus, poor old man, 1070
You and my suffering city, each a share.

IPHIS: Oimoi! Why do not mortals have this privilege,
To be young men and to be old men twice in turn?
For in our homes if anything is not in order,
By taking second thoughts we set it right again.
We can't do this with age; if we were young again
Two times and old men likewise, if a person erred,
We might correct him, having won a double life.
When I saw others begetting children, raising them,
I loved them too and by my love I was undone. 1080
If I had come to this and had begotten mine,
Had learned what fathers suffer when their children die,
I would not ever have come to this point in my grief.
I who begot a boy, the best of sons for me,
Am now bereaved; I've lost him after all my care.

So let it be. What must I do, a man bereft?
Go home again, to see the desolation there
Of many homes, to drag out life in poverty?
Or shall I go to the dwelling of this Capaneus?
How sweet it was before when daughter lived with me! 1090
But she is gone; she used to press this beard of mine
Close to her lips and take my head into her hands.
There's nothing sweeter than a girl when father's old;
The souls of men are greater but less sweet to coax.
O won't you take me home as fast as we can go?
Give me to darkness; there I'll starve and waste away.
My aged body dwindling slowly I'll destroy.
What good will it do me now to touch my daughter's bones?

Old age, so hard to fight, I hold and hate you too,
I hate you and the men who wish to lengthen life, 1100
With food and drink and spells of magic to divert
The stream, so not to die; they should have long ago,
Because they are no good on earth, have died and given
Their place to young men, vanishing away from sight.

CHORUS: Oh, oh!
Here are the bones of my dead sons;
They're carried here; take me, handmaidens,
Old, strengthless woman — there's no force
Left in me, for I grieve.

I've lived a long time, but I'm pining 1110
Away in death because of sorrow.
What greater suffering can you find
Than this for mortals,
　　To look on children dead?

BOYS: 　I bring, I bring,
Poor mother, father's bones from the fire,
A weight not light because of woes.
　　I put my all in a little space.

CHORUS: 　Oh, oh!
　　Where do you bring what calls the tears 1120
　　To a mother dear of the ones who died?
A little heap of ash instead of bodies
　　Once famous in Mycenae?

BOYS: 　Childless, childless!
And I am wretched, bereft of my poor father,
I shall be orphaned in a barren home,
　　Not cherished in my father's hands.

CHORUS: 　Oh, oh!
　　Where is my childbirth labor?
　　Where is the joy of marriages? 1130
The care a mother gives, her sleepless vigils,
　　Sweet kisses on the mouth?

BOYS: 　They're gone, they are no more; oimoi, my father!
They're gone.

CHORUS: 　　The air above us holds them now,
　　　Melted to ash of fire,
　　　They've winged their way to Hades.

BOYS: 　Father, don't you hear your children's moans?
Shall I ever, shield on arm, avenge your death?
　　May justice for my father come, god willing.

CHORUS: 　　Not yet does evil sleep. 1140
　　　Ah woes! Enough of sorrow,
　　　Enough of pain there is for me.

BOYS: The waters of Asopus will yet receive me,
A general of the Danaïds in brazen armor,
Avenger of my dead father.
I seem to see you still, father, before my eyes . . .

CHORUS: Placing a sweet kiss upon your cheek.

BOYS: And the bracing courage of your words
Is gone, borne in the air.

CHORUS: The grief of two he left his mother.   1150
But grief for your father will never leave you.

BOYS: I have so great a weight that it has killed me.

CHORUS: Come, I shall sprinkle the beloved dust around my breast.

BOYS: I weep as I hear this word,
Most hateful; it has touched my heart.

CHORUS: O child, you have gone; no more
Shall I look on you, the dear delight of a mother.

THESEUS: Adrastus and you women sprung from Argive stock,
You see these children bearing in their little hands
The bodies of their noble fathers which I gained for them: 1160
I and my city give them as a gift to you.
But you must now remember for their sake to be
Forever grateful, seeing what you've won through me.
And to the children I have whispered these same words,
To honor this city as generations follow each,
Hand down the memory of the favors you have won.
With Zeus as witness and the other gods in heaven,
How you are honored by us, take your way again.

ADRASTUS: Theseus, we know the kind deeds you've done the Argive
land,
When she had need of kindness; we shall owe to you   1170
A gratitude unaging for your noble gifts;
We must repay you, we whom you have treated well.

THESEUS: What other favors may I offer you besides?

ADRASTUS: Farewell; a worthy man you are, from a worthy city.

THESEUS: So be it; may good luck to you and yours befall.

ATHENA (*who appears unexpectedly*):
Hear, Theseus, now Athena's words and her command,

Which you must do, and when you've done, reap benefit.
Give not these bones for transfer to the Argive land
By little boys and let them go so easily,
But for your toils and for your city's helpfulness   1180
First obtain an oath. This must Adrastus swear;
He is the proper person since he's king in charge
To pledge an oath for all the land of Danaids.
This oath shall be: the Argives never shall invade
This land with armies, send in hostile armament;
If others come, they shall prevent them with the spear.
But if, breaking the oath, they come against you, then
Beseech the gods to ruin Argos utterly.
    Hear now from me the place where you must slay the beasts.
You have a tripod with brass feet inside your house,   1190
Which Heracles, when he had upset Ilium,
And was in haste to set out on another task
Told you to place before the hearth of Pythia.
When you have cut the throats of three sheep, write on this
The oath, inside the tripod's hollow vessel, and
Give it to him who'll keep it, to the Delphic god
As a remembrance of the oath for Greece to see.
But hide the sharp-edged sword with which you cut their throats
And kill the beasts within a hole deep in the earth
Beside the seven funeral pyres of the dead.   1200
For it will scare them if they come against the city,
When it is shown, and make them turn in evil flight.
When you have done this, send the bodies from the land.
But leave the precinct where they were consumed in fire
As sacred to Apollo, by his three-way road.
    I've said these words to you; to Argive sons I say:
Attack the city of Ismenus when you're of age,
Avenge your fathers' death, who fell before its gates,
You for your father, Aigialeus, as general,
A youthful leader; and you, the son of Tydeus —   1210
Your father called you Diomede — from Aetolia.
But just as soon as beard casts shade upon your chin
Send brass-armed men of Argos in their battle-dress
Against the seven-gated walls of Cadmus' land.
You'll come in bitterness against them, grown-up cubs
Of raging lions, eager to destroy the city.
There is no other way but this. You will be called
Offspring through Greece; they'll sing of you among the men
To come. Send such an army, by the grace of god.
THESEUS: Mistress Athena, I shall do what you command.   1220

You set me right so that I may not miss the mark,
And I shall bind the man to this by oath. One thing
Alone I ask: to guide me straight, for while you look
With kindness on the city, we'll dwell in safety here.

CHORUS: Let us go, Adrastus, let us swear the oath
To this man and the city; they have toiled for us
And they are worthy of this honor.

EURIPIDES

ANDROMACHE

Translated by L. R. Lind

INTRODUCTION

THE *Andromache* describes the murderous passion and remorse of a childless woman who fears that a more fruitful rival may supplant her in the affections of her husband. This, with a good deal of bluster by Peleus and an obscure intrigue by Orestes, forms the plot of the drama. Its tragedy, perhaps the one universal idea intended in it by the author, lies in the misuse of power over another human being by an unstable and neurotic personality. Force corrupts in this play, as Simone Weil, in her fine essay "The Iliad, or the Poem of Force," has shown that it corrupts in Homer's poem. There is also a kindred theme in Hermione's imminent desertion by Neoptolemus which makes of her almost a Medea in a reversed situation, the legal wife this time jealous of the helpless concubine who is a prize of war. It is the tremendous hair-pulling of Andromache and Hermione which constitutes the essential action. Andromache is one of Euripides' most attractive heroines; her self-sacrifice is almost as impressive as that of Alcestis. Yet her appearance in only the first half of the play is not sufficient to preserve the unity implied in its title. We cannot say a great deal for the remaining characters: Menelaus is a windy coward, Peleus an old faker, and Orestes a cautious and sinister bore.

The play has marked affinities with plays of several types in the *theâtre* of Euripides. If we had more than twenty of the eighty-eight plays he wrote, we might with more confidence be able to speak of the development of his art; but it is clear that the *Andromache* has in it something of *Medea* and even more of the *Suppliants* and *Iphigenia in Tauris*. The Wild West horse-opera effect so frequent in the plays of Euripides becomes almost absurd as Peleus, the railing, impotent old fellow, staggers to the scene to save a lady in distress. There is in the play much of the tear-jerking sentiment which so annoyed the contemporaries of Euripides. Nevertheless, although the construction of the play is defective (it is two plays in one; some would say even three plays in one), although its chief characters except for Andromache are unsympathetic, and its realism heightened at times to ridiculous excess, it is still a compelling drama with a good deal of sound psychology and a considerable understanding of human nature. As a picture of the aftermath of war in its effect upon noncombatants it is an ideal companion-piece to the *Suppliants*, a play chronologically close to it.

In two respects Euripides shows himself an excellent craftsman in these two plays: in passages of rhetorical argument or invective, and in the messengers' speeches, which provide unusually effective climaxes. His narrative skill cannot be too highly praised; his style is sharp and clear, full of exact details and startling images; it grows to pinnacles of suspense which must have been one of Euripides' greater attractions for the Athenian audience.

The usual critical discussions of the *Andromache* and *Suppliants* emphasize the political nature of both plays and treat them as propaganda: the *Suppliants* is an encomium of Athens, and *Andromache* a condemnation of Sparta. However true all this may have been in contemporary Athens, such interpretations leave the ordinary reader cold. What he sees in these plays is chiefly the violent action of human beings driven by their fears, passions, and weakness and suffering for their misdeeds as people still do. It is certainly the characters and their realistic movement, not any possible political interpretation of them (that Theseus, for example, represents Alcibiades) upon which the modern reader will concentrate his attention. In other words, how good is Euripides as "theater," as an analyst of human behavior, as a poet who deals in universal ideas? How does he compare in effectiveness with Shaw and Ibsen? (Hermione might well be closely compared to Hedda Gabler.) What does he have to tell us today in his commentaries on human folly? How genuine is his realism? The reader will find that Euripides, like Shaw and sometimes Ibsen, occasionally creates a realism which is not entirely authentic but colored by personal prejudice and perversity.

The play was presented between 430 and 424 B.C. Sparta, the Spartans, and the god Apollo are especially criticized in it, and the line of Achilles, in the person of his son Neoptolemus, is looked upon with sympathy. Orestes, the son of Agamemnon and the slayer of his mother, Clytemnestra, is the villain of the piece. The plot concerns particularly the question of Hermione's marriage to Neoptolemus, when she had earlier been affianced to Orestes. Andromache falls between the two contenders here, particularly under Hermione's hate. The scene is Phthia, the home of Neoptolemus to which he has brought his prize of war, Andromache.

L. R. LIND

ANDROMACHE

◨

CHARACTERS

ANDROMACHE, *slave of Neoptolemus*
SERVANT GIRL
HERMIONE, *daughter of Menelaus*
MENELAUS
BOY, *son of Andromache*
PELEUS, *grandfather of Neoptolemus*
NURSE
ORESTES, *son of Agamemnon*
MESSENGER
THETIS, *wife of Peleus, mother of Achilles*
CHORUS *of women of Phthia*

SCENE. *At the shrine of Thetis near Phthia, the home of Neoptolemus. Andromache, a suppliant, utters the prologue.*

ANDROMACHE: Pride of Asia's land, the city-state of Thebes,*
From which I came with dowry of gold and luxury
To Priam's house, the hearthstone of a sovereign king,
Given as wife to Hector, to bear boys for him,
Andromache, an envied girl in times long past,
But now the unhappiest woman that has ever lived,
I have stood by to see my Hector lying dead
Beneath Achilles' hand; the boy Astyanax

---

* In northeast Asia; not to be confused with cities of the same name in central Greece and in Egypt.

I bore my husband thrown down from the straight tall towers
Upon that day when Greeks captured the plain of Troy.   10
And I a slave, who once was member of a house
Most free, have come to Hellas; Neoptolemus
The islander has picked me from the Trojan loot.
I dwell in ground near Phthia and Pharsalia
Where the sea-goddess Thetis lived with Peleus
Apart from men; and all the folk of Thessaly
Call this place Thetideion, where she married him.
Achilles' son has taken up a dwelling here;
Pharsalian rule he gives to father Peleus.
He does not wish to take it from him while he lives.   20
And mingling with Achilles' son I bear a boy
To him and to his house; he is my master now.

     And yet before, although I lay in misery,
Hope urged me on: if my boy should be saved, grow up,
I'd find some aid, protection in my suffering.
But since my master has wed the Spartan Hermione,
Abandoning my bed (I'm nothing but a slave),
She drives me cruelly, treats me worse than any slave.
She says I've made her childless with my secret drugs
And hateful to her husband; that I wish to take   30
Her place and live here, casting out her marriage right
By force. I never wished that right from the very first,
And now I've left it! Mighty Zeus, be witness here,
I never shared his bed in willing love at all.
I can't convince her, and she wants to kill me now;
Her father Menelaus joins her in this plan.
And now he's in the house, he's come from Sparta straight
To do the deed. I'm frightened and I've come to sit
At Thetis' shrine so close beside my master's house,
If it may save my life. For Peleus and his kin   40
Respect the shrine, memorial of the wedding day
Of Nereus' daughter. Him who is my only son
I've sent away in secret to another house.
I am afraid they'll kill him, for his father's not
At hand to help me or the boy, because he's gone
To Delphi, where he will atone to Loxias
Since in his madness he once went there to demand
For his dead father satisfaction from the god;
If somehow he can beg forgiveness for his past
Mistakes, he might make Phoebus kindly from now on.   50
SERVANT GIRL: Mistress — I do not shrink at all from calling you
This name, since that is what I called you in your house

When both of us lived once upon the Trojan plain,
And I was fond of you and Hector while he lived.
But now I bring you news, although I am afraid
Some one among the masters might get wind of it.
I pity you. They're plotting fearful things for you,
Menelaus and his daughter: you must be on guard.

ANDROMACHE: O dearest fellow-slave — for that is what you are
To me who was your queen but now unfortunate — 60
What are they doing? What snares do they weave for me,
Who wish to kill me, I most miserable of all?

SERVANT: It is your boy they plan to kill, poor creature you,
The boy you sent away in secret from this house.

ANDROMACHE: Oimoi! Then she has learned I've sent my boy away?
But how and when? O wretched me, completely lost!

SERVANT: I do not know, but I learned this from their very lips:
Menelaus is gone from home, gone after him.

ANDROMACHE: I'm done for surely. O my child, they'll slaughter you,
The clawing vultures that they are! But he who's called 70
Your father happens to be still at Delphi's shrine.

SERVANT: I do not think you would fare ill like this if he
Were here, but now you haven't any friends at all.

ANDROMACHE: Has no word reached us that Peleus is coming?

SERVANT: He is too old to help you even if he came.

ANDROMACHE: And yet I've sent for him not once but many times.

SERVANT: You don't think the men you sent are really loyal?

ANDROMACHE: Why not? Will you go carry word for me to him?

SERVANT: What shall I tell them when I'm gone so long from home?

ANDROMACHE: You'll find a lot of ways to trick them; you're a woman.

SERVANT: There's danger; Hermione is no trifling guard. 81

ANDROMACHE: You see? You won't help friends when they're in
trouble.

SERVANT: That isn't true. You should not say such words to me.
I'll go: my life is not worth much, a female slave's;
It doesn't matter if I meet with danger now.

ANDROMACHE: Then go. But I'll send up the groans and cries and
tears
To which I've always yielded, up into the sky.
For women like to keep their troubles ever in
Their mouths, and always keep them on their tongues as well.
I have not one but many sorrows to bewail: 90
My native city, my dead husband Hector, and
The hard and cruel fate to which I have been yoked,
Who fell on slavery's day without deserving it.
We must not ever say a man finds happiness

Until he dies and you can see how he has spent
His final day on earth before he goes below.

To lofty Ilium Paris led Helen not as a bridegroom
 Leads a girl to his bed, but like a fury of fate;
For sake of her, O Troy, with ravening spear and with fire
 Swift Ares, a thousand boats, from Greece laid hands on you,
And my poor husband Hector the son of Thetis of ocean   101
 Dragged at his chariot wheel round and round near the walls.
But out of the bridal chamber they led me down to the seashore
 And covered my head with shame, with slavery's terrible veil.
The tears, the tears fell down my cheeks the day that I parted
 From city, from home, from you, dear husband dead in the dust.
Oimoi, I am wretched with grief; why must I look on light longer,
 A slave to Hermione now, who wears me down with her hate?
A suppliant here by her statue, I fling my arms round the goddess,
 I waste away like the water that runs in a rill from the stone.

CHORUS: O woman, you sit by the shrine and precinct of Thetis 111
   Long, and you do not leave.
  A Phthian, I come to you born of the Asian race,
   If I can in any way
   Cut up a drug that will soothe your pains.
  They have hemmed you and Hermione in with hate
   And strife, poor wretch, round the bed
   Of a double marriage: your own
   And hers with Achilles' son.
  Know your fate, think of the pass you have come to. 120
   Do you struggle with masters,
  A daughter of Troy, with offspring of Lacedaemon?
   Leave the sheep-taking home,
  The shrine of the goddess of ocean. What need
  To waste your sweet body away with an ugly woe
   At the force of your masters?
   But power will make you yield. Why suffer
   This toil? You are less than naught.
  But come now, leave the lovely shrine of the Nereid,
   Learn that you are a slave   130
   In another city, a strange
   Land where you see no friends,
   Most ill-fated of all,
    Poor wretched bride.
  Deeply pitied by me, O woman of Troy, you have come
   To the house of my masters; but I
   In my fear I am silent —

Though mourning the lot that you bear —
Lest the daughter of Zeus should discover
My pitying good will for you.   140

HERMIONE: I wear no ornament of precious gold around
  My head, no robe of richly woven stuff I wear
  As first-fruits from Achilles or from Peleus,
  Although I come straight to this place from their great home.
  But from the land of Sparta, from Laconian soil,
  My father Menelaus gave me these fine things
  With many bridal gifts so that I may speak out
  In freedom and give answer in such words as these:
      You are a slave, a woman captured by the spear,
  And yet you wish to own this house, to cast me out,   150
  And make me hated by my husband through your drugs:
  Through you my womb is barren and it wastes away.
  The mind, the soul of Asiatic women are
  Quite clever for these ends: but I shall hold you back.
  And this, the home of Thetis, will not help at all;
  No shrine, no altar will, but you shall die.
  If any mortal, any god should wish to save
  You, you must drop those haughty thoughts you had before
  And crouch submissively, fall down here at my knees,
  And sweep this house of mine, sprinkling from the gilded   160
  Vessels the dew of Achelous' stream the while.
  And know what land you're in. There is no Hector here,
  No Priam and no gold, but a Greek city-state.
  To this degree of witlessness you've come, you wretch,
  Who dare to sleep with the son of the man who killed
  Your husband and bear children to the murderer.
  That is the kind of people all barbarians are!
  Father with daughter, son with mother sleep in sin,
  Sister with brother, dearest kin kills dearest kin,
  And no law stops this. Don't bring us such hideous acts.   170
  It is not well for one man to hold reins on two
  Women, but looking at one love upon their beds
  Men are content — that's if they wish to live in peace.
CHORUS: An envious thing for sure is the female mind
  And always hateful to its rival for men's love.
ANDROMACHE: Pheu, pheu!
  An evil for mortals is youth, and in one's youth
  Evil for any man to be unjust to men.
  I fear because I am a slave that this will keep
  Me from the words I'd speak to you with perfect right.   180

Yet if I should prevail on you, I'd pay for this;
The high and mighty bear with bitterness the words,
Though more convincing, of those subject to their will.
But all the same I'll not appear to betray my cause.

  Young lady, tell me, by what word that's worth belief
Are you persuaded that I wish to seize your man?
Is it because the Spartan city's smaller than
The Phrygians', I'm in luck, and you see me free?
Or is it that my body's young and beautiful,
And I am proud of my great city and my friends   190
That I should wish to wrest your house out of your hands?
Or that I shall bear children for him in your place,
Though mine will be enslaved, a wretched drag on me?
Or that my sons will rule in Phthia if you have none?
Because the Greeks love me and for dear Hector's sake,
Though I am humble and not a queen of Phrygians?
It's not my poison that makes your husband hate you;
It's just because you're not a woman fit for him.
This too is a love-spell: it's not loveliness alone
But patient virtues that delight a man in bed.   200
To soothe your jealousy, then Sparta *is* a great
City; then Scyros is not any land at all;
You're rich among the poor, and Menelaus is
A greater than Achilles. This is why your man
Hates you. And even if a woman gets a bad
Husband, she should be glad and not keep arguing.
But if in Thrace where snow and ice flow everywhere
You had a royal husband, where men share and share
Alike their beds with many women, turn by turn,
Would you have killed the others? Then you would have brought
The charge of greediness for love on every wife.   211
It's a low habit; yet we suffer from its ill
More than the men, although we're better at hiding it.

  Hector dear, I loved your sweethearts for your sake;
If Love herself led you astray toward other loves,
I often gave my breast to your bastard children
So that I might not rouse the bitterness in you.
And acting thus I drew my husband with virtue.
But you're afraid to let a drop of dew from heaven
Fall on your husband. Do not try to beat your mother   220
At loving men, for children that have any sense
Should shun the ways that brought their mothers to disgrace.

CHORUS: Mistress, as far as you may easily be won,
 So far be now persuaded by the words she speaks.

HERMIONE: Why do you play the pedant and contend with words,
As though you're chaste alone, and I am quite unchaste?
ANDROMACHE: You are unchaste, to judge from what you've said just
now.
HERMIONE: Woman, I hope *your* mind may never dwell with me.
ANDROMACHE: You're young, and yet you talk about some shameful
things.   229
HERMIONE: You don't talk of them; you *do* them to me, all you can.
ANDROMACHE: But won't you grieve about your love-pain silently?
HERMIONE: What's that? When this is first in every woman's mind?
ANDROMACHE: Yes, when she treats love well; if not, it's only shame.
HERMIONE: We do not run our city by barbarian laws.
ANDROMACHE: Both here and there vile deeds bring on their own dis-
grace.
HERMIONE: Wise, wise, that's you; but you must perish just the same.
ANDROMACHE: Do you see Thetis' statue looking at you here?
HERMIONE: Yes, hating your country for Achilles' murder.
ANDROMACHE: Helen, your mother, murdered him; it was not I.
HERMIONE: What, will you touch upon my ills again, again?   240
ANDROMACHE: Look, I am silent and I shut my lips up tight.
HERMIONE: Speak out instead the reason why I've come to you.
ANDROMACHE: I say you haven't as much sense as you ought to have.
HERMIONE: Will you not leave the holy precinct of the nymph?
ANDROMACHE: If I'm to live; but if to die, I'll never leave.
HERMIONE: My mind's made up. I'll not wait for my man to come.
ANDROMACHE: But neither will I yield myself to you before.
HERMIONE: I'll bring you fire, I'll make you suffer terribly.
ANDROMACHE: Light up your flame. The gods will know the deeds you
do.
HERMIONE: They'll know the pains of dreadful wounds upon your
flesh.   250
ANDROMACHE: Kill me, spill blood on the goddess' altar; she'll punish
you.
HERMIONE: O barbarian creature you, bold, hard, and fierce,
You brave out death? I'll swiftly pull you off the seat
You cling to even if you will not come along.
I have a bait for you, but I shall hide my plans;
The deed itself will quickly show you what I mean.
Sit where you are, for even if around you poured
A stream of melted lead I'll snatch you from the place
Before the man you trust, Achilles' son, returns.
ANDROMACHE: I trust him. But it's strange one of the gods above   260
Has given to mortals medicine for serpent bites
But never found a cure for savage women who

Are worse than any snakes, are worse than fire itself.
So great an evil are we women to mankind.

CHORUS: Surely he caused great grief, when to Idaean
        Woods came Maia's son
        (Also the son of Zeus),
        Leading three fillies, the car
        Of three goddesses, gleaming-yoked,
   Helmeted, armed for hateful quarrel of beauty,   270
        To the herdsman's shed,
      To the shepherd, the lonely youth,
        And the deserted
      Hearth of the hut, his home.

But when they came to the mountain grove thick-grown
        With trees, they washed their gleaming
          Bodies in gushing streams;
        They came to the son of Priam
        With overstraining of speech,
 As they vied with each other: Cypris caught him with words,   280
        Guileful and pleasant to hear
      But bitter destruction of life to the Phrygian city
                  Unlucky,
        And to the towers of Troy.

Yet I wish she had dashed him to earth,
        She who bore Paris,
         Before the Idae-
        an cliff was his home;
    When beside her prophetic laurel
        Cassandra cried, "Kill him!"   290
        The ruin of Priam's great city.
   To whom did she not go? Which of the chiefs
           Did she not beg
        To kill the small baby?

So upon Ilium would no yoke have come
        Of slavery, nor would you, woman,
         Have found a home
         Among tyrants;
    She would have prevented the sorrows
        Greece suffered round Troy   300
   Where ten years long the young men roamed with their spears,
        Beds would have never been widowed,
            Nor orphaned
        Of young the old men.

MENELAUS: I come, I have your son, whom to another house
  In secret from my daughter you had sent away.
  You prayed this image of the goddess would save you,
  And they'd save him by hiding; you have been found out
  Less shrewd than this man Menelaus, O woman.
  If you don't leave this place and make it bare again,   310
  This boy of yours we'll sacrifice instead of you.
  Consider this then, whether you may wish to die
  Or let him perish for the error that is yours
  And that you've made against my daughter, against me.
ANDROMACHE: Vain glory, glory, how you've swelled their pride in life
  For countless mortals who were born nothing at all!
  I call them happy who win fame in truth alone,
  But those who win it falsely have it not, I say;
  They only seem to be wise men, and that by chance.
  Did you take Troy from Priam, vile as you now are,   320
  By leading companies of picked Greeks against his town?
  You breathe such wrath from words your daughter, a mere child,
  Has spoken, and against a helpless female slave
  You set your strength in contest? I cannot regard
  You any longer worthy of Troy or Troy of you.
  [An outward splendor shines in those who seem to be
  Wise men, but inwardly they're like all men except
  Perhaps in wealth, for money has a mighty power.]
  Come, Menelaus, let's go through our arguments:
  Suppose I'm killed: to please your daughter I'm destroyed;   330
  She'd never escape defilement for the murder.
  And you among most men would have to plead yourself
  A murderer; for as accomplice you'd be forced.
  If I don't die, and run from under that dark fate,
  Would you still murder my boy? How would his father
  Then lightly bear the killing of his only son?
  Troy will not call him such an utter coward;
  He'll take the path he ought to take; he'll show himself
  In deed the true son of Achilles and of Peleus.
  He'll drive your daughter from the house, and when you give   340
  Her to another, what will you say? That she fled,
  With her good sense, from a bad husband? What a lie!
  And who will marry her? Or will you keep her here
  At home, unwedded, white-haired, widowed? O poor man,
  Don't you see how the streams of great unhappiness
  Will flow? How many marriages, all to her pain,
  Would you desire for her, than suffer what I say?
  It is not right to bring great evils on for little
  Gain nor, if we women are a ruinous lot,

For men to make their natures seem like a woman's. 350
For if I drug your daughter, as she says I do,
And make her womb abortive, then I'll willingly
And not against my will crouch at no altars still
But suffer trial before your son-in-law myself:
I could not owe him less for his wife's childlessness.
That is my stand; but as for what is in your mind —
One thing I fear — through quarrel about a woman,
You did destroy the wretched Phrygian city-state.

CHORUS: Too much you've spoken, for a woman faced with men;
The moderation of your mind is shot and spent. 360

MENELAUS: These things are trifles, woman, of my monarchy
Unworthy, as you say, unworthy of all Greece.
But know this well: whatever any man may crave,
This need is greater for each man than to take Troy.
And I back up my daughter's cause as her ally,
Since I judge this unwise, to rob her of her rights.
The other griefs a woman might suffer take second place;
But when she loses a husband then she loses life.
And it is right that he should rule over my slaves,
And I and mine rule over him and his as well: 370
There's nothing private where friends are truly friends to each;
The goods they have are held in common, share and share.
Yet while I wait for absent ones, I'd be a fool
And not a wise man if I don't set things to rights.
But now get up and go away from the goddess' shrine
So that if you should die your boy escapes his fate;
If you refuse to die, why then I'll murder him.
One of you two will have to leave this life, I say.

ANDROMACHE: Oimoi, a bitter choice and lot of life you've set.
And if I choose, I'm wretched; if I don't, ill-starred. 380
O you who wreak great havoc for a little cause,
Hear me! Why do you kill me? What's your reason? What
City have I betrayed, which child of yours destroyed?
And which house have I burned? I've gone to bed by force
With masters; then you slaughter me, you don't kill him,
The cause of all these things? Setting aside the source
Of ill, you hasten to its very end instead?
Oimoi for woes like these, unhappy fatherland,
What dreadful pains I suffer! Why should I have borne
A child to make my burdens twice as hard to bear? 390
[But why do I wail for these things, and what's at my feet
I do not weep for * nor count up immediate ills?]

---

* Corrupt; I base my conjecture on the first meaning given in Liddell-Scott.

I who have seen my Hector slaughtered, drawn about
At chariot wheels, and Ilium burning — piteous sights!
And I a slave went down to board the Argive ship,
Dragged by the hair; and when I came to Phthia's land,
To Hector's murderer became a wedded bride.
Why then is life sweet? To what must I look ahead?
To what is present or to fortunes that are gone?
One boy I had was left to me, the eye of life; 400
They're going to kill him, they who think they're doing right.
They shall not do this for the sake of my poor life;
My hope, my all lies in him, if he should be saved;
For me disgrace if I should live and let him die.
  Look you! I quit the altar, I am in your hands,
To kill, to slaughter, bind, hang by the neck till dead.
O child, the one who bore you, so you may not die,
Goes down to Hades; if you should escape my fate
Remember mother, what I suffered, how I died,
And go to kiss your father, throw your little arms 410
Around his neck, wet him with tears, and tell him how
I acted. To all men their children are as life
Itself; the childless censures what he has not known.
He suffers less, but his joy is a misfortune.
CHORUS: I pity as I hear you; piteous are one's woes
To every mortal, even if a stranger weeps.
But, Menelaus, you must come to compromise,
Your daughter and yourself, to set this woman free.
MENELAUS: Seize me the woman, throw your hands around her here,
You servants; she will hear no friendly words from me. 420
So that you might leave free from stain the goddess' shrine
I dangled death before you, your son's death, and so
I led you on into my hands for your own death.
And understand the plight in which you find yourself.
As for this boy, my daughter shall decide his fate,
Whether to kill or not to kill him, at her wish.
But go into the house, slave that you are, and learn
Never to heap insults again on free-born people.
ANDROMACHE: Oimoi! you've tricked me by deceit, I have been fooled.
MENELAUS: Announce the fact to all; I'll not deny it's true. 430
ANDROMACHE: Are tricks like these held clever by Eurotas' folk?
MENELAUS: Yes, and by Trojans: those who suffer take revenge.
ANDROMACHE: You think the gods are not the gods and won't be just?
MENELAUS: When justice comes I'll bear it then; but you I'll kill.
ANDROMACHE: This little fledgling too, dragged from beneath my wing?
MENELAUS: Not he; I'll let my daughter kill him if she likes.
ANDROMACHE: Oimoi! How shall I mourn for you, my little boy?

MENELAUS: I'm sure no bold and confident hope awaits for him.
ANDROMACHE: O you most hateful mortals to all men alive,
    Dwellers in Sparta, crafty councillors, of lies   **440**
    The lords supreme, vile stitchers of an evil plot,
    Crooked and unsound thinkers, twisting all things up,
    Unjustly are you prosperous throughout all Greece.
    What baseness is not in you? Are not murderers,
    Lovers of gain, frequent among you? Don't you speak
    One thing with tongues but always think in other terms?
    May you be damned! My death is not so hard to bear
    As you may think, for those sorrows have destroyed me,
    When that poor Phrygian city crumbled down to ruin,
    And my famed husband died, who often with his spear   **450**
    Made you a coward sailor, not a soldier.
    Now scaring women like a bogey-soldier, you
    Kill me. Kill me then; I won't flatter you or your
    Daughter. For you are great in Sparta, but I am
    Great in Troy, and if I shall fare miserably
    Be not exalted in your pride; you may fare ill.

CHORUS: Never shall I praise the double marriage of mortals
        Nor children born of different mothers,
    Makers of quarrels at home and hateful sorrow.
        Let husbands be contented with one marriage couch,   **460**
            Unshared
        By another man.

For not in cities are twin tyrannies
        Better than one to bear;
They're burden on burden and strife for citizens.
        When two fine craftsmen create a song
            The Muses love
          To set them quarrelling too.

But when swift winds blow sailors out to sea,
        Divided wisdom of minds about the helm,   **470**
A huddled group of wise men, is a weaker guide
        Than that of a lesser mind in full control.
        The power of one is better in a home
        As in a city when men wish to find
           What is the best for both.

The Spartan child of Menelaus has shown
        This truth; she goes through fire against another wife

And kills the wretched girl who came from Troy
And her boy for the sake of hateful strife.
Godless, lawless, graceless is the murder;   480
But yet, dear mistress, a change
For the better will come.

And now I see
The closely clinging pair before the house
Destined to death by vote.
Poor woman, and you, poor boy,
You die for your mother's marriage,
Having no share
Of guilt against the kings.

ANDROMACHE: Look: with my bloody hands   490
Bound in a noose of rope
I'm sent below the earth.
BOY: Mother, mother, under your wing
I'll go down with you.
ANDROMACHE: Terrible sacrifice, O rulers,
Of Phthia's land.
BOY: O father,
Come help the ones you love.
ANDROMACHE: You'll lie there then, my darling,
Upon your mother's breasts,
A corpse under earth, with a corpse.   500
BOY: Omoi, what shall I feel?
But I'll be with you, mother.
MENELAUS: Go under earth, for you have come from
Enemy towers; die, you two,
For two good reasons: my vote slays you,
My daughter Hermione slays the boy.
It's folly to spare an enemy's child
When you can kill him
And take that fear from the house.
ANDROMACHE: O husband, husband, would I had   510
Your hand and spear to fight for me,
O son of Priam.
BOY: Poor me, what song shall I find
To turn aside my fate?
ANDROMACHE: Beseech him, cling to the knees
Of your master, my boy.
BOY: O friend,
Friend, spare me from death.

ANDROMACHE: I wet my pupils with tears,
  I drip as from the steep stone
  In a sunless spot the water, ah wretch . . .   520
BOY: Omoi for me! What healing
    For ill shall I find?
MENELAUS: Why fall before me, praying as
  To some sea-rock or ocean wave?
  I help my own, I do not help
  You, I have no cure for you;
  Since I have wasted a great part of
  My life in taking Troy and your
  Mother, whose deeds now bring
    You harm as you go to Hell.   530
CHORUS: Indeed I see old Peleus coming; he's at hand
  Shuffling an aged foot this way with all his speed.
PELEUS: I ask you all and him who stands to sacrifice,
  What's this? What goes on here? Why has the house grown ill?
  What are you doing? Planning death without a trial?
  Hold, Menelaus! Do not rush beyond the law.
  Lead me on faster, slave boy, for it does not seem
  That there is time to lose; I wish I had again
  My youthful strength, as I have never wished before.
  Just like a ship that sails to port, I'll luff my breeze   540
  Upon this woman (I'm breathless!) Say by what right
  Do these lead you, hands tied with ropes, you and your boy?
  Just like an ewe with lamb you perish in protest,*
  While I am absent and your lord's not here to help.
ANDROMACHE: Old man, they're leading me and my boy to our death,
  These people, as you see; what shall I say to you?
  I sent for you most urgently not once alone
  But many times by many messengers from here.
  You must have heard about the quarrel in this house
  Stirred up by his daughter, for whose sake I must die.   550
  Now from the shrine of Thetis, she who bore for you
  Your noble son, she whom you worship in your wonder,
  They lead me, drag me, having held no legal trial
  Nor waiting till those absent from the home come back,
  But knowing only that we are most desolate,
  They seek to kill me and my blameless boy with me.
  Now I implore you, old man, falling at your knees —
  I cannot reach your reverend beard with my bound hand —

---

* I incorporate in my translation Verrall's suggestion, given in Norwood's
note. See Norwood's edition: John Murray, London (1906), p. 80.

To save me, by the gods; for if you don't, we die:
Disgrace for you but misery for me, old man.   560
PELEUS: I order you, release her, or some one will pay
For this; take off the ropes that bind both of her hands.
MENELAUS: But I say no! I am your equal too in power,
And far more master of the woman who stands here.
PELEUS: How's that? Shall you come here and rule my house for me?
It's not enough for you to run affairs in Sparta?
MENELAUS: I took her with my spear as captive out of Troy.
PELEUS: But my boy's son it was who took her as reward.
MENELAUS: Are not the things he owns my things to own as well?
PELEUS: Yes, to take care of, not to harm nor slay by force.   570
MENELAUS: You never will take her away out of my hands.
PELEUS: Why don't I beat your head till bloody with my staff?
MENELAUS: Just touch me once, come near me, and you will find out!
PELEUS: You count yourself a man, you lowest of the low?
What right have you to be regarded as a man?
Why, you're the one whose wife a Phrygian stole away,
Who left your house unlocked, untended by the slaves,
As though you had a woman you could trust at home,
She worst of all. Not even if she wished to be
Could any Spartan wench be chaste and pure, for they   580
Abandon house and home, they go among the men
With naked thighs and dresses that are much too loose,
To race and wrestle and to hold companionship
Which shocks me. Is it any wonder then that you
In Sparta do not train up women who have sense?
You ought to ask this question of Helen, who left
Your house and love in riotous adultery
And went with her young man into another land.
And then for her sake did you gather up and send
So great a crowd of Greeks against the town of Troy?   590
You should have spit on her, not stirred a single spear,
Since she was worthless; let her stay right where she was
And paid a price never to take her home again.
But your mind never breezed along in this direction;
You went ahead, destroyed so many gallant souls,
And left old women childless in their empty homes,
And snatched from aged fathers their well-born offspring.
I'm one of those you made so wretched; I regard
You as the red-handed slayer of Achilles too.
You were the only one who came uninjured back   600
From Troy, and brought your polished weapons scratchless home
In their fine cases, just as fine as when you left.

And I advised my grandson when he married not
To join alliance with you nor take to his house
The foal of an evil woman, for they carry out
The mother's ill fame. Suitors everywhere, be sure:
Take care you marry the daughters of good mothers.
Moreover, what an insult did you bring your brother
By bidding him to sacrifice his daughter, most
Foolishly! You so feared to lose your evil wife. 610
When you took Troy — I'll go there too along with you —
You did not kill the woman when you captured her,
But when you saw her breast you threw your sword away,
You took her kisses, fondling the treacherous bitch,
Conquered, enslaved by Cypris, O you scoundrel you.
And then you come when he is gone to my son's house
To rob, to kill his wife dishonorably,
His wife and wretched boy, who though he were a child
Three times a bastard will make you and your daughter pay.
For many times seed sown in dry land has surpassed 620
That sown in deep loam; many bastards have become
Better than men of noble birth. Take out the child.
It's better for men to have an in-law who is
Poor but honest than a rich, dishonest one.
You're nothing at all.

CHORUS: From small beginnings the tongue provides a weighty cause
For quarrel to men; wise mortals are on guard against
Just this — to bring their friends excuse for hateful strife.

MENELAUS: Why should you say then that old men, and everyone
Who seemed so clever once among the Greeks, are wise? 630
When you, named Peleus, sprung from noble father,
Joined in alliance, speak words shameful to yourself
And me upon the theme of a barbarian woman
Whom you should have chased out beyond the streams of Nile,
Beyond the Phasis, should have urged I do the same,
Since she comes from the Asiatic mainland, where
So many Greeks have fallen corpses by the spear,
Who shared beside the blame for your son's bloody death.
For Paris, the man who slew your son Achilles,
Was Hector's brother, and Hector was her husband. 640
And yet you enter the same roof with her and you
See fit to live and eat together with her too;
And you allow her to bear hateful children here.
With your good and my own in mind, I wished, old man,
To kill her, but she's being snatched out of my hands.
Yet, come — for it's not shameful to argue this out —

If my child cannot bring to birth, but from this woman
Children are born, will you set them as kings to rule
In Phthia? Although they are barbarians shall
They govern Greeks? Then have I not good sense when I   650
Despise what is not just? And is there sense in you?
[Look now at this point: If you'd given your daughter
To some one citizen and she had suffered things
Like this, would you have sat in silence? I think not.
But for a stranger's sake you bark out in this way
Against your dear kins people? Yet a man and wife
Have equal rights to protest, when he injures her
And when he finds his wife unfaithful in his home.
The husband's hand is greatly strengthened by the fact
He's husband, but her cause by relatives and friends.   660
Am I not right in helping those most dear to me?]
Old, old you are. In speaking of my generalship
You help my cause more than if you'd kept your mouth shut.
For Helen suffered not by her will but through the gods,
And this it was that aided Greece the most of all
Since ignorant of arms, untrained in battle, they
Marched on to manly deeds; it is companionship
That teaches everything to mortal men.
If, when I came upon her, glimpsed my wife again,
I held my hand from murder, I showed common sense.   670
I should have wished you had not slaughtered Phocus either.*
      I've made this charge against you through good will, not anger;
If you resent it, then your wordiness will give
You greater aches; my gain lies in foresightedness.
CHORUS: Hold off now; for it's better far to interrupt
Vain arguments, so both won't make the same mistake.
PELEUS: Oimoi, how badly throughout Greece is life adjusted!
When fighting men set trophies over enemies,
They do not think these the reward of those who fought;
It is the general who reaps the glory then,   680
Who one with many thousand others shook his spear
And fought no more than one but wins the greater fame.
Solemn they sit in seats of power in the city;
They think themselves more lofty than the folk, but they
Are nothing; the people are ten thousand times more wise,
If boldness should be added to their thoughtfulness.
So you too and your brother, puffed up full of pride,
Sat down at Troy and in that campaign's generalship

---

* In jealous anger Peleus had helped to kill his half-brother Phocus.

Were raised on high by others' toil and suffering.
But I shall show you that Idaean Paris is   690
No more an enemy than Peleus ever was
If you don't get to Hell * away as fast as you
Can go from this roof, and your childless daughter too,
Before my son can clutch her hair and drag her through
The house, that barren heifer who cannot endure
That other women bear a child, because she can't!
If she's unhappy since she's childless, must we too
Be rendered childless? Servants, get away so I
Can learn if he dares stop me as I loose her hands.
　　　Raise up yourself; although I'm trembling I'll unbind   700
The twisted coils of leather thongs that hold you here.
See that, you devil, how you've raised welts on her hands?
Did you think you were tying a bull or lion?
Or did you fear she'd take a sword, protect herself?
Run here beneath my arms, my child; untie your mother.
I'll bring you up in Phthia, a great foe to these.
If Sparta had no glory in the spear or war,
Know this: you'd be no better than any one else.
CHORUS: The breed of old men is a thing without restraint
And hard to guard against, its temper is so quick.   710
MENELAUS: You're borne headlong, too ready to revile and curse.
I've come to Phthia, I propose through violence
To do or suffer nothing shabby while I'm here.
And now — I really haven't time to talk with you —
I'll go back home . . . . a certain city which before
Was friendly, threatens now: I wish to head it off
And lead my army out, force it to my hand.
But when I've settled matters there to satisfaction,
I shall return and in the presence of my son-
In-law I'll show, and I'll be shown, the reasons here.   720
And if he punishes this woman and hereafter
Acts moderately toward me, I shall do the same.
But if he's angry, I'll be angry in my turn
And give as good as I receive in fair exchange.
Your words I find it easy to endure, for you
Are but the shadow of a man, a shadow's voice,
And powerless for anything except to talk.

　　(*Exit* MENELAUS)

---

* See Norwood's note. I use the closest English equivalent to the Greek
colloquialism.

PELEUS: Lead on, my boy, come hither, stand beneath my arms,
 You too, poor wretch; you've sailed into a savage storm,
 But you have won to harbor in a quiet port.   730
ANDROMACHE: O reverend sir, may gods give gifts to you and yours,
 For saving me, poor suffering creature, and my boy.
 But take care now that these who crouch beside me here
 In a deserted place don't lead me off by force,
 Seeing you're aged, and I'm weak, and that my boy
 Is but an infant; please take care of this so we
 Who now escape may not be captured after all.
PELEUS: Don't talk like that, in timid words of woman kind.
 Go forward; who will touch you? He will pay for it
 Who touches you. By heaven's will, I have command   740
 Of many cavalry and infantry in Phthia.
 I still stand straight, and I'm no old man, as you think,
 But merely looking at a man like *that* I'll build
 A trophy over him, although I'm elderly.
 An old man, if he's brave, is better than the young.
 What need is there for cowards to be strong in body?

CHORUS: Would I had not been born, or from good parents
 Been born to share the wealth of a noble home.
  For if one suffers some ill with which he cannot cope
   No little help lies in good birth.   750
 To those whose famous ancestry is widely known
 There's honor and renown; time never takes away
  These memories of good men, but greatness shines
   Even among the dead.

Better to win without an evil name
Than overturn justice with one's hateful power
 For though it's sweet at the moment to a man,
  In time the triumph withers,
And lies among reproaches to the house.
This, this I praise; this way of life I wish to win,   760
 To wield no unjust power in the home
  Or in the city either.

 O aged son of Aeacus,
I am persuaded that with Lapithae
 You once fought Centaurs,
Using that famous spear,* and on the Argo passed

---

* The spear that Chiron, the Centaur, gave to Peleus.

The wet, unfriendly Euxine, through the Clashing Rocks,
   In glorious seamanship;
      When Zeus' illustrious son before
Surrounded Troy with massacre and death,   770
     Winning a just acclaim
       You came back to Europe.

NURSE: O dearest women, how this day has brought to us
  Evil on evil, followed one by one in turn!
  My mistress in the house, I mean Hermione,
  Bereft of father, and in consciousness as well
  Of what she did, to try to kill Andromache
  And her small boy, now wishes to die herself,
  Fearing her husband, lest in payment for her deeds
  She should be sent disgracefully away from home,   780
  Or killed for trying to kill those she should help instead.
  She wants to hang herself; the servants find it hard
  Preventing her; they snatch the sword from her right hand.
  So greatly does she grieve, and what she did before
  She knows was not done well; and I can hardly keep
  My mistress from her suicide, dear friends of mine.
  But you go in, go in to the house and set her free
  From death, for new friends can persuade more than the old.
CHORUS: Truly we hear the servants who are in the house
  Crying about the news that you have come to tell.   790
  That desperate woman seems to show how much remorse
  She has for evil deeds; she's running from the house,
  Fleeing the hands of servants in her wish for death.
HERMIONE: Io moi moi!
  I'll tear my hair and with my fingernails I will
  Scratch up my face.
NURSE: O child, what are you doing? Do you mar your body?
HERMIONE: Aiai, aiai!
  Rise into air from my tresses,
  Gossamer veil.   800
NURSE: Child, cover your bosom, bring your gown together.
HERMIONE: Why should I cover my bosom
  With dresses? Plain and clear
  And unhidden what I have done,
  To my husband.
NURSE: You grieve because you schemed death for your fellow-wife?
HERMIONE: I mourn for my dreadful
  Daring, for what I have
  Done; I'm accursed,
  Accursed among men.

NURSE: Your husband will forgive you for this one mistake.   810
HERMIONE: Why have you snatched
  The sword from my hand?
  Give it back, give it back, O friend, that I may
  Plunge it straight through! Why keep me from ropes?
NURSE: But if I set you free, insane, to kill yourself —
HERMIONE: Oimoi my fate!
  Where is the dear flame of fire?
  Where is a rock to rise up to
  By the sea or in mountain woods   820
  So that dying I'd dwell with the dead?
NURSE: Why suffer torture? Troubles sent by gods above
  Come now, come sometime to all mortal men alive.
HERMIONE: You've left me, left me, father, on the ocean beach,
  Like one alone, deserted by sea-going ships.
    He'll kill me, kill me! No more shall I live
    In the house of my husband.
    What statue shall I hasten to embrace?
    A slave, shall I fall at the knees of a slave?
    Would I were a blue-winged bird to fly   830
    From the land of Phthia,
    Or a pinetree boat
    To sail like the one that passed the Dark Blue Beaches,
    First among sailing ships.
NURSE: O child, I did not praise your wild excessive act
  When you did wrong against the Trojan woman here,
  Nor do I praise the too great fear that overpowers you.
  Your husband will not thus thrust off your marriage-bond,
  Won by the low words of a barbarous woman.
  He did not have you as a captive out of Troy   840
  But as the daughter of noblemen with many
  Bride-gifts, and from a city blessed not moderately.
  Your father will not thus desert you as you fear,
  My child, and let you be cast from this house, your home.
  But go on in and do not show yourself before
  The palace, lest you bring reproach upon you there.
CHORUS: Some strange, outlandish foreigner is coming now;
  In haste toward us he's moving, step by measured step.
ORESTES: Foreign ladies, is this place the palace of the
  Son of great Achilles, his royal roof and home?   850
CHORUS: It is; but who are you who wish to find this out?
ORESTES: I'm born of Agamemnon and Clytaemestra,
  Orestes is my name, I'm travelling to the shrine
  Of Zeus at Dodona, and since I have arrived

In Phthia, I thought I would inquire about one
Of my relations, if she lives here and fares well,
Spartan Hermione; though she lives so far away
From our land, all the same she's dear to us at home.

HERMIONE: O harbor showing up to sailors in a storm,
O son of Agamemnon, by your knees I beg,   860
Take pity on me, seeing what mischance is mine.
I am unfortunate. I fling my arms about
Your knees — I have no garlands of the suppliant.

ORESTES: Hah!
What is this? Have I wandered? Do I clearly see
The child of Menelaus, mistress of the house?

HERMIONE: I'm she the daughter of Tyndareus gave birth to,
Helen, in her father's house. You understand?

ORESTES: O Phoebus healer, may you give release from ills.
What is this? Do you suffer pain from men or gods?   870

HERMIONE: Some from myself, some from the man who married me,
Some from a god; on every side I am destroyed.

ORESTES: What mishap might befall you since you have no child,
Except misfortune to your marriage bed and right?

HERMIONE: This very ill I suffer: how you've drawn me out!

ORESTES: Your husband loves some other girl instead of you?

HERMIONE: The spear-won captive who was Hector's bed-fellow.

ORESTES: That's bad, for any man to have two wedded wives.

HERMIONE: But that's the way things are. And then I took revenge.

ORESTES: You didn't plot against the woman, as wives do?   880

HERMIONE: Yes, death to her and to her little bastard boy.

ORESTES: And did you kill her? Or did some chance hinder you?

HERMIONE: Old man Peleus, siding with the wretched things.

ORESTES: But was there some one who was partner to this crime?

HERMIONE: My father came from Sparta for that very end.

ORESTES: And then was beaten at the hands of the old man?

HERMIONE: He felt ashamed; and then he left me quite alone.

ORESTES: I understand. You fear your husband for what's done.

HERMIONE: You're right. He'll kill me justly. Need I tell you that?
I beg you, calling on the Zeus of relatives,*   890
To take me from this land as far as I can go
Or to my father's home: this dwelling seems to have
A haunting voice that drives me out, away from here.
The land of Phthia hates me. If my husband comes
From Phoebus' oracle before I can escape
He'll kill me in most shameful fashion or enslave

---

* Hermione and Orestes were cousins.

Me to a concubine whose mistress I had been.
How did you make this error? some one might inquire.
The visits of evil women it was that ruined me.
They puffed me up with vanity; they said these words: 900
"Will you endure to have that rotten slave girl here
To share your husband's bed, with you right in the house?
By Hera queen, she wouldn't look upon daylight
One moment in *my* home or wallow in my bed!"
    I lent a willing ear to all these Siren songs,
[Smart talkers, trouble-makers, gifted with their gab]
Inflated by my folly. For what need had I
To keep an eye on him who gave me everything,
Much wealth, a handsome house to make my home? I might
Have borne him children in the normal course of things,   910
While hers, unlawful, would have been half-slaves to mine.
But never, never — I shall say it many times —
Should men who have sound sense, who have a wife besides,
Allow the frequent visits coming in and out
Of women; for they teach her only wickedness.
One woman, paid to do it, will corrupt the wife,
Another wants for her the same disgrace *she* has,
And many from sheer love of sin . . . and thus the homes
Of men grow sick. Be on your guard against such tricks.
Shut up the house and lock it tight with bolts and bars.   920
There's nothing healthy in this running in and out
That women do, but many evils come from it.
CHORUS: You've let your tongue speak out too much against your sex.
One may forgive you this, but all the same it's right
For women to make the best of other women's faults.
ORESTES: A wise word that, of him who taught us mortal men
To hear with care both sides in any argument.
For, knowing this house has fallen to confusion
And strife between you and the wife of Hector, I
Have kept my watch to learn if you remain at home   930
Or, terrified because you tried to murder her,
The captive woman, you wish to go away from here.
I came, not honoring the messages you sent me;
If you should give me, as you've given, chance to speak
I'd take you from this house. Though you were mine before,
You dwell with this man through your father's crookedness.
Before he crashed beyond the boundaries of Troy,
He gave you to me, later pledging you to him
Who has you now, if he should sack the Trojan town.
But when Achilles' son came hither home again   940

I then forgave your father and I begged him * to
Release you from your marriage, mentioning my fate
And present misfortune, saying I might marry you
As kin to me, yet it was hard since I'm forced out;
A fugitive from home, I'm on the run, you see.
But he insulted me about my mother's murder,
He taunted me with the blood-faced Goddesses.
And I, made humble by misfortune in my home,
Was grieved, yes grieved, but I endured calamities;
Robbed of marriage, against my will I went away.   950
But now since fortune has swung round and given you
Unhappiness from which you cannot struggle out,
I'll lead you home and put you in your father's hands.
Relationship is strangely strong, and in our troubles
There's nothing better than to have a friend at home.

HERMIONE: My father will have charge of the second marriage;
That is his care, it's not for me to choose my own.
But take me home as quickly as you can from here,
So that my husband may not find me when he comes
Or Peleus learn that I have left the house alone   960
And come pursuing after in horse-chariots.

ORESTES: Don't fear the old man's hand; don't fear Achilles' son,
As far as the insults he has given are concerned.
For such a clever net of death I have entwined
With looping meshes! He will not escape my hand.
He'll never know, but when it's sprung, the Delphic rock
Will know; a mother-slayer, if my spear-friends hold
Firmly to oaths they've sworn to me in Pythian land,
Will teach him not to marry a girl betrothed to me.
And bloody justice for his father's death he'll ask   970
Bitterly of lord Apollo nor will change
Of mind avail him, for the god will punish him.
And through Apollo and my accusations he
Will perish evilly, will come to know my hate.
God overthrows the fortunes of our enemies;
He does not let them live in haughtiness of mind.

> (*Exeunt* ORESTES *and* HERMIONE. A *lapse of some days is*
> *indicated.*)

CHORUS: O Phoebus, who built up the towers on Troy's well-walled
   hill,
   And, Sea God, who ride with your sea-blue horses
      And chariot over the ocean,

---

* Neoptolemus.

Why did you give up to Ares   980
Spear-master the hand of the workman,
Dishonoring it and surrendering,
    Wretched, O wretched,
Why did you yield up Troy?

Many fine-horsed chariots you yoked up on banks of Simois,
You set many bloody contests
    Of men, without victor's crowns;
    And gone among the dead
        Are the kings of Ilium;
        No longer the altar-fire in Troy   990
            Shines for the gods
        Out of its fragrant smoke.

And Atrides has gone through his wife's violence,
And she in her turn has exchanged murder for death.
    At the hands of her children
    She has known the god's power.
Against her was turned the god's awful command,
Oracular word, when Agamemnon's son set out
From Argos and entered the sanctuary of the god,
    Become a mother-killer: 1000
O god, O Apollo, how shall I believe?

And many women sent up their moans in the market-places of
    Greece,
Keening the wail for their poor children, and wives
    Left their homes
To be wives to another. Not to you alone
There befell heart-aches, nor to your friends, deep grief;
A disease Greece suffered, disease; into Phrygia
    And to its fruitful fields
A lightning storm came, dripping with Hell's own blood.

PELEUS: Women of Phthia, as I make my inquiry,   1010
    Explain to me, for I have heard an unclear story
    That Menelaus' daughter, having left this house,
    Has gone away; I come in eagerness to know
    If this is true, for when one's friends are out of town
    Those who remain must work to save their interests.
CHORUS: Peleus, you've heard clearly; it's not honorable
    For me to hide the state in which I find myself.
    It's true: the queen has left this house, a fugitive.

PELEUS: What fear came over her? Go through the tale for me.

CHORUS: She feared her husband, lest he throw her from the house. 1020

PELEUS: And not because she tried to kill his infant son?

CHORUS: Yes, and because she feared the captive woman too.

PELEUS: But has she left the house with her father, or with whom?

CHORUS: The son of Agamemnon took her from the land.

PELEUS: Accomplishing what hope? He wishes to marry her?

CHORUS: Yes, and preparing to murder your son's son.

PELEUS: Lying in wait in ambush or in open fight?

CHORUS: In Loxias' holy temple with the Delphians.

PELEUS: Oimoi! But this is awful. Won't somebody go

As fast as possible to the Pythian dwelling 1030

And tell this story to our friends who live up there

Before Achilles' son is killed by enemies?

(Enter, as MESSENGER, *a servant of Neoptolemus.)*

MESSENGER: O moi moi!

Bad luck it is I come to tell you, luckless man,

To you, old fellow, and to all my master's friends.

PELEUS: Aiai! my heart's foreboding tells me something now.

MESSENGER: So you may know, old man, your grandson is no more.

Such sword-blows struck him by the Delphians and by

The stranger from Mycenae!

CHORUS: Ah, ah, what are you doing, old man? Do not fall. 1040

Raise up yourself.

PELEUS: I'm nothing; I'm completely ruined!

Gone is my voice, gone out from under me my legs.

MESSENGER: Hear what was done, if you wish to bring aid to friends;

Straighten your body.

PELEUS: O fate, upon the utmost limits of old age,

How you have compassed me about in my misfortune!

How did he die, the only son of my only son?

Explain; I wish to hear what ought not to be heard.

MESSENGER: When we had reached the famous soil of Phoebus' shrine,

For three full revolutions of the shining sun 1050

We filled our eyes sight-seeing, looked at everything.

And this was viewed suspiciously. The folk who dwelt

Within the god's enclosure formed in knots and groups.

The son of Agamemnon moving through the town

Spoke hostile words into the ears of each and all:

"You see this man who walks within the god's precinct

Among the golden treasures heaped up here by men?

He comes again for the same purpose as before;

He wishes to destroy the temple of the god."
He set an evil tumult running through the town. 1060
The rulers came a-flocking to the council halls,
And all who had in private charge the treasuries
Saw that a guard was placed around the colonnades.
We took some sheep which had been fed upon the grass
Of mount Parnassus (we suspected nothing yet)
And stood at the hearth with patrons and Pythian seers.
And someone spoke: "O young man, what is it that we
May ask the god for you? What have you come to seek?"
So he replied: "To Phoebus for my earlier
Mistake I wish to offer payment: once I asked 1070
The god for satisfaction for my father's blood."
And then Orestes' speech seemed greatly to prevail;
He said my master lied, that he had come with base
Intent. He climbed the steps that skirt the temple-hall
To pray to Phoebus and consult the oracle;
He happened to be busy with burnt-offerings.
A gang of swordsmen, laurel-shaded, awaited him.
The son of Clytaemestra, stitcher of the plot,
Was leader there. And standing in full view of them,
My master prayed. But they with keenly whetted blades 1080
Attacked Achilles' son unwarned and all unarmed.
And he fell back; a mortal blow had not been struck.
He drew the spear out; snatching up the arms that hung
From pegs upon the temple-front he took his stand
Upon the altar, a warrior fierce to see,
And shouting thus to Delphi's sons, he questioned them:
"Why do you slay me who have come to worship here,
A pilgrim from afar? For what cause do I die?"
But no one of the thousands who stood near replied
A single word; they only pelted him with stones. 1090
And pounded by the hailstorm coming from all sides,
He thrust his armor out and warded off the blows;
This way and that he stretched the shield upon his arm.
Yet nothing helped him, for together many darts
And arrows, spears, light two-pronged forks unsheathed,
Ox-sticking knives fell thick before him as he stood.
You should have seen the dreadful war-dance of the man
On guard for missiles. When they circled him about
And pinned him down, permitting him no breathing space,
He left the sheep-receiving altar and its hearth. 1100
Leaping the Trojan leap with both his feet at once
He ran against them; they, like pigeons who have seen

A hawk swoop down on them, turned tail and fled from him.
And many fell pell-mell, both those with wounds he gave
And those whose comrades trod them in the narrow path.
Ill-omened cries arose within well-omened shrines
And echoed from the cliffs. But in a calm he stood,
My master shining brightly with his shining arms,
Before some voice was heard within the holy place,
Hair-raising, awful, and stirred up the mob again,   1110
Turned it to valor. Here Achilles' son fell down,
Struck in the side with a sharp-whetted sword at last
By one of Delphi's men who cut my master down
With many helping; as he fell upon the ground,
Who did not thrust a sword? Who did not throw or hurl
A rock at him? His handsome body, all of it,
Was mutilated and laid waste by savage wounds.
When he was dead and lying near the altar-stone,
They cast him from the god's incense-receiving shrine.
We snatched him up in hand as swiftly as we could   1120
And brought him back to you, for you to mourn him here,
To wail, old man, and lay him in an earthen tomb.
> This is the way the god who gives his sacred word
To others, who is judge to all of what is right,
Has paid Achilles' son who offered to atone.
He has remembered, like a man who bears a grudge,
An ancient quarrel. How can Apollo then be wise?
CHORUS: Truly the master comes, borne shoulder-high
Upon a litter from the Delphic land,
Poor wretched sufferer; and you too, old man,   1130
For you receive Achilles' whelp into your house
Not as you wish; you've fallen, as he fell,
> And struck on one same fate.
PELEUS: Omoi for me, what evil do I look upon,
Receiving it in my hands, into my house.
Io moi moi aiai!
O city of Thessaly, I am destroyed,
I'm done for. I have no family, no children
Are left at home.
O I am wretched with my suffering. To what   1140
Friend shall I turn my eyes in joy?
O dear mouth and cheek and hands,
I wish that god had killed you at Ilium,
> On Simois' banks.
CHORUS: Old man, if he had died there, honor would be his,
As it is now, but you would be more fortunate.

PELEUS: O marriage, marriage, which destroyed this home,
    My city too! Aiai!
    Ee, ee, O son!
    I wish your marriage, ill-omened in her name,   1150
    Had not flung death upon my family and my home
    And you, because of Hermione,
    But that she had been struck before
    With lightning; nor should you have fixed
    On Phoebus for cruel bowmanship
    Which killed your father, the guilt for his
        Zeus-nourished blood!
CHORUS: Ottotototoi! My master's dead; with wails
      In the melody
  Of those below I shall begin.   1160
PELEUS: Ottotototoi! In my turn, wretched I
      An old man and
  Unfortunate, I weep.
CHORUS: It is god's fate; a god has brought this tragedy.
PELEUS: O friend,
      You left your house barren,
      O moi moi, suffering as I am,
      You've left an old man childless.
CHORUS: You should have died, have died before your children died.
PELEUS: Shall I not tear my hair,   1170
      Shall I not beat my head
      With deadly blows of fists? O city,
        Of both my sons
      Phoebus has robbed me.
CHORUS: O poor old man who've seen and suffered ills,
        What life
      Will be yours after this?
PELEUS: Childless, deserted, finding no end to sorrow,
        I'll labor through
      My grief until I die.   1180
CHORUS: In vain the gods once blessed you with a marriage.
PELEUS: Flown upward,
    All is gone, it lies

     . . . .

    Far from my empty boasting.
CHORUS: Alone you pace about in a lonely house.
PELEUS: You are no more, city, city,
        Let this my scepter be dashed to earth,
    And you, O daughter of Nereus, from your night-dark cave,
          In utter ruin

       Shall see me falling to the earth.   1190
CHORUS: Io, io!
  What's set on foot? What god do I
  See coming? Maidens, look, behold.
  Some goddess sailing on white air
  Is coming to horse-nourishing
      Pastures of Phthia.
THETIS: Peleus, for the sake of our former wedding, I,
  Thetis, have come and left the house of Nereus.
  And first of all I tell you, do not grieve too much
  Because of present sorrows, for I too who should   1200
  Have borne my children deathless, not to weep for them,
  Lost great Achilles swift-foot whom I bore to you.
  But why I came I'll tell you; and receive my words.
  Bury at Delphi Achilles' son who lies dead,
  And when you've done that go to the Pythian altar-hearth,
  So dead in his tomb he may reproach the Delphians
  Because he died by violence at Orestes' hands.
  But she, the spear-won captive named Andromache,
  Must dwell in land of the Molossians, old man,
  And consummate a legal marriage with Helenus.   1210
  Her son with her, alone of those from Aeacus,
  Is left alive. But from him will descend a king,
  Another and another, to rule Molossian land
  In happiness, for not so utterly destroyed
  Must be your race and mine as it appears, old man —
  Or Trojan race; the gods watch over it as well.
  But I, that you may know the blessings of my bed,
  [I, born a goddess who am daughter of a god,]
  Shall make you an immortal god beyond decay   1220
  And free you fully from the ills that mortals know.
  And then in the house of Nereus along with me,
  A god, you'll live with me, a goddess, evermore.
  Thence, lifting your foot unwetted from the open sea,
  You'll find your son Achilles, who is very dear
  To you and me, alive within an island home
  On the White Beach within the Euxine passage way.
  But go to Delphi, that god-founded citadel;
  Take this corpse with you; when you've laid it in the earth,
  Go to the hollow hiding place of the old Rock   1230
  Of Cuttle Fish; sit down and stay there till I come
  Out of the sea and with my band of fifty nymphs,
  The Nereids, I'll fetch you; we must follow fate
  And bring you to the ocean — Zeus has settled this.

Cease then your weeping for the son that you have lost.
Each man alive owes this one debt unto the gods:
The gods have cast their vote; and every man must die.
PELEUS: O gentle lady, noble comrade of my bed,
Daughter of Nereus, greetings! Everything you do
Is worthy of you, worthy of your children too.   1240
I'll cease my sorrow at your bidding, goddess, now;
I'll go to bury him in Pelion's folded glens,
Where once I took your lovely body in my arms.
Then ought one not to marry into noble clans,
To give in marriage to the good, if one is wise,
And not to have desire for a base-born union,
Not even if one carries home a fabulous dowry?
They never would fare ill this way by will of gods.

CHORUS: Many shapes the gods will take,
                 And many things they bring to pass   1250
                 Beyond our hope, and what we sought
                 Is not fulfilled by them; and for
                 Undreamed of things god finds a way.
                    So has this action happened here.

EURIPIDES

BACCHAE

Translated by Henry Birkhead

INTRODUCTION

THE *Bacchae* is the last and the strangest of Euripides' plays. It is as though in his old age the bitter rationalist who had scoffed at religion, had denounced the evils of warfare, slavery, and the inequality of the sexes, who had brilliantly analyzed a variety of morbid psychological conditions, and whose innovations in drama had so shocked the Athenians that they gave him only five first prizes during his entire life, should have turned to a religious theme at the end and looked beyond the veil of reality into the ecstasies of mysticism.

One of Friedrich Nietzsche's most fertile insights in his highly original essay, *The Birth of Tragedy Out of the Spirit of Music* (1872), was the development of his famous contrast between the Apollonian and the Dionysian elements in ancient Greek life. The Apollonian comprised human reason; the individual; civilized life; in drama, the dialogue; plastic art; science; and dialectics. The Dionysian, on the other hand, included the opposed elements of human emotion; the mass of mankind; nature; in drama, the chorus; music; myth; and tragedy itself.

It is this profound dichotomy which lies at the center of the *Bacchae*. In this play alone among all those we have, the god Dionysus, whom drama was created to honor, is the chief character. The play, at least in its external form, is a vindication of his position in Greek life and a hymn of praise for the primitive orgiastic sensuality of the individual caught up in hysteric worship of the god of wine and creative nature.

There are serious difficulties which hamper the interpretation of this play. Gilbert Norwood, in *The Riddle of the Bacchae* (1908), was among the first to point them out and to suggest a solution. First, Euripides as is well known did not believe in the divinity of the gods; his attitude toward popular Greek religion was one of scepticism which he demonstrated on the stage in the attempt to show his audience how the religious myths had gained mastery of their minds. He could not then have with sincerity glorified Dionysus or believed in him as a supernatural being in the *Bacchae*. Dionysus is, therefore, not a god but a mortal, a stranger from Lydia, who has hypnotized his public (the chorus) into believing that he is a god and that he can work miracles like the destruction of Pentheus' palace at Thebes, his escape from it, and the slaughter of Pentheus himself at the hands of the Bacchantes led by his mother Agave.

The play is, like the *Oedipus Rex*, one of slow inexorable revelation and foreboding disaster. Pentheus, as unbending as Creon, resists the entrance of the new god into Thebes; he soon stands alone as guardian

Dionysian

of public morals when both Cadmus and Teiresias, the wisest heads in authority beside himself, join the ranks of the intruder while the women of Thebes, lost in ecstasy upon Cithaeron, form the thiasos or band of worshippers. The chorus, in lyrical outbursts of the most exalted delight and beauty, sing the praises of the newcomer. All Pentheus, whose name means "grief-stricken," can do to restore order is to imprison the leader of the revelers and to threaten his followers, but he becomes the ritual victim, the traditional scapegoat, for the god. He is turned mad and made to attack in the stable a heifer whom he looks upon in his hallucination as Dionysus. This scene constitutes one of the play's many ambiguities, for Dionysus was indeed represented in the form of various animals. Now under the god's spell Pentheus sets out for the hills to hunt the Bacchae and is there attacked and killed. The manner of his death is ghastly. Dionysus seats Pentheus upon the bough of a tree which he releases, carrying the king up into the air. There he is spied by the Bacchantes. They strike at him with stones and with their thyrsi, reed-like spears of vine-stems. Finally they tear down the tree itself to reach him. The members of his mangled body are carried off in triumph, an arm here, a foot there. Agave herself fixes his head on her thyrsus as she runs over Mount Cithaeron, crying madly.

The aftermath of this ghoulish lynching is the agonized recovery of her senses by Agave and the horror-stricken realization of her crime. Cadmus too sinks into abased grief. Dionysus, now in a sterner mood, no longer the mocking, effeminate, unwarlike youth he has shown himself in the earlier scenes, declares that Cadmus shall become a dragon, his wife Harmonia a serpent. Thus through frightful deeds the name of Dionysus wins sinister honor at Thebes.

The play has a meaning more abstract than the hideous events of which it is composed. Nature and the forces of the darker side of humanity gain a victory here over the cold intellect exerted for the repression of orgiastic urges. The refusal to recognize the imperative needs of the lower consciousness that seeks to express itself in wild hysteric delight brings on its own punishment. If there is an implication which may be interpreted in terms of modern psychology, it is the lesson of Freud and of psychiatry: psychic repression exercises its baleful strength upon the human soul and recoils upon abnormally sustained "purity." The hybris of the prurient Pentheus, who had unjustly accused the Bacchantes of immorality both of drunkenness and of sex, lay in his failure to bow as Cadmus and Teiresias did before the divinity: the will of the gods, even of the newest god, must be obeyed.

The play was produced at Athens by Euripides' son about 405 B.C., after the death of his father in 406. It was written no doubt after Euripides left Athens in 408 to visit the court of King Archelaus, although of course he might have carried it with him in finished form. It is appropriate that the *Bacchae* should have also been presented in northern Greece where Dionysus had acquired so much prestige. It had a long literary influence; lines from it form a large part of the *Christus Patiens*, a medieval patchwork of lines from Greek drama. Euripides' reputation for skill in depicting both madness and love was certainly enhanced by the *Bacchae*. But its chief contribution to the ideas which can be discovered in his plays is the emphasis it places upon the needs of the human spirit which lie below the conventional consciousness; the fanatical excitement it generates; the wild, romantic scenery it evokes; and the long disturbing look it furnishes into one of the most fascinating aspects of Greek religion. The latter subject in its psychological effects can be well studied with the help of two recent books: E. R. Dodds, *The Greeks and the Irrational*, 1951; G. R. Levy, *The Gate of Horn*, 1948. The literature on Dionysus and the religion of Orphism and the Eleusinian mysteries is very large.

L. R. LIND

BACCHAE

CHARACTERS

DIONYSUS, *the god of wine, son of Zeus and Semele*
CHORUS *of Bacchantes, followers of Dionysus from Phrygia*
TEIRESIAS, *a blind Theban prophet*
CADMUS, *former king of Thebes, father of Semele*
PENTHEUS, *king of Thebes, grandson of Cadmus*
AGAVE, *daughter of Cadmus, mother of Pentheus*
AN OFFICER *of Pentheus' guard*
TWO MESSENGERS

SCENE. *In front of the royal palace at Thebes, the home of King Pentheus and of Cadmus, his grandfather. The speaker of the Prologue is a very young man in foreign dress.*

STRANGER: I, Dionysus, to the Theban land have come,
The son of Zeus by Cadmus' daughter, Semele,
Who was delivered of me in a lightning-flash;
My form divine discarding for a mortal shape,
I stand by Dirce's waters and Ismene's stream.
My mother's tomb I see here, whom that stroke destroyed,
Here by the houses and I see the wrecks of homes
Burning; the flame of Zeus' fire is living still.
Hera's immortal insolence my mother knew.
But I praise Cadmus, who untrodden keeps this ground   10
In memory of his daughter; I myself have hid
The place with green, sweet-scented clusters of the vine.
And I am come from Lydian fields enriched with gold,

330

From Phrygia, from Persia with its sun-struck plains, *He is a stranger*
From Bactrian ramparts, reaching then the wintry land
Of Media, passing to Arabia the blest,
And right through Asia, which beside the salty sea *thronging →crowds*
Has thronging cities finely girded round with walls,
Peopled alike by Hellenes and barbarians.
This is the first Hellenic city I have reached   **20**
And yonder started dances with my ritual,
To prove my god-head in the eyes of mortal men.
In all the land of Hellas, Thebes is first to ring
With my hallooing; fawnskins I have made them wear
And armed them with my thyrsus, ivy-knotted bolt.
Aye! for my mother's sisters, whom it least becomes,
Deny that Dionysus is the son of Zeus;
Semele, they say, was pregnant by some mortal man
And cited Zeus to cover her unchastity —
A scheme of Cadmus — Zeus, they vaunted, struck her dead,   **30**
Because her story of their wedlock was a lie.
Therefore I've stung these women out of house and home *Dionysus*
With madness; on the mountain they abide distraught,   *makes*
Under compulsion wearing Bacchanalian dress.   *madness*
And every woman of the seed that Cadmus sowed
I've driven frenzied from her home, yes, every one;
And mingling close with Cadmus' daughters, there they camp
Beneath green pine trees, under rocks without a roof. *They're out in nature*
However loth, this city must be made to learn   *not in the city*
That in my ritual Thebes is uninitiate.   **40**
And I must speak my mother Semele's defence,
Her son by Zeus, appearing now a god to men.
    Cadmus himself has ceded throne and sovereignty
To Pentheus, son of Cadmus' daughter. Pentheus wars
Against my godhead and he outlaws me by force,
And as for prayers, not a word for me in them!
And for that reason I'll display myself a god
To him and all the Thebans. To another land
I'll go when I have ordered things aright in Thebes,
Showing myself there; but if angry Thebes attempt   **50**
To drive the Bacchae from the mountain-side by arms *mortal shape*
I shall join issue, I will be their general.   *As stranger*
And with this purpose I have taken mortal shape;
For a man's nature I have changed my form divine.
        But come, my band of women, who with me have left
Mount Tmolus, Lydia's fastness, whom barbarian-born *Fellow*
I've brought as my supporters, fellow wayfarers,   *Babarians*

Up with the native kettle drums of Phrygia,
Invented for the Mother Rhea and myself.
Come! and surrounding Pentheus' royal palace here,   60
Set them a -drumming, so that Cadmus' city knows:
And I will join the Bacchae on Cithaeron's clefts.

(*The* CHORUS *of Bacchantes enters, women of Asia in the dress
described by their leader at line 34.*)

CHORUS: Asia left behind us,
                            Tmolus' holy height,
                            Easy burdens bind us,
                            Labor that is light.
                    Euoi! we call for Bacchus, god of Din.
                            Streets and habitations
                            Everyone must clear!
                            Speak no profanations,
                            Close your lips and hear!
                    Now Dionysus' ritual hymns begin . . .   70
                            Happy who's instructed
                            In the rites divine,
                            On the hills inducted
                            By the god of wine;
                            Freed of sins and devils
                            Life he can renew,
                            Find his soul in revels,
                            Find religion too.
                            Who rightly serves the Mother,
                            Cybele the Grand,
                            Bacchus and no other
                            Claims as ordinand,
                            Claims the thyrsus-bearers,   80
                            Ivy-garland wearers.
                            Come, Bacchic routs,
                            For the god who shouts!
                            Bring Dionysus home,
                    God-begotten god of Din,
                    From the Phrygian hills advancing;
                        Streets of Hellas wide for dancing,
                                Let him in!
                        Born, when Zeus's thunder quivered,
                        Before his time from his mother's womb,   90
                        In her agony delivered
                        When the lightning brought her doom;
                                There and then

Zeus Kronion saved his son,
Kept him hid from Hera's eye,
Till the appointed time was run,
Clasped with gold within his thigh.
Then a bull-horned god he bore,
Gave him serpents for a crown;   100
Just as now the Maenads wear
Twined and twisted in their hair
Snakes that they have hunted down.
Thebes, the nurse of Semele,
Wear the ivy crown today!
Riot, filled with briony,
Green of leaf with berries gay!
And the Bacchic revel rouse
Either with oak or pine-tree boughs.   110
Wear your dappled fawn-skin coats,
Fringed with white from hair of goats;
Haughtily your rods advance,
All the land today will dance.
To the mountain! to the mountain!
Forth he leads, the god of Din;
Fall in, there's room.
Forward with his band to find
All the girls who've left behind
Shuttle and loom,
Stung by Bacchus out of mind!

The Curetes' home I greet,   120
Zeus's birth-place, holy shrine,
Where the Corybants of Crete
Fashioned first this drum of mine,
Triple-crested men who rounded
In the caves a hide that sounded.
With Bacchus' drums in harmony
Sweet on Phrygian flutes they played
Tunes, and for Mother Rhea made
Music to match the Bacchic cry;
That music from the Mother passed
To frenzied Satyrs for their dance —   130
Hence the triennial feast at last,
The Dionysian ordinance.
Happy the life on the mountains racing;
Reeling to earth from the ranks is sweet,
Wearing the holy fawn-skin, chasing

> Goats for their blood and their tasty meat.
>> To the mountains of Phrygia!
>> Mountains of Lydia!
>>> Euoi, euoi!   140
> Flows the land with milk and wine, flows with nectar won
>> from bees,
>>> Incense rises of Syria;
> Follow the lead of the Noisy Boy!
> Bearing a torch of pine ablaze,
> Red on his rod, he darts about
> Stirring to races and dance the strays,
> Rousing them up with a Bacchic shout;
> Shaking skyward his flossy hair   150
> Goes our leader, Euoi! euoi!
> Shouting "Bacchae, be there, be there,
> Pride of Tmolus, the mount of gold.
> Deep let the kettle drums be rolled,
> Give Dionysus his own salute,
> Phrygian words in Phrygian voices,
> That be your joy, your god rejoices.
>>> Euoi, euoi!
> Sound the melodious, holy flute,
> Loud in a holy, gamesome way,
> Suiting the mountain vagrants' play!"   160
> And every Bacchante who hears him there
> Waltzes and frisks like a foal with a mare.

(TEIRESIAS, *the blind prophet of Thebes, enters, calling at the
palace for the old king,* CADMUS, *who comes out at the end of
Teiresias' first speech.*)

TEIRESIAS: Is there a porter on the gate? call Cadmus out,   170
Son of Agenor, who from Sidon's city came
And built this stronghold of the town of Thebes;
Let someone go and tell him that Teiresias
Is looking for him, and he knows my business,
How I arranged, an old man with an older still,
That each should hold a thyrsus, dress in fawn-skin cloaks,
And crown his temples with a wreath of ivy leaves.
CADMUS: Good friend, I heard you and your voice I recognized,
A wise man wisely speaking, for I was at home,
Dressed up and ready in the trappings of a god.   180
For have we not a duty to my daughter's son,
Dionysus, manifested now to men as god,
To pay him honor to the utmost of our power?

Bacchae · 335

Where do we go for dancing, where to plant our feet
And set our white heads shaking? you must help me out,
Old men together, for you're wise, Teiresias,
And with a thyrsus I could beat the ground all day,
All night too, never tiring; it is good to lose
That aged feeling.

TEIRESIAS: It is just the same with me!
Like you I'm in my boyhood, and I'll join the dance.

CADMUS: Then shall we get a carriage to the mountain side?

TEIRESIAS: The god would find that method less devotional.

CADMUS: Well then, old junior, I will see you to the school.

TEIRESIAS: It is no trouble for the god to lead us there.

CADMUS: Are we the only Thebans bound for Bacchus' dance?

TEIRESIAS: Yes, we're the only wise ones; all the rest are mad.

CADMUS: Delay is irksome; come, you hold my hand!

TEIRESIAS: Here is my own hand, clasp it, grip it tight.

CADMUS: I, a mere mortal, do not hold the gods in scorn.

TEIRESIAS: We do not practice subtleties towards the Powers;   200
Inherited traditions, old as Time itself,
We have in keeping; these no logic overthrows,
No! not the wisdom of the highest intellect.
And, if some critic says that I disgrace my years
By going dancing with a crown of ivy leaves,
"Discrimination as between the young and old"
I answer, "is not in the god's command to dance;
But his intention is that all should honor him
Collectively, not numbered off in dancing groups."

CADMUS: As you, Teiresias, do not see the light of day,   210
I'll be the prophet, prompting you with what I see.
Now here comes Pentheus, hurrying toward the house,
Echion's son, our sovereign, for I made him so,
Full of excitement. Well, I wonder what's his news?

(*The very young king*, PENTHEUS, *enters, with his guards.*)

PENTHEUS: By chance I happen to have been away from Thebes,
And extraordinary news of things in town
I hear; our women have deserted hearth and home
For some pretended Bacchic feast, and gone to live
Up in the mountains, worshipping the modern god
Dionysus, whoever *he* is, as his chorus girls.   220
Around full wine bowls are the band of revellers,
And to some solitary spot a woman steals
This way or that way, servicing a lover's bed;
They make pretences they are Maenad priestesses,

But over Bacchus they put Aphrodite's claim.
Those that I have arrested are in custody,
Handcuffed, detained by warders in the public jail;
Those that are absent I will capture on the hills,
Ino, Agave, my own mother, once Echion's wife,
And third, Actaeon's mother, our Autonoe. 230
I'll catch and hold them fast in traps of iron-work
And quickly end their evil Bacchic practices.
Some stranger also, they report to me, has come,
A juggler, a magician out of Lydia,
With golden ringlets on his sweetly scented head,
A fresh complexion, eyes with Aphrodite's charms,
Who under cover of some shouting ceremonies
Spends days and nights consorting with the younger girls.
But if I catch the fellow here inside our walls,
I'll stop his thyrsus-beating; he'll not toss his head 240
When from his body I have cut away the neck.
He says he's Dionysus, says that he's a god,
And he alleges he was stitched in Zeus's thigh,
Whereas the baby in the lightning flame was burnt,
The mother with him for her lie of wedding Zeus.
Does he not merit hanging, aye, and more, for this,
Outraging outrage, whosoever the stranger be?
But here's another marvel! here's the soothsayer,
Teiresias, in dappled fawn skins; here is too
My mother's father (how ridiculous he looks!) 250
Swinging a cane for Bacchus . . . Father, I'm ashamed
To see you both so senseless at your time of life.
Won't you unwind that ivy? won't you, grandfather,
Let go the thyrsus you are carrying in your hand?
        You made him do this, for you hope, Teiresias,
By bringing men this fellow as another god,
For more bird-watching, fees for more burnt sacrifices.
But that grey hairs protect you, you'd be sitting now
Fettered, surrounded by the women-celebrants,
For introducing evil rites; when women feel
Buoyant with grape juice at a feast, take this from me, 260
There's nothing wholesome in the revel afterwards.
CHORUS: What irreligion! have you no respect for gods
Or Cadmus, sower of the crop of earth-sprung men?
Son of Echion, do you shame your ancestry?
TEIRESIAS: It is not effort for a reasonable man
Who speaks with a good pretext, to continue well;
Your tongue runs smoothly, yes, we'd think you sensible,

But what you utter is without a word of sense.
A bold and able man, who's also eloquent, 270
Is a bad citizen when his judgment is awry.
This god, this new god, whom you find ridiculous,
Will reach a greatness far beyond what I can say,
Through Hellas; for, young fellow, two come first with men,
Goddess Demeter to begin with — she is also Earth
And you may call her by whichever name you please —
And she it is who nurtures living men with food.
Now corresponding to her came this son of Semele
Who has discovered grape-juice for a drink, his gift
Bestowed on mortals; he releases wretched men 280
From pain, whenever they are filled with running wine,
Gives sleep, oblivion of their daily miseries;
There is no other remedy for weariness.
In him immortal the immortals pledge themselves,
So that men gather benefits because of him.
You find it queer that he was stitched in Zeus's thigh?
There is a simple explanation I can give.
When Zeus had snatched him from the fire the lightning made
And brought the baby to Olympus as a god,
Hera intended to expel him out of heaven; 290
But Zeus to counter Hera framed a god's device.
From the encircling ether round the earth he took
A fragment, made a living hostage out of it,
And sent the real Dionysus far from Hera's rage.
And later men said he was reared in Zeus's thigh,
Changing *Homeron* into *Meron* — hence the myth,*
Because the god was goddess Hera's hostage once.
Now this god is a prophet; in the Bacchic state
And Maenad frenzy there is much of mantic art,
For, when the god has entered deeply into man 300
He makes his maniacs speak of things that are to be.
And he has some of Ares in him . . . now and then
Troops in full armor and in line of battle dressed
Are cowed by terror when no spear has yet been touched,
And of their mania Dionysus is the cause.
You soon will see him even on the Delphic crags,
Leaping with torches over the two-crested gorge,
Now throwing up the Bacchic bough, now twirling it,
Mighty through Hellas . . . Pentheus, be advised by me,
Do not go boasting, "Power alone prevails with men," 310

* In Greek "homeron" means "hostage," and "meron" means "thigh."

Nor, even if you think so (though your thinking's warped)
Deem you have any wisdom. Take the god to Thebes,
Pour out libations, join his revel, wear his crown.
No Dionysus can make women continent
In love; in all things one is continent or not
By natural instinct always. Just consider this:
A woman who is continent will not be lost
Even in Bacchic revels. Here's another point:
It makes you happy when the people crowd the gates
And all the city rings aloud with Pentheus' name;   320
So he, I take it, is delighted to be cheered.
Well, I and Cadmus, whom you find ridiculous,
Shall wear our ivy coronals and join the dance,
A grey-haired couple — all the same we'll join the dance;
Your words have not persuaded me to war with gods.
Your madness is most serious and there are no drugs
That would relieve you — drugs must be the cause of it.
CHORUS: Worthy of Phoebus are your words, sir; wisely too
   You honor Bromius, who is great among the gods.
CADMUS: My son, Teiresias gives you excellent advice;   330
   Stay with us, try to think as others think.
   Now you have flights of fancy, you have witless wits.
   Suppose, as you say, there is no such god as this.
   Proclaim him, tell the noble lie that he exists,
   Get Semele acknowledged mother of a god
   And thereby honor comes to all the family.
   Remember how Actaeon met a dreadful end,
   How his flesh-eating hounds, the ones he reared,
   Tore him to pieces boasting in the meadow lands
   That he was greater at the hunt than Artemis.   340
   You must not perish like him; come you here, I'll crown
   Your head with ivy — come, adore the god with us.
PENTHEUS: Keep your hands off me, go and play your Bacchic game,
   Don't taint me with a folly which is all your own.
   And this instructor of your sheer insanity
   I'll put to justice . . . Someone must go off at once —
   Yes, you! go to his station where he watches birds
   And prise it with a crow-bar, turn it inside out,
   Turn upside down in rubble everything you find,
   Throw his prophetic garlands to the winds and storms,   350
   For that's the way I'll bite him most effectively.
   Be off, you others, search the city thoroughly
   And find the girlish stranger who has introduced
   Corruption for our women and defiles our beds;

And, if you catch him, bring him here with handcuffs on,
So, when he's sentenced to be stoned, before he dies
He'll see a bitter Bacchanalian feast in Thebes.

TEIRESIAS: A hard case! for you know not when and where you speak.
Now you are raving; you already were deranged.
    Cadmus, let's hurry, you and I, to win the god   360
For Pentheus, savage as he is, and for the town,
Asking him not to visit them with something strange.
Follow my foot-steps, ivy-headed staff and all,
Try to support me, I will do the same to you;
Two old men tumbling look disgraceful — never mind!
The service of the Bacchic god, the son of Zeus,
Demands us . . . as for Pentheus, may he bring your house
No penalty — I say this, Cadmus, not with mantic art
But facts to guide me; foolish words come from a fool.

CHORUS: Right, whom gods divine revere,   370
                Right, whose golden pinions fly
                Through the world, do you not hear
                Pentheus' uprighteous blasphemy,
                Challenging Bromius, who presides
                In crownéd gods' festivity,
                Semele's son, and holds besides
                Choruses with revelry?
                With his flute the laughs begin,   380
                Buoyancy to care succeeds
                When the grape-juice once comes in
                To the rooms where heaven feeds;
      So on men-revellers ivy-crowned
      His cup brings slumber that wraps them round.

                When to his utterance man gives rein,
                When he madly to Law says No!
                Then the end of the man is woe;
                But the quiet, the wise remain,
                They and their houses alike, unshaken: 390
                For the divinities of the skies,
                Though in the ether afar, have eyes
                Watching the ways that men have taken.
                Wisdom is often foolishness;
                Thinkers of thoughts too high for man
                End their life with a shorter span:
                Loss of the little they possess
                Visits ambitious men; to me

[handwritten annotation: Pentheus as a Intellectual]

Here it seems are a mad man's ways,
Here are the evil-doer's days . . .   400
Cyprus is where I'd wish to be!
O for the city whence loves are sent us,
Paphos, in Aphrodite's isle,
Coming to mortals to content us!
O for the hundred streams of Nile!
O for that land where the harvest giver
Is the barbarous rainless river!

O for Pieria the enchanting,   410
Holy spur of Olympus high;
To the seat of the Muses' haunting
Go before with the Bacchic cry,
Bromius! take me to those places,
Take me where Love is with the Graces!
There no orders our sport deny.

Zeus's son, the god, has pleasure
Not alone in revels wild;
Peace he loves, who gives us treasure,
Goddess Peace who rears the child.   420
The rich and the poor (it is his gift to both)
He refreshes with wine's delight;
Hatred he feels for the man who's loth
To live in happiness day and night.
Words to the wise I speak aloud:
"Hold aloof from the over-clever,
Keep head and heart for the humble crowd —   430
Follow its laws and uses ever."

(*Some of the guards return with the young* STRANGER *in hand-cuffs.*)

A GUARD: Here we are, Pentheus, with the prey we've hunted down
On your instructions; our dispatch was well repaid.
Tame was this quarry, never ran from us,
But willingly surrendered, did not even show
Pallor; his fresh complexion never left his cheeks.
No, laughingly he let us bind and take him off,
Stood still and made things easy for himself and me. 440
In very shame I told him, "Sir, unwillingly
I bind you, but my orders Pentheus gave himself."
As for the Bacchae, those you caught and dragged away
And bound in fetters in the public prison house,

They've vanished; to their orgies they are frisking off
Untrammelled, hailing Bromius by name as god;
Their fetters loosened of themselves to free their feet,
And keys, untouched by human hands, unlocked the doors.
The miracles are many that this man has brought
With him to Thebes; be wary of what are to come.   450
PENTHEUS: Take off his handcuffs; now that he is in my toils
He must be nimbler than he is to get away.
Well, friend, you're not unhandsome outwardly;
You must appeal to women . . . hence you came to Thebes.
Your hair is long, for wrestling quite unsuitable,
Over your features falling most attractively;
No doubt the whiteness of your skin's intentional,
To sun rays unaccustomed, but preferring shade,
Pursuing Aphrodite with a studied charm.
However, tell me first about your parentage.   460
STRANGER: Nothing to boast of; it's an easy thing to tell.
You know perhaps of Tmolus, where the flowers are?
PENTHEUS: I do: the mountain that encircles Sardis town.
STRANGER: That's where I come from: Lydia's my fatherland.
PENTHEUS: What makes you bring these ceremonies into Greece?
STRANGER: It was Dionysus sent us here, the son of Zeus.
PENTHEUS: Is there a Zeus there, one who brings new gods to birth?
STRANGER: Oh no! the one who married Semele in Thebes.
PENTHEUS: At night time did he force you to it or by day?
STRANGER: We saw each other when he gave his secret rites.   470
PENTHEUS: What is the nature of these secret rites of yours?
STRANGER: The uninitiated must not know the Bacchic lore.
PENTHEUS: And what advantage comes to those who sacrifice?
STRANGER: Some things worth knowing, not revealable to *you*.
PENTHEUS: A neat invention! just to make me curious.
STRANGER: The sinful liver Dionysus' rites repel.
PENTHEUS: This god you say you clearly saw; what was he like?
STRANGER: Like what he chose to look like, not what I arranged.
PENTHEUS: Side stepping neatly as before — you tell me nothing.
STRANGER: Speakers of wisdom to the ignorant are fools.   480
PENTHEUS: Is this the first place where you've brought the deity?
STRANGER: No! all barbarians dance according to his rites.
PENTHEUS: Because their sense is much inferior to the Greeks'.
STRANGER: In this, superior; but their laws are not the same.
PENTHEUS: By night or day light do you hold your services?
STRANGER: Mostly at night time; darkness has solemnity.
PENTHEUS: That is for cheating women and corrupting them.
STRANGER: In open day light baseness can be practiced too.

PENTHEUS: You must be punished for your evil sophistries.
STRANGER: You, to our god unrighteous, for your ignorance.   490
PENTHEUS: Bold is our Bacchant and athletic . . . in his words.
STRANGER: Tell me my fate; what horror will you do to me?
PENTHEUS: First I will cut this tender, flowing hair of yours.
STRANGER: That lock is sacred, and I grow it for the god.
PENTHEUS: Next hand to me the thyrsus that you carry now.
STRANGER: You take it from me; this is Dionysus' property.
PENTHEUS: Then I shall hold your person in confinement here.
STRANGER: The god himself will free me when I want it done.
PENTHEUS: Aye, when you call him, standing with the Bacchic girls.
STRANGER: No, here and now he watches what I undergo.   500
PENTHEUS: But where? he's not apparent to my eyes at least.
STRANGER: With me. You'd see him but for your unrighteousness.
PENTHEUS: Arrest him! he's affronted both myself and Thebes.
STRANGER: I tell you not to bind me; I am wise, you're not.
PENTHEUS: Bind him, I order; I am master here, not you.
STRANGER: You know not what your life is, see not who you are.
PENTHEUS: Pentheus, Agave's son; Echion was my sire.
STRANGER: For evil fortune you're appropriately named.
PENTHEUS: Off with you! guard him by the horses' stable there,
 With nothing for him visible but dark and gloom.   510
 Go you and dance there, and the women that you've brought,
 Accomplices in evil, I will sell abroad,
 Or, when I've stopped their noisy drums and tambourines,
 Keep them as servants held to labor at the loom.
STRANGER: I'll go; one surely must not feel what must not be.
 But you will make atonement for this insolence
 To Dionysus, who, you say, does not exist;
 For when you wrong me, *he* is made the prisoner.

CHORUS: Lady Dirce, will you not know us?
        Why do you turn your face away?
        Virgin daughter of Achelous!   520
        It was not so in another day,
 When your stream was the first to lave him,
 Bacchus, the babe from his father's thigh;
 Zeus in the lightning came to save him;
 Zeus then spoke with a father's cry,
 "Dithyrambus! so Thebes shall name you,
 Twice-born, once from a mother's womb."
 Happy Dirce! we shall not shame you,   530
 Garlanded for our feast we come.
 Soon, on my oath by the cluster-bearing

Vine tree that Dionysus gives,
Soon for Bromius you'll be caring . . .
Meanwhile the dragon's offspring lives,
Pentheus, a monster rude, defiant,   540
Born, as his father was, from a clod,
Less like a man than a murderous giant
Ready for battle against a god.
Rope he has sent for to hold us faster,
Followers of the god of Din,
He has imprisoned our revel-master,
Holds him in dungeons black within.
Do you not see us with force contending,
Dionysus, who preached you wide?
Zeus-born sovereign, come, descending   550
Mount Olympus; your golden-eyed
Thyrsus brandish and make an ending
Of this murderous fellow's pride.

Is it on Nysa, the wild things' cover,
Dionysus, our prayer should seek
You with your thyrsus ruling over
Revels or on a Corycian peak?
Is it not in an Olympian hollow,   560
Densely-wooded, where Orpheus drew
Trees with his zither-play to follow,
Drew with his music the wild things too?
        Happy Pieria!
Honored by Evius, who will bring
Dances and Bacchic revelling;
Over Axius, the swirling,
He will bring the Maenads whirling;   570
Over Lydia, made to bless
Men with happy fruitfulness,
Over the father-stream renowned,
        Where fairest waters
Feed the finest horses' ground.

VOICE FROM WITHIN: Io! Hear my voice; hear! Io Bacchae! Io Bacchae!
CHORUS: What and whence is this voice that summons me for Evius?
VOICE: Io! Io! again I call, the son of Semele, Zeus's son.   580
CHORUS: Io! Io!
  Master, master, come now to our revel-band!
  O! Bromius, Bromius!

    (*The palace shakes. Lightning follows.*)

HALF-CHORUS: Ah! the ground . . . ah! the earthquake!
Surely Pentheus' palace will be rocked down in ruins.
Dionysus is in the palace. Worship him! 590
HALF-CHORUS: We worship him! did you see the stone architraves
Above the pillars shaking? Bromius is calling from inside.
VOICE: Zeus! set the lightning's flaming lamp
To Pentheus' palace; burn it, burn it out.
CHORUS: Ah . . . ah . . . watch and see the fire round Semele's holy tomb,
The flame she left when stricken by Zeus's thunder-bolt! 599
On the ground, on the ground fling your trembling bodies, Maenads,
For our king is coming, Zeus's son, who is overturning the palace.

(*The lightning ceases, the young* STRANGER *re-enters from the palace, which remains standing.*)

STRANGER: Women, new to Hellas, are you so beside yourselves with fear?
Fallen, have you? But you noticed very likely how the god
Shook and shivered Pentheus' palace — now, I beg you, raise yourselves,
Summon up your courage, end these quivering infirmities.
CHORUS: Brightest light of Bacchic revels, leader of our Bacchic cry,
With what ecstasy we see you, in our loneliness forlorn.
STRANGER: Then you fell into depression when they marched me off indoors, 610
Thinking they would truly throw me into Pentheus' dungeon-cells?
CHORUS: Could we help it? who'd protect us if disaster fell on you?
How did you obtain your freedom? on a wicked man you chanced.
STRANGER: Easily! It took no trouble; I was my own rescuer.
CHORUS: But he bound your hands together, he imprisoned you with ropes.
STRANGER: Herein I outmocked the mocker. He had got me fast, he thought,
But in fact he never touched me, though he made a meal of hopes,
Found a bullock in the stables where he took and locked me up.
This it was he started roping, binding round its hocks and hooves,
Breathing out his soul in fury, dripping everywhere with sweat,
Biting on his lips; I watched him, comfortably looking on 621
From a front seat I had taken. In the meantime Bacchus came,
Set the royal palace rocking, set his mother's tomb alight.
Pentheus, when at last he noticed, thought the palace was on fire,
Rushed first this way, then the other, ordering the staff to bring
Water; every slave got working, toiling at a futile task.
Thinking then that I'd escaped him, Pentheus gave the struggle up,
Off he goes inside the palace with a rusty sword he'd snatched;

Bromius next, as I imagine — this is only what I think —
Made a phantom in the courtyard; Pentheus made a dash at this,
Stabbing only air that glistened, thinking he was killing me.   631
Lost is everything of Pentheus', ruined by the Bacchic god;
To the ground he's razed the palace, left it all a shattered wreck,
My imprisonment resenting . . . Pentheus, being tired out,
Handed in his sword and yielded, for to battle with a god,
Being but a man, was daring. Quietly I slipped away,
Left the palace, came to join you; Pentheus does not trouble me.
But I fancy there are footsteps in the house at any rate:
He'll be coming any moment out in front; what *will* he say?
I can manage him — no trouble — even in his pompous mood;
For the motto of the wise man is to keep his temper cool.   641

(PENTHEUS *enters from the palace.*)

PENTHEUS: I have been made a victim, for the stranger, tied
In bonds inextricable, has got clear away.
Ho! Ho!
This is the fellow! What is this? how came you here,
Here on the palace terrace? how did you escape?
STRANGER: Stand still! don't let your temper run away with you.
PENTHEUS: By what contrivance came you out of prison here?
STRANGER: Someone, I told you — did you hear — would set me free.
PENTHEUS: Who, pray? New riddles come with every word you
speak.   650
STRANGER: He who for mortals grows the many-clustered vine.
PENTHEUS: [*line 652 is missing.*]
STRANGER: To Dionysus that reproach of yours is praise.
PENTHEUS: Let every gate tower round the city wall be barred!
STRANGER: Why so? are even walls impassable for gods?
PENTHEUS: Except where wisdom's needed, you are very wise.
STRANGER: Wisdom I have by nature when it's needed most.
But there's a man here, listen to his story first;
He's from the mountain with some news for you from there.
I will await your pleasure; I will not escape.

(*During the last speech a* COWMAN *from Mount Cithaeron has
entered.*)

COWMAN: Pentheus, the royal sovereign of this Theban land,   660
I come from Mount Cithaeron, where there never cease
The white, pellucid snow showers . . .
PENTHEUS: Yes, but what urgent message did you come to bring?
COWMAN: The women Bacchae who went hurtling out of Thebes,
Stung into madness — with their white limbs bare — I saw

On Mount Cithaeron; I must tell you, sire, and Thebes,
What heinous things they practise, far beyond belief.
But first assure me; may I openly declare
What's going on there or omit to speak the whole?
For, sire, I'm in some terror of your hastiness,   670
Your bitter temper and your over-royal mind.

PENTHEUS: Speak out! I give you a complete indemnity;
Against the law-abiding anger must not hold.
But the more heinous are the things the Bacchae do
With the more rigor of the law I'll prosecute
This man, the instigator of the women's tricks.

COWMAN: The grazing cattle I was driving to the rock,
The Calves' Rock, up the mountain, when the sun came out,
Radiant, striking heat into the ground below,
And then I saw three revel-bands of women: one   680
Autonoe commanded and the second one
Agave, your own mother; Ino's was the third.
And there they all were sleeping, with their limbs relaxed,
Some of them leaning with their backs on fir tree boughs,
Some among oak leaves with their heads upon the ground
Fallen haphazard, decently (not, as you say,
Drunken with wine cups or, to music of the flute,
Hunting the forest for the love that they had lost.)
     And then your mother gave a cry; she stood among
The Bacchae, calling them to shake themselves from sleep,   690
When first she heard the lowing of the horned beasts.
Then gentle slumber from their eyes they put away
And stood bolt upright; it was a marvellous piece of drill,
Young women, old ones, maidens who were not yet wed.
Over their shoulders firstly they arranged their hair,
And those whose fawnskin tunics had their knots undone
Tied them together; round the dappled skins they put
Serpents for girdles and the creatures licked their cheeks.
And some of them were nursing fawns or lion cubs —
Wild ones — and suckling them with milk, for these had left   700
At home their new-born infants and their breasts were full.
Then they put on their garlands: ivy leaves they wore,
But some had oak leaves, some had flowering briony.
And one would take a thyrsus up and beat the rock
And there a spring of dewy water spurted out;
Into the earthy soil another thrust a cane,
There the god sent a fountain welling up with wine;
And those who had a craving for a whiter drink
Scratched on the surface of the ground with finger tips

And milk in plenty followed. From their ivy-twined 710
Thyrsi came honey, dripping in delicious streams.
Had you been there to see this, you'd pursue with prayers
The very god that now you rate with contumely.

We herdsmen drew together and the shepherds too,
To pool our stories, each competing with the rest,
Of what the Bacchae did, how strange and wonderful.
And one, a city-goer trained in words, spoke out
To all: "You dwellers in the holy mountain clefts,
Is it your pleasure that we hunt Agave down, 720
Snatch the king's mother from the Bacchic rites and earn
Pentheus' approval?" And his words, we thought, were right.
So, in some leafy brushwood, out of sight, we laid
An ambush; and the Bacchae, at the time arranged,
Began to shake the thyrsus for the Bacchic rites,
With one voice calling on Iacchus, son of Zeus,
Naming him Bromius; all the mountain joined the rites,
And all the wild life; with the running all things shook.
Agave's leaping brought her near to me, and I
Jumped forward with intent to capture her; I left
Empty the ambush where our bodies lay concealed, 730
And she cried loudly, "Here, you running hounds of mine,
These men are out to hunt us down; but follow me,
Follow! your weapon is the thyrsus in your hands."

Now we ourselves, by taking to our heels, escaped
From being rent to pieces, but the Bacchae fell
Upon the grazing heifers — not a knife had they.
You could have seen Agave holding in two parts
A heifer near to milking and it lowed the while;
And the young cattle others tore to bits and shreds.
You could have seen here, there, and everywhere the ribs, 740
The cloven hooves, all scattered; hanging pieces dripped
Under the pine trees with a mingled mess of blood.
And bulls of mettle, but a while ago prepared
For angry tossings, there were sprawling on the ground,
Put there by tens of thousand maiden hands.
Less time was spent in stripping carcasses of flesh
Than it would take you, sire, to shut your royal eyes.
Then they went racing, with the flight of birds, across
The stretching lowlands that along Asopus stream
Yield for the Thebans goodly reaping crops of grain, 750
And they assaulted Hysiae and Erythrae,
Under Cithaeron's mountain, like an enemy;
Here, there, and everywhere they scattered all there was;

They snatched up children from their homes; and what they put
On to their shoulders, though they did not bind it on,
Stayed there and never fell upon the earthy soil,
Not even brass or iron; on their clustered hair
They carried fire that burnt not. Then the folk enraged
And harassed by the Bacchae, rushed to take up arms;
On this there followed, sire, the strangest spectacle.   760
The pointed arrows did not draw a drop of blood
Out of the Bacchae; they but threw their thyrsus wands,
With these they wounded, turned their adversaries back,
Women with men contending, not without some god.

And now they came returning to the starting point,
The very fountains that the god had raised for them,
And washed the blood off, then the serpents with their tongues
Cleaned up their streaming cheeks.

As for this god, my master, whosoever he be,
Receive him in this city, for he is a mighty god,   770
And, above all, they say of him, as I've been told,
He gave the vine to mortals, easing them of pain.
And if wine ceases there will be an end of Love,
An end of every pleasure in the life of man.

CHORUS: To give my thoughts free utterance I hesitate
Before a tyrant; all the same, this shall be said:
Second to none is Dionysus of the gods.

PENTHEUS: Near us already is the Bacchic insolence,
Like fire that kindles, making us the shame of Greece;
Delay we must not; go you to Electra's gate,   780
And give the troops the order, those who carry shields,
And all who ride swift footed horses, all who swing
The targe, and every one who with his hands can set
The bow string sounding, say our army will proceed
Against the Bacchae, for there is no end to this
If we endure from women what we now endure.

* STRANGER: Nothing, O Pentheus, if you listened to my words,
Would you endure. Enduring much from you yourself,
I still advise you: take not arms against the god,
But rest in quiet. Bromius will not allow   790
You to dislodge the Bacchae from his mountain haunts.

PENTHEUS: You shall not lecture me! bear this in mind,
You broke from prison; shall I reinforce the law?

STRANGER: Oblations would I give the god, not obloquy,

---

* There is in this passage a play on Pentheus' name, as meaning a "sufferer."

And, a mere human, would not kick against the pricks.
PENTHEUS: Oblations be it! female victims, as their due,
I'll offer up in numbers on Cithaeron's crest.
STRANGER: You'll all be routed; it will be ignominious
When Bacchic thyrsi make the brazen shields retreat.
PENTHEUS: This stranger has me knotted in a hopeless case,   800
For, doing or enduring, he must always speak.
STRANGER: Good sir, it's open to you still to set this right.
PENTHEUS: If to my subjects I subject myself, perhaps?
STRANGER: No! without weapons I will bring the women here.
PENTHEUS: Ah! you're contriving now to play a trick on me.
STRANGER: Trick? if I'm willing by my arts to rescue you?
PENTHEUS: You planned this with them to perpetuate your rights.
STRANGER: That I admit to planning, mark you, with the god.
PENTHEUS: Bring me my arms, attendants! and stop talking, you!
* STRANGER: So!   810
You want to see them on the mountains in their camp?
PENTHEUS: Yes, I'd give any quantity of gold for that.
STRANGER: Why has this sudden passion seized you for the sight?
PENTHEUS: It would be painful if I had to see them drunk.
STRANGER: And yet you'd see with pleasure what would cause you pain?
PENTHEUS: I mean, from somewhere silent underneath the pines.
STRANGER: But they will track you, even if you go there secretly.
PENTHEUS: I'll go there in the open; what you say is right.
STRANGER: Am I to take you? shall I help you on the way?
PENTHEUS: At once! I grudge you all the time we're wasting here.   820
STRANGER: Just go and dress up in a flowing linen gown.
PENTHEUS: What's that for? do I enter on the women's roll?
STRANGER: Because they'll kill you if you're seen to be a man.
PENTHEUS: Well spoken! somehow you have good, old-fashioned wits.
STRANGER: In these things Dionysus was my schoolmaster.
PENTHEUS: How can we do what you advise successfully?
STRANGER: I'll be your dresser; let us go inside the house.
PENTHEUS: What dress? a woman's? No, I couldn't face the thing!
STRANGER: You're less enthusiastic for the Maenad show.
PENTHEUS: What kind of costume do you say you'll make me wear?   830
STRANGER: Well, first I'll make you wear a wig of flowing hair.
PENTHEUS: And what's the second item in my beautifying?
STRANGER: A gown to reach your ankles; for your head, a hat.
PENTHEUS: Anything further has my outfitter for me?
STRANGER: Only a thyrsus and a dappled fawnskin cloak.

---

* At this point the conversation takes a different tone, as if Pentheus fell
gradually under hypnotic influence.

PENTHEUS: I simply cannot dress myself in women's clothes.
STRANGER: You'll want some different dressings if you go to war.
PENTHEUS: You're right, the first thing needed is reconnaissance.
STRANGER: At least that's wiser than pursuing harm with harm.
PENTHEUS: And how, pray, can I cross the city unobserved?
STRANGER: We'll go by unfrequented streets; I'll lead the way.   840
PENTHEUS: Anything rather than the Bacchae's mockery;
    We'll go inside the palace and concert our plans.
STRANGER: Agreed! I'm at your service any way you choose.
PENTHEUS: I'm going; either I proceed there under arms,
    Or else I follow the advice you've given me.

      (He goes into the palace.)

STRANGER: Women, the man is swimming well inside the net.
    He'll join the Bacchae, death will be his punishment.
    Dionysus, now it rests with you, not far away,
    To take our vengeance. First, then, drive him mad,   850
    Make him light-headed, for, if he retains his wits,
    Assuredly he'll never wear a woman's dress;
    He'll wear it only if he is beside himself.
    Now I intend him for the laughing-stock of Thebes,
    Female-impersonator, through the city led,
    No more a threatener — he excelled in threats just now.
    I go now to fit Pentheus with the clothes he'll wear,
    When from his mother's hands he passes into Death,
    By those hands slaughtered. Zeus's son he then will know,
    Dionysus; at the end he is the fiercest god,   860
    Though very gentle in his ways with humankind.

      (He goes into the palace.)

CHORUS: In the revels shall I be there,
      Night-long dancing,
      White feet glancing,
      Tossing my head in the dewy air?
      Just as the roe that in terror risks
        Hunters' ambushes, nets and snares,
      Free at last in the meadow frisks
        Glad in the green, though the hunter spares   870
      Neither his voice nor his hounds in pressing —
      Straining, but swift as the storm winds blow,
      There, by a leap the lawn possessing,
      Over the river exults the roe;
      No man comes to her meadow where
      Woods in spring have shadowy hair.

What thing wiser and what more glorious
Gift can the gods on man bestow
 Than to triumph with hand victorious
Over the head of a fallen foe? 880
 Glory is sweet and that I know.

Slow is the heavenly strength to motion,
Steadfast in purpose, it comes to school
Him who gives Ignorance devotion,
Slighting the gods like a crazy fool;
Long is the foot of Time, but they
Skillfully hiding themselves away 890
Make the unholy at last their prey:
Rightly! because there are limits set
To what we should either know or do;
And there's another lesson yet
Costing little, but it is true,
That for ever the gods endure
And the sanctions of Time are sure.

 What thing wiser and what more glorious
Gift can the gods on man bestow
 Than to triumph with hand victorious
Over the head of a fallen foe? 900
 Glory is sweet and that I know.

Happy is the man who sails
Into port from storms at sea,
And he's happy who prevails
Over troubles, though there be
Richer, poorer, weak, and strong;
And to ten thousand men belong
Ten thousand plans; some have success,
Some fail; if a man has happiness
In what comes to him day by day, 910
"All good luck to him" I say.

(*The* STRANGER *comes out of the palace, followed by* PENTHEUS.)

STRANGER: Come out, you sight-seer of the things you should not see,
 Pentheus, I mean, desirous of the undesirable,
 Come forward from the palace! let me look at you
 Dressed like a girl, a Maenad and a Bacchanal,
 Would-be observer of your mother and her band!
 You might be one of Cadmus' daughters by your looks.

PENTHEUS: What's this? I fancy I can see two suns at once,
  Two cities, each of them with seven gates;
  And you, my leader, at a close view, are a bull   920
  And on your forehead you have grown a pair of horns.
  Were you an animal all the time? for bull you are!
STRANGER: The god is with us; he was not so pleased before,
  But now he is our partner; now you see aright.
PENTHEUS: What do I look like? have I Ino's stance and poise,
  Or am I like my mother, as is natural?
STRANGER: I see them both in person when I look at you.
  One of your ringlets, though, has fallen out of place,
  Not as I tucked it nicely underneath your hat.
PENTHEUS: My fault! I disarranged it, when indoors just now   930
  I shook it up and forward in the Bacchic dance.
STRANGER: All right! this duty as your dresser falls to me,
  I'll re-adjust it; hold your head up, if you please.
PENTHEUS: There then; you fix it — see how much I lean on you.
STRANGER: Your sashes are not tight enough; your gown besides
  Over the ankles does not fall in even folds.
PENTHEUS: I see that, by the right foot in particular.
  This side it reaches to the instep perfectly.
STRANGER: You'll call me dearest friend, when once you realize
  The Bacchae are more modest than you thought before.   940
PENTHEUS: About the thyrsus — is my right hand or my left
  The one for me to carry it in Bacchic style?
STRANGER: The right hand; lift it when your right foot takes a step;
  Congratulations on your pleasant change of heart.
PENTHEUS: Think you that I could carry all Cithaeron's clefts
  Upon my shoulders with the Bacchic crew as well?
STRANGER: By all means, if you willed it, for your heart is sound
  Just as we like it — it was not so good before.
PENTHEUS: Shall we take levers? do I prise it with my hands?
  Do I put arm or shoulder underneath the peaks?   950
STRANGER: Be careful not to wreck the grottoes of the Nymphs
  And Pan-god's private building where he keeps his pipes.
PENTHEUS: That is well spoken; strength must not be used to quell
  These women; I will hide myself among the pines.
STRANGER: Yes! you will get the hiding that you ought to get
  For cunning observation of the Maenad girls.
PENTHEUS: Already I can see them in the brakes like birds
  Caught in their nests and happy in attractive snares.
STRANGER: Your mission is to guard against this very thing;
  Perhaps you'll get them, if they do not get you first.   960
PENTHEUS: Now pray conduct me through the heart of Thebes;
  I am the only man with courage for this act.

STRANGER: The only man who does not spare himself for Thebes,
    The only one; adventures worthy of you wait.
    Now follow! I will be safe-conduct for you there,
    But someone else will bring you home . . .
PENTHEUS: My mother? Yes!
STRANGER: Displayed to everybody
PENTHEUS: That is why I go.
STRANGER: You will be carried
PENTHEUS: Very comfortably, too
STRANGER: By your own mother
PENTHEUS: Luxury you force on me
STRANGER: A luxury of sorts
PENTHEUS: I only get what I deserve.   970
STRANGER: You are not ordinary and your lot will be
    Not ordinary. Fame will lift you to the skies.
    Stretch out your hands, Agave, and your sisters too,
    Daughters of Cadmus! I am leading on this youth
    To great adventure, but the victory will be
    With me and Bromius. And the rest events will show.

CHORUS: Hounds of madness, forward spring!
        Find the Bacchic gathering;
        On the mountains find and harry
        Cadmus' daughters; do not tarry.   980
        Set them on this mad spectator,
        On the flounced impersonator.
        Him his mother first will see
        By a boulder or a tree
        Lurking; to the Maenad rout
        "Who has come here?" she will shout,
        "Searching for us mountain-rangers?
        Ours is Cadmus' blood, the stranger's . . .
  Bacchae! O Bacchae! to our mountain who has come?
        Women's issue he is not;
        On a lioness begot
        Maybe, or from Libyan seed
        Such a spawn as Gorgons breed."   990

        Now let open Justice heed,
        Come with killing sword to smite
        One who knows no law, no right,
        Knows not god, Echion's son —
        Through his throat the blade shall run,
        For that creature of the soil
        Sets his mind and will to foil,

Bacchus, Lord, the ritual due 1000
To your Mother and to you.
Lawless anger rules his thought,
Justice still he sets at naught;
He is mad in heart and brain,
For the thrust of might and main
On the invincible is vain.

Man to the gods must make submission,
And for the painless life his vow
Must be acceptance without condition;
Only so far as the gods allow,
Follow wisdom! I try to practise
Deeds that are always great and fine;
Plain and eternal the daily act is,
If it but honors the life divine,
From the unrighteous holding clear.

Now let open Justice hear, 1010
Come with killing sword to smite
One who knows no law, no right,
Knows not god, Echion's son —
Through his throat the blade shall run.
Bacchus, on that earthly scion
Come you like a flaming lion,
Like a bull or like a snake,
Many-headed, come to take
In a noose the man who'd mock 1020
All the deadly Maenad flock;
Hunt the Bacchae's hunter down.

(*The* MESSENGER *enters, one of Pentheus' household staff.*)

MESSENGER: O royal household, once most prosperous in Greece,
The old Sidonian's, who produced the Men of Earth
For harvest when he sowed in earth the dragon's teeth,
I make my lamentation for you, though a slave;
Good slaves are with their masters in catastrophe.
CHORUS: What is it? from the Bacchae have you further news?
MESSENGER: Pentheus has perished, he who was Echion's son. 1030
CHORUS: All hail to Bromius! now you are a god indeed!
MESSENGER: What's that? what made you say it? does it give you joy,
Women, to have my masters in calamity?
CHORUS: Euoi! I sing my foreign strains,
Freed from the terror of the chains!

MESSENGER: Is Thebes so short of manhood, do you think? ...
CHORUS: I do not own your Theban sway —
  It is Dionysus we obey.
MESSENGER: You may be pardoned, but there's nothing fine, my friends,
  In exultation over evil so complete.   1040
CHORUS: Tell me, speak plainly, how the villain came to death,
  Unrighteous and purveyor of unrighteousness.
MESSENGER: When we had left the outskirts of the town of Thebes,
  We crossed the river of Asopus, then we made
  A thrust toward Cithaeron's rocky fastnesses,
  Pentheus and I — I followed where my master went —
  The stranger with us as our guide to see the sight.
     First then we found and halted in a grassy dell,
  Silently treading, keeping silence with our lips,
  Intent on seeing while we kept ourselves unseen.   1050
  A ghyll, with cliffs around it and a water fall,
  There was, and fir trees shaded it; the Maenads there
  Were sitting, busy with their pleasant handiwork.
  Some were renewing chaplets on their thyrsus-tops
  With ivy where the old had fallen in decay;
  And some, like fillies from the colored harness free,
  Sang to each other alternating Bacchic songs.
     Unhappy Pentheus did not see this crowd of girls
  And told the stranger, "From the place we're standing in
  I cannot see the Maenads at their vicious dance;   1060
  If I went up a hillock or a lofty pine,
  The Maenads' degradation would be plain to see."
  And then the stranger seemed to work a miracle;
  For, grasping at a pine tree's skyward pointing branch,
  He drew it downward, downward, downward to the earth,
  And like a bow it rounded or maybe an arc
  Someone is drawing with a pair of compasses;
  Just so the stranger held that mountain-shoot in hand,
  And to the earth he drew it, not a mortal's deed.
  And, perching Pentheus there among the pine tree boughs,   1070
  He slipped the tree trunk through his hands till it was straight,
  Without a quiver, lest it throw my master off,
  And there the tree stood upright to the upright sky,
  With Pentheus seated much as if he sat a horse,
  More to the Maenads visible than they to him.
  While yet he could not be distinguished sitting there,
  The stranger in the meantime being out of sight,
  A voice from ether sounded — as it seems to me,
  It was Dionysus — shouting, "Maenads, here I bring

The man that makes of you and me a mockery 1080
And of our ritual; now avenge yourselves on him!"

And while the voice was speaking there arose a light,
Skyward and earthward — it was a light of holy fire.
The air kept silent; in the pasture land the dell
Silenced its leaves; no wild thing uttered any sound.
Now they, not clearly taking in the voice they heard,
Stood upright, looking all about them. Then again
He gave the order; when the Maenads recognized
The clear command of Bacchus, Cadmus' daughters first
Rushed forward with the swiftness of a flock of doves, 1090
Running their hardest, with their racing feet astrain,
Agave, Pentheus' mother, and her sisters too,
And all the Bacchae; through the dell, the river bed
They leapt and over fissures, by the god inspired.
      Now, when they saw my master seated on the pine,
They started hurling stones at him with all their force,
And they had climbed up on a rock to press the siege,
And some were using boughs of pine for javelins.
And others sent their thyrsi flying through the air
At Pentheus, their ill-fated target, but they failed. 1100
For he, poor wretch, was higher than their zeal could reach,
Seated above them, prisoner to hopelessness.
Last, with some branches stripped from oaks as lightning strips,
They tore with timber levers at the fir tree roots.
And, when their efforts never seemed to reach an end,
Agave ordered: "Round the sapling make a ring,
Hold on to it and get it, Maenads; so we'll catch
The climbing creature — it shall not proclaim abroad
The god's mysterious revels!" Then ten thousand hands
Grasped at the pine tree and uprooted it from earth. 1110
And he who sat there up aloft came crashing down,
Pentheus, and with ten thousand groans he met the earth.
I, who was near it, witnessed the catastrophe.
      And first his mother, priestess of the sacrifice,
Fell on him; Pentheus threw the hat from off his head,
That poor Agave, recognizing him, should stay
Her hand from putting him to death; he touched her cheek
And said, "You know me, mother, for the son you bore,
Pentheus, within Echion's palace; pity me,
My mother, do not visit my iniquities 1120
On me by putting me, a son of yours, to death."
      But she, with foaming at the mouth and rolling eyes
In frenzy, thinking as a mind should never think,

Was held by Bacchus; his entreaty touched her not.
She took his wrist, the left one, in her hands and stood
With her feet pressing on his ribs, poor helpless man,
And wrenched his shoulder from its socket — not by strength,
But the god gave it to her hands an easy prey.
The other side was Ino, finishing the work,
Tearing his flesh asunder and Autonoe   1130
With all the Bacchic horde attacked: there was a cry,
One sound from all together; Pentheus, while he breathed,
Groaned, but the others cheered. A fore-arm one had got,
The feet another, with the shoes; his ribs were stripped
Piece-meal; those women, every one, with bloody hands
Joined in a ball-game, using bits of Pentheus' flesh.

    The body lies in different places, part below
Sharp rocks and part in thickets deep in undergrowth,
Not easy to discover, but the wretched head
His mother chanced on and she took it in her hands
And fixed it on her thyrsus, thinking it to be   1140
A mountain lion's — through Cithaeron this she bears,
Leaving her sisters in the Maenad choruses.
Inside these walls, rejoicing in her luckless prey,
She comes, acclaiming as her comrade in the hunt
Bacchus, participator with her in the kill,
The glorious victor — victory to her of tears.

    But I, for my part, will not face this tragedy
Or meet Agave coming to our palace gates.
All glory rests on moderation and respect for gods,
And, as I judge, the mortal who possesses these   1150
Is also wisest if he turns the gifts to use.

CHORUS: Let us dance in Bacchus' name,
                    Let us with a shout acclaim
                    Pentheus' fate, the serpent's seed,
                    Who, in women's clothes parading,
                    Went to death with no evading,
                    Carrying the thyrsus-reed,
                    Went to fate, a bull before him.   1160
                    Theban Bacchae! she who bore him
                    Wins a victor's song, begun
                    With a triumph, but it stops
                    On a note of tears and wails;
                    On her arms her nursling son
                    Spatters out his blood in drops;
                    Fine the match was — she prevails.

But now I see her to the palace rushing on,
Agave, Pentheus' mother with her rolling eyes —
Take up the revel of the god who calls 'Euoi'.

(AGAVE *enters, carrying* PENTHEUS' *head.*)

AGAVE: Bacchae from Asia!

CHORUS: What do you want of me?

AGAVE: I bring from the mountain a new-cut spray for the 1170
house, a lucky find.

CHORUS: I see and I welcome you to join our revel.

AGAVE: I caught this young lion without snares; you see what it is.

CHORUS: Where in the wilds?

AGAVE: Cithaeron . . .

CHORUS: Cithaeron?

AGAVE: . . . killed him.

CHORUS: Which of you hit him first?

AGAVE: Mine was the honor. They call me lucky Agave at our gatherings.

CHORUS: Who helped?

AGAVE: Cadmus's . . .

CHORUS: Cadmus's? 1180

AGAVE: His daughters after *me*, after *me*, wounded this creature.

CHORUS: You are lucky in your catch.

AGAVE: Share the banquet.

CHORUS: How can I?

AGAVE: The calf is young, only just growing soft down on his face below
his hair.

CHORUS: (*aside*): In truth it might be hair of some wild animal.

AGAVE: Bacchus, himself a cunning hunter, cunningly
Directed us, the Maenads, to the animal. 1190

CHORUS: He's the Hunter-King.

AGAVE: You praise me?

CHORUS: Of course.

AGAVE: So will the people of Cadmus very soon!

CHORUS: Especially your son Pentheus.

AGAVE: He'll praise his mother for taking this lion's whelp.

CHORUS: Unusual prey!

AGAVE: Unusually taken.

CHORUS: You are glad?

AGAVE: Glad to have dealt with this prey greatly, yes, greatly and conspicuously.

CHORUS: Well, miserable woman, show the spoils you've brought,
A victor's trophies, to the citizens of Thebes. 1201

AGAVE: You who live in the city with the splendid walls,

Thebans, come hither, come and see what I have caught,
The beast that Cadmus' daughters captured, all of us,
Not with the pointed javelins of Thessaly,
Not with nets either, but with women's hands ungloved.
What need to go on boasting of the arms you bear
And vainly buying weapons of the spear makers?
For with this very hand I took this victim here
And with our hands we severed all the joints apart.   1210
Where is my honored father? let him come and see.
And my son Pentheus, where is he? for he must take
A set of ladders, lean them up against the house,
And on the triglyphs he must nail this head I hold,
Head of a lion that I hunted down myself.

    (CADMUS *enters with bearers who carry* PENTHEUS' *body on a bier.*)

CADMUS: Follow behind me with your pitiable load,
Follow, bear Pentheus, servants, here before his house.
I bring the body as it is, for that I found
With countless toilsome searches in Cithaeron's clefts,
In shreds dismembered, nothing in one place I took,   1220
And in a wood it was lying, difficult to search.
I heard from someone of my daughters' outrages
When I already was inside the city walls,
Returning from the revel with our old Teiresias.
Back to the mountain then I went and here convey
The boy who suffered death at Maenads' hands. The one
Who bore Actaeon to Aristaeus long ago,
Autonoe, I saw with Ino in their wretched plight
There in the wood land stung with Bacchic frenzy still,
And someone told me that the third, with reeling gait,   1230
Was coming here — Agave — and he spoke the truth,
For here I see her, not the most propitious sight.
AGAVE: Father, you have the greatest opportunity to boast
That no one had such daughters, no one in the world;
For all of us I claim this, but my claim is first,
Since I, who left the shuttles idle on the loom,
Have found a great vocation, hunting beasts unarmed.
And, as you see, a trophy in my arms I bear
Ready for hanging up against your palace walls;   1240
Take it, dear father, in your hands and wish me joy
Over my hunting exploits; summon friends to come
And join a banquet; now congratulate yourself;
Congratulations you have earned by what I've done.

CADMUS: Immeasurable sorrow and unbearable
  To look on murder by those wretched hands of yours!
  Magnificently to the gods you've sacrificed
  Before inviting to the banquet Thebes . . . and me.
  Woe for the evil touching both, but chiefly you!
  He has destroyed us, justly, but too thoroughly,
  The god, Lord Bromius, has destroyed the kin he claims.   1250
AGAVE: Old age is always peevish in the life of man
  And always scowling. How I wish that son of mine
  Were a good hunter, following his mother's ways
  When he goes hunting with the other youth of Thebes.
  But he's no good for anything but fighting gods.
  He needs a scolding; father, you must give it him.
  Isn't there someone who will call him here to me?
  He ought to see me at the height of my success.
CADMUS: Alas! when you can reason over what you've done,
  You and your sisters will have fearful suffering.   1260
  But if you stay for ever as you are, your minds
  Will never tell you whether fortune's good or bad.
AGAVE: But what is wrong or painful in the thing we've done?
CADMUS: Now first look upward — turn your eyes toward the sky.
AGAVE: There! for what reason do you make me look at it?
CADMUS: Is it as usual? do you notice any change?
AGAVE: It's brighter and more shining than it was before.
CADMUS: You still have flights of fancy in that mind of yours.
AGAVE: I do not know your meaning, but I somehow feel
  Quite sane, my mind is different from what it was.   1270
CADMUS: I'll ask you something: can you hear and answer right?
AGAVE: Yes! I've forgotten, father, what I said just now.
CADMUS: Whose household did you enter on your wedding day?
AGAVE: You gave me to Echion, Sown-Man of the myth.
CADMUS: And to your husband in his house, what son was born?
AGAVE: Pentheus, in wedlock, to his father and myself.
CADMUS: Whose head then, tell me, are you holding in your arms?
AGAVE: A lion's . . . I was told so by the huntresses.
CADMUS: Hold it before you! look! it will not take you long.
AGAVE: Ah! . . . what *is* this I am holding in my hands?   1280
CADMUS: Look at it closely and too clearly you will know.
AGAVE: I see the greatest agony I've ever known.
CADMUS: Surely it is not like a lion to you now?
AGAVE: No! I am holding Pentheus' head, and I am lost.
CADMUS: He's had his lamentations . . . before you knew the truth!
AGAVE: Who killed him? tell me how he came into my hands.
CADMUS: Unhappy Truth! your visits are not timed aright.
AGAVE: Tell me! my heart is leaping for what is to come.

CADMUS: It was you who killed him and your sisters joined with you.
AGAVE: Where did he die then? in the house? or where was it? 1290
CADMUS: The place where once Actaeon was devoured by dogs.
AGAVE: Cithaeron! how did the unhappy boy come there?
CADMUS: To mock the god he went there — and your Bacchic rites.
AGAVE: But we? What happened to us that we climbed up there?
CADMUS: Madness. And all the city had the Bacchic craze.
AGAVE: Dionysus wrought our ruin; that I know at last.
CADMUS: Yes, for an insult, since his godhead you denied.
AGAVE: Father, where is the dear, dead body of my boy?
CADMUS: It was hard to find it, but I searched and have it here.
AGAVE: Are all the limbs together fitted in one piece? 1300

. . . .

But Pentheus! in my folly how was he concerned?
CADMUS: He followed your example, he decried the god,
Who therefore joined you all in one calamity,
You and your sisters and this boy, destroyed my line
And myself with it, for I never had a son,
And now, poor girl, the scion of your womb I see
Here in a most revolting, most disastrous death.
It was he we looked to, for you held together, boy,
The house of Cadmus, being of my daughter born.
In awe the city held you; no one ever thought 1310
Of throwing insults at the old, when he could see
Your face, for justice came to those who earned it then.
Now in dishonor from my house I shall be cast,
The mighty Cadmus, sower of the Theban race
And reaper of the finest harvest man has seen.
Dearest of men folk — for, although you are no more,
To me you'll always be among the dearest youth —
No longer, as you used to, will you touch my cheek,
Whispering, as you hold your mother's father close,
"Grandsire, who wrongs you? who dishonors you? 1320
What cruel fellow is there who disturbs your heart?
Tell me, my father, I will punish him who does you wrong."
Now I am wretched and your fate is misery,
Your mother piteous; miserable are your kin.
Who now despises spirits of the world unseen
Look at this death and thenceforth worship them as gods!
CHORUS: Your suffering grieves me, Cadmus, but your daughter's son
Was justly punished, though his fate is grief to you.
AGAVE: You see, my father, how much things have changed for me . . .

[*The rest of* AGAVE'S *speech is lost, as also is the opening of*
DIONYSUS' *speech, which is made not from the stage but from*

the platform above it, the "machina" used by gods in their manifestations at the end of Greek tragedy.]

DIONYSUS (*addressing* CADMUS): . . . You shall become a serpent and
    Harmonia, 1330
    Daughter of Ares, whom you wedded as your wife,
    Though but a mortal, to a snake shall be transformed;
    And you a yoke of oxen, with your wife, will drive
    To rule barbarians; so the oracle of Zeus proclaims.
    And with an army numberless you will erase
    Cities, but after Loxias' prophetic seat
    Has fallen to them, they will have a sad return.
    But Ares, having saved Harmonia and you,
    Will give you dwelling in the Kingdom of the Blest.
    I, Dionysus, not of mortal father born, 1340
    But son of Zeus declare it! had you learnt the ways
    Of wisdom, as you would not, prosperous today
    You would be living, in alliance with the son of Zeus.
AGAVE: Receive our worship, Dionysus, we have done you wrong.
DIONYSUS: Too late you know me; when you ought, you would not learn.
AGAVE: That we acknowledge, but your blow is too severe.
DIONYSUS: Not when you were insulting me, who am a god.
AGAVE: The gods in anger should not copy mortal men.
DIONYSUS: My sanction came from Zeus, my father, long ago.
AGAVE: Alas! a wretched exile, father, is our doom. 1350
DIONYSUS: Why do you tarry over things that have to be?
CADMUS: My daughter, we have come to dire extremity,
    All! you, poor creature, and your sisters with you too;
    And I among barbarians shall find myself
    Wretched and old, a stranger. Then it is decreed
    That I to Hellas lead a mixed barbarian host.
    And with Harmonia (Ares' daughter and my wife),
    Both changed to savage serpents in our outward form,
    Against Hellenic altars and Hellenic graves
    I shall command the spear-men. Evil shall I have 1360
    Unending; wretched, never peaceful even when
    I cross the downward falling flood of Acheron.
AGAVE: And into exile I shall go, deprived of you.
CADMUS: Why cling to me, my daughter, in your misery,
    Like the grey cygnet nestling to the helpless swan?
AGAVE: Where shall I wander, banished from my native land?
CADMUS: My child, I know not; as a helper I am weak.
AGAVE: Goodbye, our palace, and goodbye,
    Dear city of my father's hands!

Father, from our home I fly
In hopelessness to other lands.
CADMUS: To Aristaeus' palace going . . .
AGAVE: Father, I lament for you.
CADMUS: And for you my tears are flowing,
Daughter, — for your sisters too.
AGAVE: But when from Dionysus, king,
Upon your house this ruin came,
He surely wrought an evil thing.
CADMUS: You wrought him cruel suffering;
In Thebes unhonored was his name.
AGAVE: Farewell, my father!
CADMUS: Take 'farewell' from me,
Poor child, if welfare yours can be.
AGAVE: Bring here my sisters, guards, that I may go
With fellow exiles sharing in my woe:
                    Only let me find a spot
                    Where Cithaeron sees me not!
                    Foul Cithaeron, never blot
                    Eyes of mine, but be forgot!
                    Be to other Bacchae yielded
                    With the thyrsus that I wielded.

CHORUS: Many forms has the Unseen:
                    Gods' surprises intervene
                    And our plans are not perfected: 1390
                    Gods achieve the unexpected . . .
                    So this tragedy has been.

ARISTOPHANES

LYSISTRATA

□

Translated by Charles T. Murphy

INTRODUCTION

COMEDY was presented at the same festivals and under the same general conditions as was tragedy. The origins of the form are the subject of an endless debate; but whether the immediate predecessor of comedy was the phallic song (as Aristotle says) or a "beast-comos" with a chorus of revelers disguised as animals is a question which need not be argued here. For our purposes it is sufficient to note two facts which are important in explaining the nature of the earliest Greek comedies which have come down to us. The first of these is that the ultimate ancestor of comedy was undoubtedly some sort of fertility rite; the second is that comedy, as we know it, developed in fifth-century Athens with the encouragement of the growing democracy.

The first statement serves to explain the presence of the constant and startling indecency in early comedy. Primitive man, in his attempts to control nature, often makes use of "sympathetic magic," in which acts performed on or by one object are supposed to affect some other object which the first object symbolizes. Representations of the reproductive organs, the most obvious symbols of fertility, are constantly used in such rites; and the ceremony often includes ribald jests and obscene remarks, as if to stimulate nature to do her utmost. The connection of comedy at Athens with the festival of Dionysus, the god of fertility and wine, helped to preserve the tradition of indecency in comic productions.

Comedy was officially recognized by the state and admitted to the City Dionysia at Athens in 487 B.C., and there is little doubt that it was recognized and encouraged as a democratic measure. Early comedy is filled with outspoken abuse and satire of prominent individuals; it is, of course, characteristic of comedy in all ages to ridicule those who deviate from accepted social standards or who unjustifiably exalt themselves above their fellows, but early Athenian comedy is unrivaled in its freedom of abuse and mockery of real, living persons. Such attacks were, perhaps, found useful in the leveling process which took place in ancient democracies; at any rate, early comedy always tended to represent the views of the average citizen — the "little fellow" — against all abnormal and outstanding individuals, most of whom are presented by the comic poet as charlatans and impostors. Besides this liberty of personal abuse, early comedy assumed for itself the right to discuss and comment on all aspects of civic life, including politics, education, and art. Here the reader should remember that the audience which listened to these comic discussions was the same group of citizens who had, perhaps a day or two before, seriously debated these same questions in the popular assembly, and nothing delighted them more than a witty burlesque of one of the leading issues of the day.

Aristophanes is the only poet of this early comedy whose works have been preserved. We know very little about his life; he was born about 447 B.C., produced his first play in 427 and his last in 386. He thus lived through one of the most critical periods of Athenian history, for which his plays provide a wonderful store of information and a somewhat biased, partisan commentary. The best known of his comedies are the *Clouds*, an attack on the educational theories of the Sophists with a not too unpleasant caricature of Socrates; the *Birds*, a charming fantasy of a Utopia established in the clouds by two nimble-witted Athenians; the *Lysistrata*; and the *Frogs*, a burlesque descent to Hades where we find Aeschylus and Euripides debating over the merits of their tragedies. The comedies of Aristophanes reveal to us a man of tremendous creative powers with a facility in comic invention which is unapproached in literature, a dramatist careless or impatient of dramatic consistency and probability, a poet of great lyric gifts, and a buffoon with an unbounded delight in horseplay and ribald jests.

The *Lysistrata*, one of the best comedies in respect to dramatic structure, was produced in 411 B.C., at a moment when Athens' fortunes were at their lowest point: the disaster of the Sicilian Expedition in 413 had stripped the city of a large part of its manpower, many of the strongest allies had revolted, the Spartans were striving for control of the Aegean Sea with Persian support, and internally the city was on the verge of a revolution. In the midst of this situation Aristophanes produced his last and best plea for peace. The plot of the comedy is extremely simple: the women of Greece, led by the Athenian Lysistrata, unite and agree on a sex-strike to force their husbands to make a just and reasonable peace; despite the frailty of some of the women, the plan succeeds admirably: the strike has the desired effect on the men, as we see in a scene that leaves nothing to the imagination, and the play ends in general rejoicing. The Rabelaisian nature of the plot scarcely conceals the earnestness and anxiety which Aristophanes must have felt; although peace with honour was impossible for Athens at this time, and therefore the play can hardly be considered as a serious piece of political reasoning, none the less the *Lysistrata* reveals a sincere belief that the Greeks must come to terms somehow or be completely ruined. It is important to observe that at the very outset Lysistrata says that her purpose is "to save all Greece," and this note of Panhellenism is splendidly developed at the end of the comedy. The *Lysistrata* is an excellent play with which to begin one's reading of Aristophanes, since its theme and broad humour are readily comprehended by the modern reader without any detailed commentary on the situation which inspired the comedy; a highly successful production which ran in New York for several months in 1930 demonstrated that Aristophanes can speak to moderns as directly as any contemporary playwright.

From Whitney Jennings Oates and Charles Theophilus Murphy, *Greek Literature in Translation* (New York: Longmans, Green and Co., 1944), pp. 383–384.

LYSISTRATA

□

CHARACTERS *

LYSISTRATA
CALONICE } *Athenian women*
MYRRHINE
LAMPITO, *a Spartan woman*
LEADER *of the Chorus of Old Men*
CHORUS *of Old Men*
LEADER *of the Chorus of Old Women*
CHORUS *of Old Women*
ATHENIAN MAGISTRATE
THREE ATHENIAN WOMEN
CINESIAS, *an Athenian, husband of Myrrhine*
SPARTAN HERALD
SPARTAN AMBASSADORS
ATHENIAN AMBASSADORS
TWO ATHENIAN CITIZENS
CHORUS *of Athenians*
CHORUS *of Spartans*

---

* As is usual in ancient comedy, the leading characters have significant names. LYSISTRATA is "She who disbands the armies"; MYRRHINE's name is chosen to suggest *myrton*, a Greek word meaning *pudenda muliebria*; LAMPITO is a celebrated Spartan name; CINESIAS, although a real name in Athens, is chosen to suggest a Greek verb *kinein, to move,* then *to make love, to have intercourse,* and the name of his deme, Paionidai, suggests the verb *paiein,* which has about the same significance.

SCENE. *In Athens, beneath the Acropolis. In the center of the stage is the Propylaea, or gate-way to the Acropolis; to one side is a small grotto, sacred to Pan. The Orchestra represents a slope leading up to the gate-way.*

It is early in the morning. LYSISTRATA *is pacing impatiently up and down.*

LYSISTRATA: If they'd been summoned to worship the God of Wine, or Pan, or to visit the Queen of Love, why, you couldn't have pushed your way through the streets for all the timbrels. But now there's not a single woman here — except my neighbour; here she comes.

(*Enter* CALONICE.)

Good day to you, Calonice.

CALONICE: And to you, Lysistrata. (*Noticing* LYSISTRATA'S *impatient air*) But what ails you? Don't scowl, my dear; it's not becoming to you to knit your brows like that.

LYSISTRATA (*sadly*): Ah, Calonice, my heart aches; I'm so annoyed at us women. For among men we have a reputation for sly   10
trickery —

CALONICE: And rightly too, on my word!

LYSISTRATA: — but when they were told to meet here to consider a matter of no small importance, they lie abed and don't come.

CALONICE: Oh, they'll come all right, my dear. It's not easy for a woman to get out, you know. One is working on her husband, another is getting up the maid, another has to put the baby to bed, or wash and feed it.

LYSISTRATA: But after all, there are other matters more im-   20
portant than all that.

CALONICE: My dear Lysistrata, just what is this matter you've summoned us women to consider? What's up? Something big?

LYSISTRATA: Very big.

CALONICE (*interested*): Is it stout, too?

LYSISTRATA (*smiling*): Yes indeed — both big and stout.

CALONICE: What? And the women still haven't come?

LYSISTRATA: It's not what you suppose; they'd have come soon enough for *that.* But I've worked up something, and for many a sleepless night I've turned it this way and that.

CALONICE (*in mock disappointment*): Oh, I guess it's pretty fine and slender, if you've turned it this way and that.

LYSISTRATA: So fine that the safety of the whole of Greece lies   30
in us women.

CALONICE: In us women? It depends on a very slender reed then.

LYSISTRATA: Our country's fortunes are in our hands; and whether the Spartans shall perish —

CALONICE: Good! Let them perish, by all means.

LYSISTRATA: — and the Boeotians shall be completely annihilated.

CALONICE: Not completely! Please spare the eels.

LYSISTRATA: As for Athens, I won't use any such unpleasant words. But you understand what I mean. But if the women will meet here — the Spartans, the Boeotians, and we Athenians — 40 then all together we will save Greece.

CALONICE: But what could women do that's clever or distinguished? We just sit around all dolled up in silk robes, looking pretty in our sheer gowns and evening slippers.

LYSISTRATA: These are just the things I hope will save us: these silk robes, perfumes, evening slippers, rouge, and our chiffon blouses.

CALONICE: How so?

LYSISTRATA: So never a man alive will lift a spear against the foe —

CALONICE: I'll get a silk gown at once.

LYSISTRATA: — or take up his shield — 50

CALONICE: I'll put on my sheerest gown!

LYSISTRATA: — or sword.

CALONICE: I'll buy a pair of evening slippers.

LYSISTRATA: Well then, shouldn't the women have come?

CALONICE: Come? Why, they should have *flown* here.

LYSISTRATA: Well, my dear, just watch: they'll act in true Athenian fashion — everything too late! And now there's not a woman here from the shore or from Salamis. 60

CALONICE: They're coming, I'm sure; at daybreak they were laying — to their oars to cross the straits.

LYSISTRATA: And those I expected would be the first to come — the women of Acharnae — they haven't arrived.

CALONICE: Yet the wife of Theagenes means to come: she consulted Hecate about it. (*Seeing a group of women approaching*) But look! Here come a few. And there are some more over here. Hurrah! Where do they come from?

LYSISTRATA: From Anagyra.

CALONICE: Yes indeed! We've raised up quite a stink from Anagyra anyway.

(*Enter* MYRRHINE *in haste, followed by several other women.*)

MYRRHINE (*breathlessly*): Have we come in time, Lysistrata? What do you say? Why so quiet? 70

LYSISTRATA: I can't say much for you, Myrrhine, coming at this hour on such important business.

MYRRHINE: Why, I had trouble finding my girdle in the dark. But if it's so important, we're here now; tell us.

LYSISTRATA: No. Let's wait a little for the women from Boeotia and the Peloponnesus.

MYRRHINE: That's a much better suggestion. Look! Here comes Lampito now.

(*Enter* LAMPITO *with two other women.*)

LYSISTRATA: Greetings, my dear Spartan friend. How pretty you look, my dear. What a smooth complexion and well-developed   80 figure! You could throttle an ox.

LAMPITO: Faith, yes, I think I could. I take exercises and kick my heels against my bum. (*She demonstrates with a few steps of the Spartan "bottom-kicking" dance.*)

LYSISTRATA: And what splendid breasts you have.

LAMPITO: La! You handle me like a prize steer.

LYSISTRATA: And who is this young lady with you?

LAMPITO: Faith, she's an Ambassadress from Boeotia.

LYSISTRATA: Oh yes, a Boeotian, and blooming like a garden too.

CALONICE (*lifting up her skirt*): My word! How neatly her garden's weeded!

LYSISTRATA: And who is the other girl?   90

LAMPITO: Oh, she's a Corinthian swell.

MYRRHINE (*after a rapid examination*): Yes indeed. She swells very nicely (*pointing*) here and here.

LAMPITO: Who has gathered together this company of women?

LYSISTRATA: I have.

LAMPITO: Speak up, then. What do you want?

MYRRHINE: Yes, my dear, tell us what this important matter is.

LYSISTRATA: Very well, I'll tell you. But before I speak, let me ask you a little question.

MYRRHINE: Anything you like.

LYSISTRATA (*earnestly*): Tell me: don't you yearn for the fathers of your children, who are away at the wars? I know you all   100 have husbands abroad.

CALONICE: Why, yes; mercy me! my husband's been away for five months in Thrace keeping guard on — Eucrates.

MYRRHINE: And mine for seven whole months in Pylus.

LAMPITO: And mine, as soon as ever he returns from the fray, re-adjusts his shield and flies out of the house again.

LYSISTRATA: And as for lovers, there's not even a ghost of one left. Since the Milesians revolted from us, I've not even seen an eight-inch dingus to be a leather consolation for us widows. Are you   110 willing, if I can find a way, to help me end the war?

MYRRHINE: Goodness, yes! I'd do it, even if I had to pawn my dress and — get drunk on the spot!

CALONICE: And I, even if I had to let myself be split in two like a flounder.

LAMPITO: I'd climb up Mt. Taygetus if I could catch a glimpse of peace.

LYSISTRATA: I'll tell you, then, in plain and simple words. My friends, if we are going to force our men to make peace, we must   120 do without —

MYRRHINE: Without what? Tell us.

LYSISTRATA: Will you do it?

MYRRHINE: We'll do it, if it kills us.

LYSISTRATA: Well then, we must do without sex altogether. (*General consternation.*) Why do you turn away? Where go you? Why turn so pale? Why those tears? Will you do it or not? What means this hesitation?

MYRRHINE: I won't do it! Let the war go on.   130

CALONICE: Nor I! Let the war go on.

LYSISTRATA: So, my little flounder? Didn't you say just now you'd split yourself in half?

CALONICE: Anything else you like. I'm willing, even if I have to walk through fire. Anything rather than sex. There's nothing like it, my dear.

LYSISTRATA (*to* MYRRHINE): What about you?

MYRRHINE (*sullenly*): I'm willing to walk through fire, too.

LYSISTRATA: Oh vile and cursed breed! No wonder they make tragedies about us: we're naught but "love-affairs and bassinets." But you, my dear Spartan friend, if you alone are with me, our   140 enterprise might yet succeed. Will you vote with me?

LAMPITO: 'Tis cruel hard, by my faith, for a woman to sleep alone without her nooky; but for all that, we certainly do need peace.

LYSISTRATA: O my dearest friend! You're the only real woman here.

CALONICE (*wavering*): Well, if we do refrain from — (*shuddering*) what you say (God forbid!), would that bring peace?

LYSISTRATA: My goodness, yes! If we sit at home all rouged and powdered, dressed in our sheerest gowns, and neatly depilated,   150 our men will get excited and want to take us; but if you don't come to them and keep away, they'll soon make a truce.

LAMPITO: Aye; Menelaus caught sight of Helen's naked breast and dropped his sword, they say.

CALONICE: What if the men give us up?

LYSISTRATA: "Flay a skinned dog," as Pherecrates says.

CALONICE: Rubbish! These make-shifts are no good. But suppose they grab us and drag us into the bedroom?   160

LYSISTRATA: Hold on to the door.

CALONICE: And if they beat us?

LYSISTRATA: Give in with a bad grace. There's no pleasure in it for them when they have to use violence. And you must torment them in every possible way. They'll give up soon enough; a man gets no joy if he doesn't get along with his wife.

MYRRHINE: If this is your opinion, we agree.

LAMPITO: As for our own men, we can persuade them to make a just and fair peace; but what about the Athenian rabble? Who will persuade them not to start any more monkey-shines?   170

LYSISTRATA: Don't worry. We guarantee to convince them.

LAMPITO: Not while their ships are rigged so well and they have that mighty treasure in the temple of Athene.

LYSISTRATA: We've taken good care for that too: we shall seize the Acropolis today. The older women have orders to do this, and while we are making our arrangements, they are to pretend to make a sacrifice and occupy the Acropolis.

LAMPITO: All will be well then. That's a very fine idea.   180

LYSISTRATA: Let's ratify this, Lampito, with the most solemn oath.

LAMPITO: Tell us what oath we shall swear.

LYSISTRATA: Well said. Where's our Policewoman? (*to a Scythian slave*) What are you gaping at? Set a shield upside-down here in front of me, and give me the sacred meats.

CALONICE: Lysistrata, what sort of an oath are we to take?

LYSISTRATA: What oath? I'm going to slaughter a sheep over the shield, as they do in Aeschylus.

CALONICE: Don't, Lysistrata! No oaths about peace over a shield.   190

LYSISTRATA: What shall the oath be, then?

CALONICE: How about getting a white horse somewhere and cutting out its entrails for the sacrifice?

LYSISTRATA: White horse indeed!

CALONICE: Well then, how shall we swear?

MYRRHINE: I'll tell you: let's place a large black bowl upside-down and then slaughter — a flask of Thasian wine. And then let's swear — not to pour in a single drop of water.

LAMPITO: Lord! How I like that oath!

LYSISTRATA: Someone bring out a bowl and a flask.

(A *slave brings the utensils for the sacrifice*.)

CALONICE: Look, my friends! What a big jar! Here's a cup   200 that 'twould give me joy to handle. (*She picks up the bowl*.)

LYSISTRATA: Set it down and put your hands on our victim. (*As CALONICE places her hands on the flask*) O Lady of Persuasion and dear Loving Cup, graciously vouchsafe to receive this sacrifice from us women. (*She pours the wine into the bowl.*)

CALONICE: The blood has a good colour and spurts out nicely.

LAMPITO: Faith, it has a pleasant smell, too.

MYRRHINE: Oh, let me be the first to swear, ladies!

CALONICE: No, by our Lady! Not unless you're allotted the first turn.

LYSISTRATA: Place all your hands on the cup, and one of you repeat on behalf of all what I say. Then all will swear and ratify   210 the oath. *I will suffer no man, be he husband or lover,*

CALONICE: *I will suffer no man, be he husband or lover,*

LYSISTRATA: *To approach me all hot and horny.* (*As* CALONICE *hesitates*) Say it!

CALONICE (*slowly and painfully*): *To approach me all hot and horny.* O Lysistrata, I feel so weak in the knees!

LYSISTRATA: *I will remain at home unmated,*

CALONICE: *I will remain at home unmated,*

LYSISTRATA: *Wearing my sheerest gown and carefully adorned,*

CALONICE: *Wearing my sheerest gown and carefully adorned,*   220

LYSISTRATA: *That my husband may burn with desire for me.*

CALONICE: *That my husband may burn with desire for me.*

LYSISTRATA: *And if he takes me by force against my will,*

CALONICE: *And if he takes me by force against my will,*

LYSISTRATA: *I shall do it badly and keep from moving.*

CALONICE: *I shall do it badly and keep from moving.*

LYSISTRATA: *I will not stretch my slippers toward the ceiling,*

CALONICE: *I will not stretch my slippers toward the ceiling,*   230

LYSISTRATA: *Nor will I take the posture of the lioness on the knife-handle.*

CALONICE: *Nor will I take the posture of the lioness on the knife-handle.*

LYSISTRATA: *If I keep this oath, may I be permitted to drink from this cup,*

CALONICE: *If I keep this oath, may I be permitted to drink from this cup,*

LYSISTRATA: *But if I break it, may the cup be filled with water.*

CALONICE: *But if I break it, may the cup be filled with water.*

LYSISTRATA: Do you all swear to this?

ALL: I do, so help me!

LYSISTRATA: Come then, I'll just consummate this offering.

(*She takes a long drink from the cup.*)

CALONICE (*snatching the cup away*): Shares, my dear! Let's drink to our continued friendship.

(*A shout is heard from off-stage.*)

LAMPITO: What's that shouting?

LYSISTRATA: That's what I was telling you: the women have   240
just seized the Acropolis. Now, Lampito, go home and arrange
matters in Sparta; and leave these two ladies here as hostages. We'll
enter the Acropolis to join our friends and help them lock the gates.

CALONICE: Don't you suppose the men will come to attack us?

LYSISTRATA: Don't worry about them. Neither threats nor fire will
suffice to open the gates, except on the terms we've stated.   250

CALONICE: I should say not! Else we'd belie our reputation as un-
manageable pests.

> (LAMPITO *leaves the stage. The other women retire and enter
> the Acropolis through the Propylaea.*)
> (*Enter the* CHORUS OF OLD MEN, *carrying fire-pots and a load of
> heavy sticks.*)

LEADER OF MEN: Onward, Draces, step by step, though your shoulder's
aching.

Cursèd logs of olive-wood, what a load you're making!

FIRST SEMI-CHORUS OF OLD MEN (*singing*):

Aye, many surprises await a man who lives to a ripe old age;

For who could suppose, Strymodorus my lad, that the women
we've nourished (alas!),   260

  Who sat at home to vex our days,

  Would seize the holy image here,

  And occupy this sacred shrine,

  With bolts and bars, with fell design,

  To lock the Propylaea?

LEADER OF MEN: Come with speed, Philourgus, come! to the temple
hast'ning.

There we'll heap these logs about in a circle round them,

And whoever has conspired, raising this rebellion,

Shall be roasted, scorched, and burnt, all without exception,

Doomed by one unanimous vote — but first the wife of Lycon.   270

SECOND SEMI-CHORUS (*singing*):

No, no! by Demeter, while I'm alive, no woman shall mock at me.

Not even the Spartan Cleomenes, our citadel first to seize,

  Got off unscathed; for all his pride

  And haughty Spartan arrogance,

  He left his arms and sneaked away,

  Stripped to his shirt, unkempt, unshav'd,

  With six years' filth still on him.   280

LEADER OF MEN: I besieged that hero bold, sleeping at my station,

Marshalled at these holy gates sixteen deep against him.
Shall I not these cursèd pests punish for their daring,
Burning these Euripides-and-God-detested women?
Aye! or else may Marathon overturn my trophy.

FIRST SEMI-CHORUS (*singing*): There remains of my road
  Just this brow of the hill;
  There I speed on my way.

Drag the logs up the hill, though we've got no ass to help.   290
  (God! my shoulder's bruised and sore!)
  Onward still must we go.
  Blow the fire! Don't let it go out
  Now we're near the end of our road.

ALL (*blowing on the fire-pots*): Whew! Whew! Drat the smoke!

SECOND SEMI-CHORUS (*singing*): Lord, what smoke rushing forth
  From the pot, like a dog
  Running mad, bites my eyes!

This must be Lemnos-fire. What a sharp and stinging smoke!   300
  Rushing onward to the shrine
  Aid the gods. Once for all
  Show your mettle, Laches my boy!
  To the rescue hastening all!

ALL (*blowing on the fire-pots*): Whew! Whew! Drat the smoke!

> (*The chorus has now reached the edge of the Orchestra nearest the stage, in front of the Propylaea. They begin laying their logs and fire-pots on the ground.*)

LEADER OF MEN: Thank heaven, this fire is still alive. Now let's first put down these logs here and place our torches in the pots to catch; then let's make a rush for the gates with a battering-ram. If the women don't unbar the gate at our summons, we'll have to   310 smoke them out.

Let me put down my load. Ouch! That hurts! (*to the audience*) Would any of the generals in Samos like to lend a hand with this log? (*Throwing down a log*) Well, *that* won't break my back any more, at any rate. (*Turning to his fire-pot*) Your job, my little pot, is to keep those coals alive and furnish me shortly with a red-hot torch.

O mistress Victory, be my ally and grant me to rout these audacious women in the Acropolis.

> (*While the men are busy with their logs and fires, the CHORUS OF OLD WOMEN enters, carrying pitchers of water.*)

LEADER OF WOMEN: What's this I see? Smoke and flames? Is that a
  fire ablazing?   319
Let's rush upon them. Hurry up! They'll find us women ready.

FIRST SEMI-CHORUS OF OLD WOMEN (*singing*):
    With wingèd foot onward I fly,
    Ere the flames consume Neodice;
    Lest Critylla be overwhelmed
  By a lawless, accurst herd of old men.
  I shudder with fear. Am I too late to aid them?
  At break of the day filled we our jars with water
 Fresh from the spring, pushing our way straight through the crowds.
    Oh, what a din!
  Mid crockery crashing, jostled by slave-girls,   330
  Sped we to save them, aiding our neighbours,
  Bearing this water to put out the flames.
SECOND SEMI-CHORUS OF OLD WOMEN (*singing*):
    Such news I've heard; doddering fools
    Come with logs, like furnace-attendants,
    Loaded down with three hundred pounds,
  Breathing many a vain, blustering threat,
  That all these abhorred sluts will be burnt to charcoal.   340
  O goddess, I pray never may they be kindled;
 Grant them to save Greece and our men, madness and war help
    them to end.
  With this as our purpose, golden-plumed Maiden,
  Guardian of Athens, seized we thy precinct.
  Be my ally, Warrior-maiden,
  'Gainst these old men, bearing water with me.

(*The women have now reached their position in the Orchestra, and their* LEADER *advances toward the* LEADER OF THE MEN.)

LEADER OF WOMEN: Hold on there! What's this, you utter   350 scoundrels? No decent, God-fearing citizens would act like this.

LEADER OF MEN: Oho! Here's something unexpected: a swarm of women have come out to attack us.

LEADER OF WOMEN: What, do we frighten you? Surely you don't think we're too many for you. And yet there are ten thousand times more of us whom you haven't even seen.

LEADER OF MEN: What say, Phaedria? Shall we let these women wag their tongues? Shan't we take our sticks and break them over their backs?

LEADER OF WOMEN: Let's set our pitchers on the ground; then if any-one lays a hand on us, they won't get in our way.

LEADER OF MEN: By God! If someone gave them two or three   360 smacks on the jaw, like Bupalus, they wouldn't talk so much!

LEADER OF WOMEN: Go on, hit me, somebody! Here's my jaw! But no other bitch will bite a piece out of you before me.

LEADER OF MEN: Silence! or I'll knock out your — senility!

LEADER OF WOMEN: Just lay one finger on Stratyllis, I dare you!

LEADER OF MEN: Suppose I dust you off with this fist? What will you do?

LEADER OF WOMEN: I'll tear the living guts out of you with my teeth.

LEADER OF MEN: No poet is more clever than Euripides: "There is no beast so shameless as a woman."

LEADER OF WOMEN: Let's pick up our jars of water, Rhodippe.   370

LEADER OF MEN: Why have you come here with water, you detestable slut?

LEADER OF WOMEN: And why have you come with fire, you funeral vault? To cremate yourself?

LEADER OF MEN: To light a fire and singe your friends.

LEADER OF WOMEN: And I've brought water to put out your fire.

LEADER OF MEN: What? You'll put out my fire?

LEADER OF WOMEN: Just try and see!

LEADER OF MEN: I wonder: shall I scorch you with this torch of mine?

LEADER OF WOMEN: If you've got any soap, I'll give you a bath.

LEADER OF MEN: Give *me* a bath, you stinking hag?

LEADER OF WOMEN: Yes — a bridal bath!

LEADER OF MEN: Just listen to her! What crust!

LEADER OF WOMEN: Well, I'm a free citizen.

LEADER OF MEN: I'll put an end to your bawling.

(*The men pick up their torches.*)

LEADER OF WOMEN: You'll never do jury-duty again.   380

(*The women pick up their pitchers.*)

LEADER OF MEN: Singe her hair for her!

LEADER OF WOMEN: Do your duty, water!

(*The women empty their pitchers on the men.*)

LEADER OF MEN: Ow! Ow! For heaven's sake!

LEADER OF WOMEN: Is it too hot?

LEADER OF MEN: What do you mean "hot"? Stop! What are you doing?

LEADER OF WOMEN: I'm watering you, so you'll be fresh and green.

LEADER OF MEN: But I'm all withered up with shaking.

LEADER OF WOMEN: Well, you've got a fire; why don't you dry yourself?

(*Enter an Athenian* MAGISTRATE, *accompanied by four Scythian policemen.*)

MAGISTRATE: Have these wanton women flared up again with their timbrels and their continual worship of Sabazius? Is this another Adonis-dirge upon the roof-tops — which we heard not   390 long ago in the Assembly? That confounded Demostratus was urging us to sail to Sicily, and the whirling women shouted, "Woe for Adonis!" And then Demostratus said we'd best enroll the infantry from Zacynthus, and a tipsy woman on the roof shrieked, "Beat your breasts for Adonis!" And that vile and filthy lunatic forced his measure through. Such license do our women take.

LEADER OF MEN: What if you heard of the insolence of these women here? Besides their other violent acts, they threw water all 400 over us, and we have to shake out our clothes just as if we'd leaked in them.

MAGISTRATE: And rightly, too, by God! For we ourselves lead the women astray and teach them to play the wanton; from these roots such notions blossom forth. A man goes into the jeweler's shop and says, "About that necklace you made for my wife, goldsmith: last night, while she was dancing, the fastening-bolt slipped out of the hole. I have to sail over to Salamis today; if you're free, do 410 come around tonight and fit in a new bolt for her." Another goes to the shoe-maker, a strapping young fellow with manly parts, and says, "See here, cobbler, the sandal-strap chafes my wife's little — toe; it's so tender. Come around during the siesta and stretch it a little, so she'll be more comfortable." Now we see the results of such treatment: here I'm a special Councillor and need 420 money to procure oars for the galleys; and I'm locked out of the Treasury by these women.

But this is no time to stand around. Bring up crow-bars there! I'll put an end to their insolence. (*To one of the policemen*) What are you gaping at, you wretch? What are you staring at? Got an eye out for a tavern, eh? Set your crow-bars here to the gates and force them open. (*Retiring to a safe distance*) I'll help from over here.

(*The gates are thrown open and* LYSISTRATA *comes out followed by several other women.*)

LYSISTRATA: Don't force the gates; I'm coming out of my own 430 accord. We don't need crow-bars here; what we need is good sound common-sense.

MAGISTRATE: Is that so, you strumpet? Where's my policeman? Officer, arrest her and tie her arms behind her back.

LYSISTRATA: By Artemis, if he lays a finger on me, he'll pay for it, even if he is a public servant.

(*The policeman retires in terror.*)

MAGISTRATE: You there, are you afraid? Seize her round the waist — and you, too. Tie her up, both of you!

FIRST WOMAN (*as the second policeman approaches* LYSISTRATA): By
Pandrosus, if you but touch her with your hand, I'll kick the stuff-
ings out of you.   440

(*The second policeman retires in terror.*)

MAGISTRATE: Just listen to that: "kick the stuffings out." Where's
another policeman? Tie *her* up first, for her chatter.

SECOND WOMAN: By the Goddess of the Light, if you lay the tip of
your finger on her, you'll soon need a doctor.

(*The third policeman retires in terror.*)

MAGISTRATE: What's this? Where's my policeman? Seize *her* too.
I'll soon stop your sallies.

THIRD WOMAN: By the Goddess of Tauros, if you go near her, I'll tear
out your hair until it shrieks with pain.

(*The fourth policeman retires in terror.*)

MAGISTRATE: Oh, damn it all! I've run out of policemen. But women
must never defeat us. Officers, let's charge them all to-   450
gether. Close up your ranks!

(*The policemen rally for a mass attack.*)

LYSISTRATA: By heaven, you'll soon find out that we have four companies of warrior-women, all fully equipped within!

MAGISTRATE (*advancing*): Twist their arms off, men!

LYSISTRATA (*shouting*): To the rescue, my valiant women!
O sellers-of-barley-green-stuffs-and-eggs,
O sellers-of-garlic, ye keepers-of-taverns, and vendors-of-bread,
   Grapple! Smite! Smash!
Won't you heap filth on them? Give them a tongue-lashing!   460

(*The women beat off the policemen.*)

Halt! Withdraw! No looting on the field.

MAGISTRATE: Damn it! My police-force has put up a very poor show.

LYSISTRATA: What did you expect? Did you think you were attacking
slaves? Didn't you know that women are filled with passion?

MAGISTRA E: Aye, passion enough — for a good strong drink!

LEADER OF MEN: O chief and leader of this land, why spend your
words in vain?
Don't argue with these shameless beasts. You know not how we've
   fared: 469
A soapless bath they've given us; our clothes are soundly soaked.

LEADER OF WOMEN: Poor fool! You never should attack or strike a
   peaceful girl.

But if you do, your eyes must swell. For I am quite content
To sit unmoved, like modest maids, in peace and cause no pain;
But let a man stir up my hive, he'll find me like a wasp.

CHORUS OF MEN (*singing*):
O God, whatever shall we do with creatures like Womankind?
This can't be endured by any man alive. Question them!
  Let us try to find out what this means.
  To what end have they seized on this shrine,   480
    This steep and rugged, high and holy,
      Undefiled Acropolis?

LEADER OF MEN: Come, put your questions; don't give in, and probe her every statement.
For base and shameful it would be to leave this plot untested.

MAGISTRATE: Well then, first of all I wish to ask her this: for what purpose have you barred us from the Acropolis?

LYSISTRATA: To keep the treasure safe, so you won't make war on account of it.

MAGISTRATE: What? Do we make war on account of the treasure?

LYSISTRATA: Yes, and you cause all our other troubles for it, too. Peisander and those greedy office-seekers keep things stirred   490 up so they can find occasions to steal. Now let them do what they like: they'll never again make off with any of this money.

MAGISTRATE: What will you do?

LYSISTRATA: What a question! We'll administer it ourselves.

MAGISTRATE: *You* will administer the treasure?

LYSISTRATA: What's so strange in that? Don't we administer the household money for you?

MAGISTRATE: That's different.

LYSISTRATA: How is it different?

MAGISTRATE: We've got to make war with this money.

LYSISTRATA: But that's the very first thing: you mustn't make war.

MAGISTRATE: How else can we be saved?

LYSISTRATA: We'll save you.

MAGISTRATE: *You?*

LYSISTRATA: Yes, we!

MAGISTRATE: God forbid!

LYSISTRATA: We'll save you, whether you want it or not.

MAGISTRATE: Oh! This is terrible!

LYSISTRATA: You don't like it, but we're going to do it none the less.

MAGISTRATE: Good God! it's illegal!   500

LYSISTRATA: We *will* save you, my little man!

MAGISTRATE: Suppose I don't want you to?

LYSISTRATA: That's all the more reason.

MAGISTRATE: What business have you with war and peace?

LYSISTRATA: I'll explain.

MAGISTRATE (*shaking his fist*): Speak up, or you'll smart for it.

LYSISTRATA: Just listen, and try to keep your hands still.

MAGISTRATE: I can't. I'm so mad I can't stop them.

FIRST WOMAN: Then you'll be the one to smart for it.

MAGISTRATE: Croak to yourself, old hag! (*To* LYSISTRATA) Now then, speak up.

LYSISTRATA: Very well. Formerly we endured the war for a good long time with our usual restraint, no matter what you men did. You wouldn't let us say "boo," although nothing you did suited us. But we watched you well, and though we stayed at home we'd   510 often hear of some terribly stupid measure you'd proposed. Then, though grieving at heart, we'd smile sweetly and say, "What was passed in the Assembly today about writing on the treaty-stone?" "What's that to you?" my husband would say. "Hold your tongue!" And I held my tongue.

FIRST WOMAN: But I wouldn't have — not I!

MAGISTRATE: You'd have been soundly smacked, if you hadn't kept still.

LYSISTRATA: So I kept still at home. Then we'd hear of some plan still worse than the first; we'd say, "Husband, how could you pass such a stupid proposal?" He'd scowl at me and say, "If you don't mind your spinning, your head will be sore for weeks. *War shall be the concern of men.*"   520

MAGISTRATE: And he was right, upon my word!

LYSISTRATA: Why right, you confounded fool, when your proposals were so stupid and we weren't allowed to make suggestions?
"There's not a *man* left in the country," says one. "No, not one," says another. Therefore all we women have decided in council to make a common effort to save Greece. How long should we have waited? Now, if you're willing to listen to our excellent proposals and keep silence for us in your turn, we still may save you.

MAGISTRATE: We men keep silence for you? That's terrible; I won't endure it!

LYSISTRATA: Silence!

MAGISTRATE: Silence for *you*, you wench, when you're wearing   530 a snood? I'd rather die!

LYSISTRATA: Well, if that's all that bothers you — here! take my snood and tie it round your head. (*During the following words the women dress up the* MAGISTRATE *in women's garments.*) And *now* keep quiet! Here, take this spinning-basket, too, and card your wool with robes tucked up, munching on beans. *War shall be the concern of Women!*

LEADER OF WOMEN: Arise and leave your pitchers, girls; no time is this to falter.   539

We too must aid our loyal friends; our turn has come for action.

CHORUS OF WOMEN (*singing*):
I'll never tire of aiding them with song and dance; never may
Faintness keep my legs from moving to and fro endlessly.
   For I yearn to do all for my friends;
   They have charm, they have wit, they have grace,
      With courage, brains, and best of virtues —
         Patriotic sapience.

LEADER OF WOMEN: Come, child of manliest ancient dames, offspring
of stinging nettles,   549
Advance with rage unsoftened; for fair breezes speed you onward.

LYSISTRATA: If only sweet Eros and the Cyprian Queen of Love shed
charm over our breasts and limbs and inspire our men with amorous
longing and priapic spasms, I think we may soon be called Peace-
makers among the Greeks.

MAGISTRATE: What will you do?

LYSISTRATA: First of all, we'll stop those fellows who run madly about
the Marketplace in arms.

FIRST WOMAN: Indeed we shall, by the Queen of Paphos.

LYSISTRATA: For now they roam about the market, amid the pots and
greenstuffs, armed to the teeth like Corybantes.

MAGISTRATE: That's what manly fellows ought to do!

LYSISTRATA: But it's so silly: a chap with a Gorgon-emblazoned shield
buying pickled herring.   560

FIRST WOMAN: Why, just the other day I saw one of those long-haired
dandies who command our cavalry ride up on horseback and pour
into his bronze helmet the egg-broth he'd bought from an old dame.
And there was a Thracian slinger too, shaking his lance like Tereus;
he'd scared the life out of the poor fig-peddler and was gulping
down all her ripest fruit.

MAGISTRATE: How can you stop all the confusion in the various states
and bring them together?

LYSISTRATA: Very easily.

MAGISTRATE: Tell me how.

LYSISTRATA: Just like a ball of wool, when it's confused and snarled:
we take it thus, and draw out a thread here and a thread there with
our spindles; thus we'll unsnarl this war, if no one prevents us, and
draw together the various states with embassies here and embassies
there.

MAGISTRATE: Do you suppose you can stop this dreadful business with
balls of wool and spindles, you nit-wits?   570

LYSISTRATA: Why, if *you* had any wits, you'd manage all affairs of
state like our wool-working.

MAGISTRATE: How so?

LYSISTRATA: First you ought to treat the city as we do when we wash the dirt out of a fleece: stretch it out and pluck and thrash out of the city all those prickly scoundrels; aye, and card out those who conspire and stick together to gain office, pulling off their heads. Then card the wool, all of it, into one fair basket of goodwill, mingling in the aliens residing here, any loyal foreigners,   580 and anyone who's in debt to the Treasury; and consider that all our colonies lie scattered round about like remnants; from all of these collect the wool and gather it together here, wind up a great ball, and then weave a good stout cloak for the democracy.

MAGISTRATE: Dreadful! Talking about thrashing and winding balls of wool, when you haven't the slightest share in the war!

LYSISTRATA: Why, you dirty scoundrel, we bear more than twice as much as you. First, we bear children and send off our sons as soldiers.

MAGISTRATE: Hush! Let bygones be bygones!   590

LYSISTRATA: Then, when we ought to be happy and enjoy our youth, we sleep alone because of your expeditions abroad. But never mind us married women: I grieve most for the maids who grow old at home unwed.

MAGISTRATE: Don't men grow old, too?

LYSISTRATA: For heaven's sake! That's not the same thing. When a man comes home, no matter how grey he is, he soon finds a girl to marry. But woman's bloom is short and fleeting; if she doesn't grasp her chance, no man is willing to marry her and she sits at home a prey to every fortune-teller.

MAGISTRATE (*coarsely*): But if a man can still get it up —

LYSISTRATA: See here, you: what's the matter? Aren't you dead yet? There's plenty of room for you. Buy yourself a shroud and   600 I'll bake you a honey-cake. (*Handing him a copper coin for his passage across the Styx*) Here's your fare! Now get yourself a wreath.

(*During the following dialogue the women dress up the* MAGISTRATE *as a corpse.*)

FIRST WOMAN: Here, take these fillets.

SECOND WOMAN: Here, take this wreath.

LYSISTRATA: What do you want? What's lacking? Get moving; off to the ferry! Charon is calling you; don't keep him from sailing.

MAGISTRATE: Am I to endure these insults? By God! I'm going straight to the magistrates to show them how I've been treated.   610

LYSISTRATA: Are you grumbling that you haven't been properly laid out? Well, the day after tomorrow we'll send around all the usual offerings early in the morning.

(*The* MAGISTRATE *goes out still wearing his funeral decorations.* LYSISTRATA *and the women retire into the Acropolis.*)

LEADER OF MEN: Wake, ye sons of freedom, wake! 'Tis no time for sleeping. Up and at them, like a man! Let us strip for action.

(*The* CHORUS OF MEN *remove their outer cloaks.*)

CHORUS OF MEN (*singing*):
  Surely there is something here greater than meets the eye;
  For without a doubt I smell Hippias' tyranny.
  Dreadful fear assails me lest certain bands of Spartan men,   620
  Meeting here with Cleisthenes, have inspired through treachery
  All these god-detested women secretly to seize
  Athens' treasure in the temple, and to stop that pay
    Whence I live at my ease.

LEADER OF MEN: Now isn't it terrible for them to advise the state and chatter about shields, being mere women?

    And they think to reconcile us with the Spartans — men who hold nothing sacred any more than hungry wolves. Surely this is a web of deceit, my friends, to conceal an attempt at tyranny. But   630 they'll never lord it over me; I'll be on my guard and from now on,
    "The blade I bear   A myrtle spray shall wear."
I'll occupy the market under arms and stand next to Aristogeiton.

    Thus I'll stand beside him. (*He strikes the pose of the famous statue of the tyrannicides, with one arm raised.*) And here's my chance to take this accurst old hag and — (*striking the* LEADER OF WOMEN) smack her on the jaw!

LEADER OF WOMEN: You'll go home in such a state your Ma won't recognize you!
Ladies all, upon the ground let us place these garments.

(*The* CHORUS OF WOMEN *remove their outer garments.*)

CHORUS OF WOMEN (*singing*):
  Citizens of Athens, hear useful words for the state.
  Rightly; for it nurtured me in my youth royally.   640
  As a child of seven years carried I the sacred box;
  Then I was a Miller-maid, grinding at Athene's shrine;
  Next I wore the saffron robe and played Brauronia's Bear;
  And I walked as a Basket-bearer, wearing chains of figs,
    As a sweet maiden fair.

LEADER OF WOMEN: Therefore, am I not bound to give good advice to the city?

    Don't take it ill that I was born a woman, if I contribute something better than our present troubles. I pay my share; for   650

I contribute MEN. But you miserable old fools contribute nothing, and after squandering our ancestral treasure, the fruit of the Persian Wars, you make no contribution in return. And now, all on account of you, we're facing ruin.

What, muttering, are you? If you annoy me, I'll take this hard, rough slipper and — (*striking the* LEADER OF MEN) smack you on the jaw!

CHORUS OF MEN (*singing*):

This is outright insolence! Things go from bad to worse.   660
If you're men with any guts, prepare to meet the foe.
Let us strip our tunics off! We need the smell of male
Vigour. And we cannot fight all swaddled up in clothes.

   (*They strip off their tunics.*)

Come then, my comrades, on to the battle, ye once to
    Leipsydrion came;
Then ye were MEN. Now call back your youthful vigour.
    With light, wingèd footstep advance,
    Shaking old age from your frame.   670

LEADER OF MEN: If any of us give these wenches the slightest hold, they'll stop at nothing; such is their cunning.

They will even build ships and sail against us, like Artemisia. Or if they turn to mounting, I count our Knights as done for: a woman's such a tricky jockey when she gets astraddle, with a good firm seat for trotting. Just look at those Amazons that Micon painted, fighting on horseback against men!

But we must throw them all in the pillory — (*seizing*   680 *and choking the* LEADER OF WOMEN) grabbing hold of yonder neck!

CHORUS OF WOMEN (*singing*):

'Ware my anger! Like a boar 'twill rush upon you men.
Soon you'll bawl aloud for help, you'll be so soundly trimmed!
Come, my friends, let's strip with speed, and lay aside these robes;
Catch the scent of women's rage. Attack with tooth and nail!

   (*They strip off their tunics.*)

Now then, come near me, you miserable man! you'll never eat garlic
   or black beans again.   690
And if you utter a single hard word, in rage I will "nurse" you as
   once
   The beetle requited her foe.

LEADER OF WOMEN: For you don't worry me; no, not so long as my Lampito lives and our Theban friend, the noble Ismenia.

You can't do anything, not even if you pass a dozen — decrees! You miserable fool, all our neighbours hate you. Why, just the other day when I was holding a festival for Hecate, I invited as playmate from our neighbours the Boeotians a charming, wellbred Copaic — eel. But they refused to send me one on account of your decrees. 700

And you'll never stop passing decrees until I grab your foot and — (*tripping up the* LEADER OF MEN) toss you down and break your neck!

> (*Here an interval of five days is supposed to elapse.* LYSISTRATA *comes out from the Acropolis.*)

LEADER OF WOMEN (*dramatically*): Empress of this great emprise and undertaking,
Why come you forth, I pray, with frowning brow?

LYSISTRATA: Ah, these cursèd women! Their deeds and female notions make me pace up and down in utter despair.

LEADER OF WOMEN: Ah, what sayest thou? 710

LYSISTRATA: The truth, alas! the truth.

LEADER OF WOMEN: What dreadful tale hast thou to tell thy friends?

LYSISTRATA: 'Tis shame to speak, and not to speak is hard.

LEADER OF WOMEN: Hide not from me whatever woes we suffer.

LYSISTRATA: Well then, to put it briefly, we want — laying!

LEADER OF WOMEN: O Zeus, Zeus!

LYSISTRATA: Why call on Zeus? That's the way things are. I can no longer keep them away from the men, and they're all deserting. I caught one wriggling through a hole near the grotto of 720 Pan, another sliding down a rope, another deserting her post; and yesterday I found one getting on a sparrow's back to fly off to Orsilochus, and had to pull her back by the hair. They're digging up all sorts of excuses to get home. Look, here comes one of them now.

> (*A woman comes hastily out of the Acropolis.*)

Here you! Where are you off to in such a hurry?

FIRST WOMAN: I want to go home. My very best wool is being devoured by moths.

LYSISTRATA: Moths? Nonsense! Go back inside. 730

FIRST WOMAN: I'll come right back; I swear it. I just want to lay it out on the bed.

LYSISTRATA: Well, you won't lay it out, and you won't go home, either.

FIRST WOMAN: Shall I let my wool be ruined?

LYSISTRATA: If necessary, yes.

> (*Another woman comes out.*)

SECOND WOMAN: Oh dear! Oh dear! My precious flax! I left it at home all unpeeled.

LYSISTRATA: Here's another one, going home for her "flax." Come back here!

SECOND WOMAN: But I just want to work it up a little and then I'll be right back.

LYSISTRATA: No indeed! If you start this, all the other women   740 will want to do the same.

     (*A third woman comes out.*)

THIRD WOMAN: O Eilithyia, goddess of travail, stop my labour till I come to a lawful spot!

LYSISTRATA: What's this nonsense?

THIRD WOMAN: I'm going to have a baby — right now!

LYSISTRATA: But you weren't even pregnant yesterday.

THIRD WOMAN: Well, I am today. O Lysistrata, do send me home to see a midwife, right away.

LYSISTRATA: What are you talking about? (*Putting her hand on her stomach*) What's this hard lump here?

THIRD WOMAN: A little boy.

LYSISTRATA: My goodness, what have you got there? It seems hollow; I'll just find out. (*Pulling aside her robe*) Why, you silly   750 goose, you've got Athene's sacred helmet there. And you said you were having a baby!

THIRD WOMAN: Well, I *am* having one, I swear!

LYSISTRATA: Then what's this helmet for?

THIRD WOMAN: If the baby starts coming while I'm still in the Acropolis, I'll creep into this like a pigeon and give birth to it there.

LYSISTRATA: Stuff and nonsense! It's plain enough what you're up to. You just wait here for the christening of this — helmet.

THIRD WOMAN: But I can't sleep in the Acropolis since I saw the sacred snake.

FIRST WOMAN: And I'm dying for lack of sleep: the hooting of   760 the owls keep me awake.

LYSISTRATA: Enough of these shams, you wretched creatures. You want your husbands, I suppose. Well, don't you think they want us? I'm sure they're spending miserable nights. Hold out, my friends, and endure for just a little while. There's an oracle that we shall conquer, if we don't split up. (*Producing a roll of paper*) Here it is.

FIRST WOMAN: Tell us what it says.

LYSISTRATA: Listen.   769

"When in the length of time the Swallows shall gather together,
Fleeing the Hoopoe's amorous flight and the Cockatoo shunning,
Then shall your woes be ended and Zeus who thunders in heaven
Set what's below on top — "

FIRST WOMAN: What? Are we going to be on top?

LYSISTRATA: "But if the Swallows rebel and flutter away from the
temple,
Never a bird in the world shall seem more wanton and worthless.

FIRST WOMAN: That's clear enough, upon my word!

LYSISTRATA: By all that's holy, let's not give up the struggle now.
Let's go back inside. It would be a shame, my dear friends, to disobey the oracle. 780

(*The women all retire to the Acropolis again.*)

CHORUS OF MEN (*singing*):
I have a tale to tell,
Which I know full well.
It was told me
In the nursery.

Once there was a likely lad,
Melanion they name him;
The thought of marriage made him mad,
For which I cannot blame him.

So off he went to mountains fair;
(No women to upbraid him!)
A mighty hunter of the hare, 790
He had a dog to aid him.

He never came back home to see
Detested women's faces.
He showed a shrewd mentality.
With him I'd fain change places!

ONE OF THE MEN (*to one of the women*): Come here, old dame; give
me a kiss.

WOMAN: You'll ne'er eat garlic, if you dare!

MAN: I want to kick you — just like this!

WOMAN: Oh, there's a leg with bushy hair! 800

MAN: Myronides and Phormio
Were hairy — and they thrashed the foe.

CHORUS OF WOMEN (*singing*):
I have another tale,
With which to assail
Your contention
'Bout Melanion.

    Once upon a time a man
      Named Timon left our city,
    To live in some deserted land.
      (We thought him rather witty.)   810

    He dwelt alone amidst the thorn;
      In solitude he brooded.
    From some grim Fury he was born:
      Such hatred he exuded.

    He cursed you men, as scoundrels through
      And through, till life he ended.
    He couldn't stand the sight of you!
      But women he befriended.   820

WOMAN (*to one of the men*): I'll smash your face in, if you like.
MAN: Oh no, please don't! You frighten me.
WOMAN: I'll lift my foot — and thus I'll strike.
MAN: Aha! Look there! What's that I see?
WOMAN: Whate'er you see, you cannot say
    That I'm not neatly trimmed today.

      (LYSISTRATA *appears on the wall of the Acropolis.*)

LYSISTRATA: Hello! Hello! Girls, come here quick!

    (*Several women appear beside her.*)

WOMAN: What is it? Why are you calling?   830
LYSISTRATA: I see a man coming: he's in a dreadful state. He's mad
    with passion. O Queen of Cyprus, Cythera, and Paphos, just keep
    on this way!
WOMAN: Where is the fellow?
LYSISTRATA: There, beside the shrine of Demeter.
WOMAN: Oh yes, so he is. Who is he?
LYSISTRATA: Let's see. Do any of you know him?
MYRRHINE: Yes indeed. That's my husband, Cinesias.
LYSISTRATA: It's up to you, now: roast him, rack him, fool him, love
    him — and leave him! Do everything, except what our   840
    oath forbids.
MYRRHINE: Don't worry; I'll do it.
LYSISTRATA: I'll stay here to tease him and warm him up at bit. Off
    with you.

    (*The other women retire from the wall. Enter* CINESIAS *followed by a slave carrying a baby.* CINESIAS *is obviously in great pain and distress.*)

CINESIAS (*groaning*): Oh-h! Oh-h-h! This is killing me! O God, what tortures I'm suffering!

LYSISTRATA (*from the wall*): Who's that within our lines?

CINESIAS: Me.

LYSISTRATA: A *man*?

CINESIAS (*pointing*): A *man*, indeed!

LYSISTRATA: Well, go away!

CINESIAS: Who are you to send me away?

LYSISTRATA: The captain of the guard.

CINESIAS: Oh, for heaven's sake, call out Myrrhine for me.   850

LYSISTRATA: Call Myrrhine? Nonsense! Who are you?

CINESIAS: Her husband, Cinesias of Paionidai.

LYSISTRATA (*appearing much impressed*): Oh, greetings, friend. Your name is not without honour here among us. Your wife is always talking about you, and whenever she takes an egg or an apple, she says, "Here's to my dear Cinesias!"

CINESIAS (*quivering with excitement*): Oh, ye gods in heaven!

LYSISTRATA: Indeed she does! And whenever our conversations turn to men, your wife immediately says, "All others are mere rubbish compared with Cinesias."   860

CINESIAS (*groaning*): Oh! Do call her for me.

LYSISTRATA: Why should I? What will you give me?

CINESIAS: Whatever you want. All I have is yours — and you see what I've got.

LYSISTRATA: Well then, I'll go down and call her. (*She descends.*)

CINESIAS: And hurry up! I've had no joy of life ever since she left home. When I go in the house, I feel awful: everything seems so empty and I can't enjoy my dinner. I'm in such a state all the time!

MYRRHINE (*from behind the wall*): I do love him so. But he won't let me love him. No, no! Don't ask me to see him!   870

CINESIAS: O my darling, O Myrrhine honey, why do you do this to me?

(MYRRHINE *appears on the wall.*)

Come down here!

MYRRHINE: No, I won't come down.

CINESIAS: Won't you come, Myrrhine, when *I* call *you*?

MYRRHINE: No; you don't want me.

CINESIAS: *Don't want you?* I'm in agony!

MYRRHINE: I'm going now.

CINESIAS: Please don't. At least, listen to your baby. (*To the baby*) Here you, call your mamma! (*Pinching the baby*)

BABY: Ma-ma! Ma-ma! Ma-ma!

CINESIAS (*to* MYRRHINE): What's the matter with you? Have you no

pity for your child, who hasn't been washed or fed for five 880
whole days?

MYRRHINE: Oh, poor child; your father pays no attention to you.

CINESIAS: Come down then, you heartless wretch, for the baby's sake.

MYRRHINE: Oh, what it is to be a mother! I've got to come down, I
suppose.

 (*She leaves the wall and shortly reappears at the gate.*)

CINESIAS (*to himself*): She seems much younger, and she has such a
sweet look about her. Oh, the way she teases me! And her pretty,
provoking ways make me burn with longing.

MYRRHINE (*coming out of the gate and taking the baby*): O my sweet
little angel. Naughty papa! Here, let Mummy kiss you, Mamma's
little sweetheart! 890

 (*She fondles the baby lovingly.*)

CINESIAS (*in despair*): You heartless creature, why do you do this?
Why follow these other women and make both of us suffer so?

 (*He tries to embrace her.*)

MYRRHINE: Don't touch me!

CINESIAS: You're letting all our things at home go to wrack and ruin.

MYRRHINE: I don't care.

CINESIAS: You don't care that your wool is being plucked to pieces by
the chickens?

MYRRHINE: Not in the least.

CINESIAS: And you haven't celebrated the rites of Aphrodite for ever so
long. Won't you come home?

MYRRHINE: Not on your life, unless you men make a truce and stop
the war. 900

CINESIAS: Well then, if that pleases you, we'll do it.

MYRRHINE: Well then, if that pleases *you*, I'll come home — afterwards! Right now I'm on oath not to.

CINESIAS: Then just lie down here with me for a moment.

MYRRHINE: No — (*in a teasing voice*) and yet, I won't say I don't love
you.

CINESIAS: You love me? Oh, do lie down here, Myrrhine dear!

MYRRHINE: What, you silly fool! in front of the baby?

CINESIAS (*hastily thrusting the baby at the slave*): Of course not.
Here — home! Take him, Manes! (*The slave goes off with the
baby.*) See, the baby's out of the way. Now won't you lie down?

MYRRHINE: But where, my dear? 910

CINESIAS: Where? The grotto of Pan's a lovely spot.

MYRRHINE: How could I purify myself before returning to the shrine?

CINESIAS: Easily: just wash here in the Clepsydra.

MYRRHINE: And then, shall I go back on my oath?

CINESIAS: On my head be it! Don't worry about the oath.

MYRRHINE: All right, then. Just let me bring out a bed.

CINESIAS: No, don't. The ground's all right.

MYRRHINE: Heavens, no! Bad as you are, I won't let you lie on the bare ground.

(*She goes into the Acropolis.*)

CINESIAS: Why, she really loves me; it's plain to see.

MYRRHINE (*returning with a bed*): There! Now hurry up and lie down. I'll just slip off this dress. But — let's see: oh yes, I must fetch a mattress. 920

CINESIAS: Nonsense! No mattress for me.

MYRRHINE: Yes indeed! It's not nice on the bare springs.

CINESIAS: Give me a kiss.

MYRRHINE (*giving him a hasty kiss*): There!

(*She goes.*)

CINESIAS (*in mingled distress and delight*): Oh-h! Hurry back!

MYRRHINE (*returning with a mattress*): Here's the mattress; lie down on it. I'm taking my things off now — but — let's see: you have no pillow.

CINESIAS: I don't *want* a pillow!

MYRRHINE: But I do.

(*She goes.*)

CINESIAS: Cheated again, just like Heracles and his dinner!

MYRRHINE (*returning with a pillow*): Here, lift your head. (*to herself, wondering how else to tease him*) Is that all?

CINESIAS: Surely that's all! Do come here, precious! 930

MYRRHINE: I'm taking off my girdle. But remember: don't go back on your promise about the truce.

CINESIAS: Hope to die, if I do.

MYRRHINE: You don't have a blanket.

CINESIAS (*shouting in exasperation*): I don't want one! I WANT TO —

MYRRHINE: Sh-h! There, there, I'll be back in a minute.

(*She goes.*)

CINESIAS: She'll be the death of me with these bed-clothes.

MYRRHINE (*returning with a blanket*): Here, get up.

CINESIAS: I've got *this* up!

MYRRHINE: Would you like some perfume?

CINESIAS: Good heavens, no! I won't have it!

MYRRHINE: Yes, you shall, whether you want it or not.

(*She goes.*)

CINESIAS: O lord! Confound all perfumes anyway!   940

MYRRHINE (*returning with a flask*): Stretch out your hand and put some on.

CINESIAS (*suspiciously*): By God, I don't much like this perfume. It smacks of shilly-shallying, and has no scent of the marriage-bed.

MYRRHINE: Oh dear! This is Rhodian perfume I've brought.

CINESIAS: It's quite all right, dear. Never mind.

MYRRHINE: Don't be silly!

(*She goes out with the flask.*)

CINESIAS: Damn the man who first concocted perfumes!

MYRRHINE (*returning with another flask*): Here, try this flask.

CINESIAS: I've got another one all ready for you. Come, you wretch, lie down and stop bringing me things.

MYRRHINE: All right; I'm taking off my shoes. But, my dear,   950
see that you vote for peace.

CINESIAS (*absently*): I'll consider it.

(MYRRHINE *runs away to the Acropolis.*)

I'm ruined! The wench has skinned me and run away! (*chanting, in tragic style*) Alas! Alas! Deceived, deserted by this fairest of women, whom shall I — lay? Ah, my poor little child, how shall I nurture thee? Where's Cynalopex? I needs must hire a nurse!

LEADER OF MEN (*chanting*): Ah, wretched man, in dreadful wise beguiled, bewrayed, thy soul is sore distressed. I pity thee,   960
alas! alas! What soul, what loins, what liver could stand this strain? How firm and unyielding he stands, with naught to aid him of a morning.

CINESIAS: O lord! O Zeus! What tortures I endure!

LEADER OF MEN: This is the way she's treated you, that vile and cursèd wanton.

LEADER OF WOMEN: Nay, not vile and cursèd, but sweet and dear.   970

LEADER OF MEN: Sweet, you say? Nay, hateful, hateful!

CINESIAS: Hateful indeed! O Zeus, Zeus!
Seize her and snatch her away,
Like a handful of dust, in a mighty,
Fiery tempest! Whirl her aloft, then let her drop
Down to the earth, with a crash, as she falls —
On the point of this waiting
Thingummybob!

(*He goes out.*)
(*Enter a Spartan* HERALD, *in an obvious state of excitement, which he is doing his best to conceal.*)

HERALD: Where can I find the Senate or the Prytanes? I've   980
got an important message.

(*The Athenian* MAGISTRATE *enters.*)

MAGISTRATE: Say there, are you a man or Priapus?

HERALD (*in annoyance*): I'm a herald, you lout! I've come trom Sparta about the truce.

MAGISTRATE: Is that a spear you've got under your cloak?

HERALD: No, of course not!

MAGISTRATE: Why do you twist and turn so? Why hold your cloak in front of you? Did you rupture yourself on the trip?

HERALD: By gum, the fellow's an old fool.

MAGISTRATE (*pointing*): Why, you dirty rascal, you're all excited.

HERALD: Not at all. Stop this tom-foolery.   990

MAGISTRATE: Well, what's that I see?

HERALD: A Spartan message-staff.

MAGISTRATE: Oh, certainly! That's just the kind of message-staff I've got. But tell me the honest truth: how are things going in Sparta?

HERALD: All the land of Sparta is up in arms — and our allies are up, too. We need Pellene.

MAGISTRATE: What brought this trouble on you? A sudden Panic?

HERALD: No, Lampito started it and then all the other women in Sparta with one accord chased their husbands out of their   1000
beds.

MAGISTRATE: How do you feel?

HERALD: Terrible. We walk around the city bent over like men lighting matches in a wind. For our women won't let us touch them until we all agree and make peace throughout Greece.

MAGISTRATE: This is a general conspiracy of the women; I see it now. Well, hurry back and tell the Spartans to send ambassadors here with full powers to arrange a truce. And I'll go tell the   1010
Council to choose ambassadors from here; I've got a little something here that will soon persuade them!

HERALD: I'll fly there; for you've made an excellent suggestion.

(*The* HERALD *and the* MAGISTRATE *depart on opposite sides of the stage.*)

LEADER OF MEN: No beast or fire is harder than womankind to tame,
Nor is the spotted leopard so devoid of shame.

LEADER OF WOMEN: Knowing this, you dare provoke us to attack?
  I'd be your steady friend, if you'd but take us back.
LEADER OF MEN: I'll never cease my hatred keen of womankind.
LEADER OF WOMEN: Just as you will. But now just let me help you find
  That cloak you threw aside. You look so silly there   1020
  Without your clothes. Here, put it on and don't go bare.
LEADER OF MEN: That's very kind, and shows you're not entirely bad.
  But I threw off my things when I was good and mad.
LEADER OF WOMEN: At last you seem a man, and won't be mocked,
  my lad.
  If you'd been nice to me, I'd take this little gnat
  That's in your eye and pluck it out for you, like that.
LEADER OF MEN: So that's what's bothered me and bit my eye so long!
  Please dig it out for me. I own that I've been wrong.
LEADER OF WOMEN: I'll do so, though you've been a most ill-natured
  brat.   1030
  Ye gods! See here! A huge and monstrous little gnat!
LEADER OF MEN: Oh, how that helps! For it was digging wells in me.
  And now it's out, my tears can roll down hard and free.
LEADER OF WOMEN: Here, let me wipe them off, although you're such
  a knave,
  And kiss me.
LEADER OF MEN: No!
LEADER OF WOMEN: Whate'er you say, a kiss I'll have.

  (*She kisses him.*)

LEADER OF MEN: Oh, confound these women! They've a coaxing way
  about them.
  He was wise and never spoke a truer word, who said,
  "We can't live with women, but we cannot live without them."
  Now I'll make a truce with you. We'll fight no more; instead,   1040
  I will not injure you if you do me no wrong.
  And now let's join our ranks and then begin a song.
COMBINED CHORUS (*singing*):
  Athenians, we're not prepared,
  To say a single ugly word
  About our fellow-citizens.
  Quite the contrary: we desire but to say and to do
  Naught but good. Quite enough are the ills now on hand.

            Men and women, be advised:
              If anyone requires
            Money — minae two or three —   1050
              We've got what he desires.

My purse is yours, on easy terms:
  When Peace shall reappear,
Whate'er you've borrowed will be due.
  So speak up without fear.

You needn't pay me back, you see,
  If you can get a cent from me!

We're about to entertain
  Some foreign gentlemen;   1060
We've soup and tender, fresh-killed pork.
  Come round to dine at ten.

Come early; wash and dress with care,
  And bring the children, too.
Then step right in, no "by your leave."
  We'll be expecting you.

Walk in as if you owned the place.
  You'll find the door — shut in your face!   1070

(*Enter a group of* SPARTAN AMBASSADORS; *they are in the same desperate condition as the Herald in the previous scene.*)

LEADER OF CHORUS: Here come the envoys from Sparta, sprouting long beards and looking for the world as if they were carrying pig-pens in front of them.

    Greetings, gentlemen of Sparta. Tell me, in what state have you come?

SPARTAN: Why waste words? You can plainly see what state we've come in!

LEADER OF CHORUS: Wow! You're in a pretty high-strung condition, and it seems to be getting worse.

SPARTAN: It's indescribable. Won't someone please arrange   1080 a peace for us — in any way you like.

LEADER OF CHORUS: Here come our own, native ambassadors, crouching like wrestlers and holding their clothes in front of them; this seems an athletic kind of malady.

(*Enter several* ATHENIAN AMBASSADORS.)

ATHENIAN: Can anyone tell us where Lysistrata is? You see our condition.

LEADER OF CHORUS: Here's another case of the same complaint. Tell me, are the attacks worse in the morning?

ATHENIAN: No, we're always afflicted this way. If someone 1090
doesn't soon arrange this truce, you'd better not let me get my hands
on — Cleisthenes!

LEADER OF CHORUS: If you're smart, you'll arrange your cloaks so none
of these fellows who smashed the Hermae can see you.

ATHENIAN: Right you are; a very good suggestion.

SPARTAN: Aye, by all means. Here, let's hitch up our clothes.

ATHENIAN: Greetings, Spartan. We've suffered dreadful things.

SPARTAN: My dear fellow, we'd have suffered still worse if one of those
fellows had seen us in this condition.

ATHENIAN: Well, gentlemen, we must get down to business. 1100
What's your errand here?

SPARTAN: We're ambassadors about peace.

ATHENIAN: Excellent; so are we. Only Lysistrata can arrange things
for us; shall we summon her?

SPARTAN: Aye, and Lysistratus too, if you like.

LEADER OF CHORUS: No need to summon her, it seems. She's coming
out of her own accord.

    (*Enter* LYSISTRATA *accompanied by a statue of a nude female
figure, which represents Reconciliation.*)

Hail, noblest of women; now must thou be
A judge shrewd and subtle, mild and severe,
Be sweet yet majestic: all manners employ.
The leaders of Hellas, caught by thy love-charms, 1110
Have come to thy judgment, their charges submitting.

LYSISTRATA: This is no difficult task, if one catch them still in amorous
passion, before they've resorted to each other. But I'll soon find out.
Where's Reconciliation? Go, first bring the Spartans here, and
don't seize them rudely and violently, as our tactless husbands used
to do, but as befits a woman, like an old, familiar friend; if they
won't give you their hands, take them however you can. Then go
fetch these Athenians here, taking hold of whatever they 1120
offer you. Now then, men of Sparta, stand here beside me, and you
Athenians on the other side, and listen to my words.

    I am a woman, it is true, but I have a mind; I'm not badly off in
native wit, and by listening to my father and my elders, I've had a
decent schooling.

    Now I intend to give you a scolding which you both deserve.
With one common font you worship at the same altars, 1130
just like brothers, at Olympia, at Thermopylae, at Delphi — how
many more might I name, if time permitted; — and the Barbarians
stand by waiting with their armies; yet you are destroying the men
and towns of Greece.

ATHENIAN: Oh, this tension is killing me!

LYSISTRATA: And now, men of Sparta, — to turn to you — don't you remember how the Spartan Pericleidas came here once as a suppliant, and sitting at our altar, all pale with fear in his   1140 crimson cloak, begged us for an army? For all Messene had attacked you and the god sent an earthquake too? Then Cimon went forth with four thousand hoplites and saved all Lacedaemon. Such was the aid you received from Athens, and now you lay waste the country which once treated you so well.

ATHENIAN (*hotly*): They're in the wrong, Lysistrata, upon my word, they are!

SPARTAN (*absently, looking at the statue of Reconcilation*): We're in the wrong. What hips! How lovely they are!

LYSISTRATA: Don't think I'm going to let you Athenians off. Don't you remember how the Spartans came in arms when you   1150 were wearing the rough, sheepskin cloak of slaves and slew the host of Thessalians, the comrades and allies of Hippias? Fighting with you on that day, alone of all the Greeks, they set you free and instead of a sheepskin gave your folk a handsome robe to wear.

SPARTAN (*looking at* LYSISTRATA): I've never seen a more distinguished woman.

ATHENIAN (*looking at Reconciliation*): I've never seen a more voluptous body!

LYSISTRATA: Why then, with these many noble deeds to think of, do you fight each other? Why don't you stop this villainy?   1160 Why not make peace? Tell me, what prevents it?

SPARTAN (*waving vaguely at Reconciliation*): We're willing, if you're willing to give up your position on yonder flank.

LYSISTRATA: What position, my good man?

SPARTAN: Pylus; we've been panting for it for ever so long.

ATHENIAN: No, by God! You shan't have it!

LYSISTRATA: Let them have it, my friend.

ATHENIAN: Then what shall we have to rouse things up?

LYSISTRATA: Ask for another place in exchange.

ATHENIAN: Well, let's see: first of all (*Pointing to various parts of Reconciliation's anatomy*) give us Echinus here, this Maliac Inlet in back there, and these two Megarian legs.   1170

SPARTAN: No, by heavens! You can't have *everything*, you crazy fool!

LYSISTRATA: Let it go. Don't fight over a pair of legs.

ATHENIAN (*taking off his cloak*): I think I'll strip and do a little planting now.

SPARTAN (*following suit*): And I'll just do a little fertilizing, by gosh!

LYSISTRATA: Wait until the truce is concluded. Now if you've decided on this course, hold a conference and discuss the matter with your allies.

ATHENIAN: Allies? Don't be ridiculous! They're in the same state we

are. Won't all our allies want the same thing we do — to jump in
bed with their women? 1180

SPARTAN: Ours will, I know.

ATHENIAN: Especially the Carystians, by God!

LYSISTRATA: Very well. Now purify yourselves, that your wives may
feast and entertain you in the Acropolis; we've provisions by the
basketfull. Exchange your oaths and pledges there, and then each
of you may take his wife and go home.

ATHENIAN: Let's go at once.

SPARTAN: Come on, where you will.

ATHENIAN: For God's sake, let's hurry!

(*They all go into the Acropolis.*)

CHORUS (*singing*):

Whate'er I have of coverlets 1190
And robes of varied hue
And golden trinkets, — without stint
I offer them to you.

Take what you will and bear it home,
Your children to delight,
Or if your girl's a Basket-maid;
Just choose whate'er's in sight.

There's naught within so well secured
You cannot break the seal
And bear it off; just help yourselves;
No hesitation feel.

But you'll see nothing, though you try, 1200
Unless you've sharper eyes than I!

If anyone needs bread to feed
A growing family,
I've lots of wheat and full-grown loaves;
So just apply to me.

Let every poor man who desires
Come round and bring a sack
To fetch the grain; my slave is there
To load it on his back. 1210

But don't come near my door, I say:
Beware the dog, and stay away!

(*An* ATHENIAN *enters carrying a torch; he knocks at the gate.*)

ATHENIAN: Open the door! (*To the* CHORUS, *which is clustered around the gate*) Make way, won't you! What are you hanging around for? Want me to singe you with this torch? (*To himself*) No; it's a stale trick, I won't do it! (*To the audience*) Still if I've go to do it to please *you*, I suppose I'll have to take the   1220 trouble.

(*A* SECOND ATHENIAN *comes out of the gate.*)

SECOND ATHENIAN: And I'll help you.

FIRST ATHENIAN (*waving his torch at the* CHORUS): Get out! Go bawl your heads off! Move on there, so the Spartans can leave in peace when the banquet's over.

(*They brandish their torches until the* CHORUS *leaves the Orchestra.*)

SECOND ATHENIAN: I've never seen such a pleasant banquet: the Spartans are charming fellows, indeed they are! And we Athenians are very witty in our cups.

FIRST ATHENIAN: Naturally: for when we're sober we're never at our best. If the Athenians would listen to me, we'd always get a little tipsy on our embassies. As things are now, we go to Sparta   1230 when we're sober and look around to stir up trouble. And then we don't hear what they say — and as for what they *don't* say, we have all sorts of suspicions. And then we bring back varying reports about the mission. But this time everything is pleasant; even if a man should sing the Telamon-song when he ought to sing "Cleitagorus," we'd praise him and swear it was excellent.

(*The two* CHORUSES *return, as a* CHORUS OF ATHENIANS *and a* CHORUS OF SPARTANS.)

Here they come back again. Go to the devil, you scoundrels!   1240

SECOND ATHENIAN: Get out, I say! They're coming out from the feast.

(*Enter the Spartan and Athenian envoys, followed by* LYSISTRATA *and all the women.*)

SPARTAN (*to one of his fellow-envoys*): My good fellow, take up your pipes; I want to do a fancy two-step and sing a jolly song for the Athenians.

ATHENIAN: Yes, do take your pipes, by all means. I'd love to see you dance.

SPARTAN (*singing and dancing with the* CHORUS OF SPARTANS):
    These youths inspire
To song and dance, O Memory;
Stir up my Muse, to tell how we
And Athens' men, in our galleys clashing   **1250**
At Artemisium, 'gainst foemen dashing
    In godlike ire.
Conquered the Persian and set Greece free.

    Leonidas
Led on his valiant warriors
Whetting their teeth like angry boars.
Abundant foam on their lips was flow'ring,
A stream of sweat from their limbs was show'ring.
    The Persian was
Numberless as the sand on the shores.   **1260**

O Huntress who slayest the beasts in the glade,
O Virgin divine, hither come to our truce,
Unite us in bonds which all time will not loose.
Grant us to find in this treaty, we pray,
An unfailing source of true friendship today,
And all of our days, helping us to refrain
From weaseling tricks which bring war in their train.
    Then hither, come hither! O huntress maid.   **1270**

LYSISTRATA: Come then, since all is fairly done, men of Sparta, lead away your wives, and you, Athenians, take yours. Let every man stand beside his wife, and every wife beside her man, and then, to celebrate our fortune, let's dance. And in the future, let's take care to avoid these misunderstandings.

CHORUS OF ATHENIANS (*singing and dancing*):
        Lead on the dances, your graces revealing.
        Call Artemis hither, call Artemis' twin,   **1280**
        Leader of dances, Apollo the Healing,
        Kindly God — hither! let's summon him in!

        Nysian Bacchus call,
        Who with his Maenads, his eyes flashing fire,
        Dances, and last of all
        Zeus of the thunderbolt flaming, the Sire,
        And Hera in majesty,
        Queen of prosperity.

Come, ye Powers who dwell above
Unforgetting, our witnesses be
Of Peace with bonds of harmonious love —
The Peace which Cypris has wrought for me.   1290
Alleluia! Io Paean!
Leap in joy — hurrah! hurrah!
'Tis victory — hurrah! hurrah!
Euoi! Euoi! Euai! Euai!

LYSISTRATA (*to the Spartans*): Come now, sing a new song to cap ours.

CHORUS OF SPARTANS (*singing and dancing*):
Leaving Taygetus fair and renown'd,
Muse of Laconia, hither come:
Amyclae's god in hymns resound,
Athene of the Brazen Home,   1300
And Castor and Pollux, Tyndareus' sons,
Who sport where Eurotas murmuring runs.

On with the dance! Heia! Ho!
All leaping along,
Mantles a-swinging as we go!
Of Sparta our song.
There the holy chorus ever gladdens,
There the beat of stamping feet,
As our winsome fillies, lovely maidens,
Dance, beside Eurotas' banks a-skipping, —   1310
Nimbly go to and fro
Hast'ning, leaping feet in measures tripping,
Like the Bacchae's revels, hair a-streaming.
Leda's child, divine and mild,
Leads the holy dance, her fair face beaming.
On with the dance! as your hand
Presses the hair
Streaming away unconfined.
Leap in the air
Light as the deer; footsteps resound
Aiding our dance, beating the ground.
Praise Athene, Maid divine, unrivalled in her might,
Dweller in the Brazen Home, unconquered in the fight.   1320

(*All go out singing and dancing.*)

Biographical Notes: The Translators

Richard Aldington, the well-known English poet, novelist, and anthologist, lives at Les Rosiers, Montpellier, France.

Henry Birkhead, of Pembroke, South Wales, is an M. A. from Oxford and formerly a scholar of Trinity College; he has published in *Punch* and other British periodicals. Benn Brothers, of London, have recently published his translation of the Fourth Pythian Ode of Pindar as one of their shilling Books of Modern Poetry.

Albert Cook, a Harvard graduate, has published a discussion of the meaning of comedy and tragedy, *The Dark Voyage and the Golden Mean* (Harvard University Press, 1949). His version of *Oedipus Rex* was produced in February, 1948, by the Tributary Theater of Boston. He now teaches English at the University of California.

Kathleen Freeman, a teacher of the Classics, whose acting version of Sophocles' *Philoctetes* was first performed in 1939 at the University College of South Wales and Monmouthshire, has published translations from the Greek, studies of Greek philosophy and politics, English history, current affairs, and a novel. Among her most useful productions are *The Pre-socratic Philosophers, a Companion to Diels, Fragmente der Vorsokratiker* (1949) and *Ancilla to the Pre-Socratic Philosophers, a Complete Translation of Diels* (1948).

L. R. Lind, professor of Latin and Greek and chairman of the Department at the University of Kansas, and a fellow of the American Council of Learned Societies, has published articles, reviews, notes, and poems in many magazines. Among his books are *The Epitome of Vesalius Translated from the Latin* (Macmillan, 1949); an edition of the *Vita Sancti Malchi* of Reginald of Canterbury (University of Illinois Press, 1942); an edition of the *Ecclesiale* of Alexander of Villa Dei (University of Kansas Press, 1957); and two anthologies, *Lyric Poetry of the Italian Renaissance* (Yale University Press, 1954) and *Latin Poetry in Verse Translation* (Houghton Mifflin, 1957).

Louis MacNeice has published poetry, criticism, and travel sketches. He is a prominent member of the group of British poets which includes W. H. Auden, C. Day Lewis, and Stephen Spender.

CHARLES THEOPHILUS MURPHY is professor of Classics at Oberlin College and co-editor with Whitney J. Oates of *Greek Literature in Translation* (Longmans, Green, 1944).

SHAEMAS O'SHEEL, who died recently at his home near New York City, is the author of the famous poem "They Went Forth to Battle But They Always Fell" and of several books of poetry. He earned his living for many years as a professional writer. His version of Sophocles' *Antigone* was presented by The Atticans, a student group of the Department of Speech, Brooklyn College.

REX WARNER is the British poet and essayist among whose works are a translation of Euripides' *Medea, Poems and Contradictions, The Wild Goose Chase, The Professor, The Aerodrome,* and *The Cult of Power.*

The Divisions of the Plays

Agamemnon
Prologue 1–39
Parodos 40–104
First Stasimon 105–257
First Episode 258–354
Second Stasimon 355–474
Second Episode 475–680
Third Stasimon 681–781
Third Episode 782–974
Fourth Stasimon 975–1033
Fourth Episode 1034–1071
Kommos 1072–1177
Fifth Episode 1178–1405
Exodus 1406–1673

Prometheus Bound
Prologue 1–128
Parodos 129–193
First Episode 194–387
First Stasimon 388–435
Second Episode 436–528
Second Stasimon 529–560
Third Episode 561–886
Third Stasimon 887–906
Exodus 907–1093

Antigone
Prologue 1–99
Parodos 100–155
First Episode 156–330
First Stasimon 331–370
Second Episode 371–582
Second Stasimon 583–630
Third Episode 631–780
Third Stasimon 781–800
Fourth Episode (includes Kommos, 801–880) 801–945
Fourth Stasimon 946–988
Fifth Episode 989–1112

Hyporchema (chorus dance) 1113–1155
Exodus 1156–1352

Oedipus Rex
Prologue 1–150
Parodos 151–214
First Episode 215–461
First Stasimon 462–511
Second Episode 512–862
Second Stasimon 863–910
Third Episode 911–1084
Third Stasimon 1085–1109
Fourth Episode 1110–1186
Fourth Stasimon 1187–1222
Exodus 1223–1530

Philoctetes
Prologue 1–135
Parodos 136–219
First Episode, with choral songs, one a hyporchema 220–675
First Stasimon 676–729
Second Episode 730–828
First Kommos 829–865
Third Episode 866–1080
Second Kommos 1081–1218
Exodus 1219–1471

Alcestis
Prologue 1–76
Parodos 77–135
First Episode 136–212
First Stasimon 213–238
Second Episode 239–436
Second Stasimon 437–475
Third Episode 476–565 (2 scenes)
Third Stasimon 566–608
Fourth Episode 609–962 (3 scenes)
Fourth Stasimon 963–1004
Exodus 1005–1163

Andromache

Prologue 1–110
Parodos 111–140
First Episode 141–264
First Stasimon 265–304
Second Episode 305–456
Second Stasimon 457–482
Third Episode (includes Kommos, 490–530) 483–746
Third Stasimon 747–772
Fourth Episode 773–976
Fourth Stasimon 977–1009
Exodus (Kommos 1134–1196) 1010–1254

Bacchae

Prologue 1–62
Parodos 63–162
First Episode 163–369
First Stasimon 370–431
Second Episode 432–517
Second Stasimon 518–577
Third Episode (Kommos 578–601) 578–861
Third Stasimon 862–911
Fourth Episode 912–976
Fourth Stasimon 977–1022
Fifth Episode 1023–1151
Hyporchema (chorus dance) 1152–1168
Exodus 1169–1392

Suppliants

Prologue 1–39
Parodos 40–86
First Episode 87–362
First Stasimon 363–380
Second Episode 381–595
Second Stasimon 596–629
Third Episode 630–769
Third Stasimon 770–827
Fourth Episode 828–944
Fourth Stasimon 945–981
Fifth Episode (Evadne, Iphis) 982–1104
Fifth Stasimon (Kommos) 1105–1157
Exodus 1158–1227

Lysistrata

Prologue 1–253
Parodos, or Entrance of the Chorus 254–386
Scene (or Pro-agon) 387–475
Agon, or Debate 476–613
Parabasis of the Chorus 614–705
First Episode 706–780
First Stasimon 781–828
Second Episode (954–979, Kommos) 829–1013
Second Stasimon 1014–1071
Third Episode 1072–1188
Third Stasimon 1189–1215
Exodus 1216–1321

Glossary of Proper Names

ABAE: a town of Phocis, near Boeotia, seat of an oracle of Apollo.

ACASTUS: son of Pelias and brother of Alcestis, of Iolcus; an Argonaut.

ACHERON: one of the rivers of Hades, near which the shades gathered.

ACHILLES: the chief hero of Homer's *Iliad*, son of Peleus of Phthia in Thessaly.

ACTAEON: son of Aristaeus and Autonoë, destroyed by Artemis because he saw her bathing; he was turned to a stag and killed by his dogs.

ADRASTEIA: a title of Nemesis, the goddess of retribution.

AEACUS: the father of Peleus and grandfather of Achilles.

AEGEUS: son of Pandion, father of Theseus, and king of Athens.

AEGIPLANCTUS: a mountain in Megaris, near the Gulf of Corinth.

AGAMEMNON: son of Atreus, grandson of Pelops, and brother of Menelaus of Sparta; he later acquired control of Mycenae and of Argos when he usurped the throne of Thyestes, his uncle.

AGENOR: son of Poseidon and Libya, and father of Europa and of Cadmus of Thebes; he seems to have come originally from Phoenicia.

AIGIALEUS: son of Adrastus, leader of the Seven against Thebes.

AITHIOPS: Ethiopian, "Burnt-face." The Scholiast to *Prometheus Bound* explains this as the Nile river.

ALCMENE: daughter of Electryon of Tiryns, wife of Amphitryon, and mother of Hercules by Zeus.

AMAZONS: mythical female warriors in Asia Minor; literally "breastless."

AMMON: an Egyptian god identified by the Greeks with Zeus and by the Romans with Jupiter; he had a temple and oracle in the oasis of Siwah in Libya.

AMPHIAREUS: also spelled Amphiaraus; son of Oicleus. He tried to dissuade Adrastus from the expedition of the Seven against Thebes and was swallowed up by the earth near Thebes.

AMPHION: son of Zeus and Antiope, brother of Zethus; he helped kill Lycus and Dirce of Thebes, because they had mistreated Amphion's mother.

AMPHITRITE: a Nereid or Oceanid, wife of Poseidon, god of the sea, and mother of Triton.

ANAGYRA: a deme of Attica, thus a district of Athens.

ANDROMACHE: wife of Hector of Troy.

ANTILOCHOS: a son of Nestor of Pylos, a character in the *Iliad*.

ARACHNAEAN: referring to Mt. Arachnaios in Argolis, one of the seven beacon-stations in Aeschylus' *Agamemnon*.

ARES: the Greek god of war.

ARGO: the boat built by Argus which carried the fifty heroes (the Argonauts) in search of the golden fleece.

ARGOS: a city in the western Peloponnesus, home of Agamemnon.

ARIA: a region near the Caucasus mountains; hence "Aryan."

ARIMASPIA: a land north of Scythia in the Ural region.

ARISTAEUS: husband of Autonoë, father of Actaeon, and grandson of Cadmus of Thebes.

ARTEMIS: the Greek goddess of the hunt.

ARTEMISIA: queen of Halicarnassus in Caria, Asia Minor; she helped Xerxes invade Greece and fought well at Salamis (480 B.C.).

ARTEMISIUM: the north coast of Euboea where the fleet of Xerxes was defeated by the Greeks, 480 B.C.

ASCLEPIUS: also Aesculapius; the Greek god of medicine.

ASOPUS: the name of three rivers in Sicyon, Boeotia, and Thessaly in Greece.

ATHOS: the mountain which forms the southeast promontory of the peninsula of Chalcidice, one of the beacon-stations in Aeschylus' *Agamemnon.*

ATLAS: a Titan, the brother of Prometheus, condemned after his defeat by Zeus to hold up the earth on his shoulders.

ATREUS: grandson of Tantalus, son of Pelops, and father of Agamemnon and Menelaus; his brother was Thyestes.

AULIS: a harbor in Boeotia where the Greek fleet assembled before sailing to Troy.

AXIUS: a river in Macedonia, now called the Vardar.

BACCHUS: son of Zeus and Semele of Thebes, the Greek god of wine. He is also called Dionysus.

BIBLINE: referring to Byblos, a city in Phoenicia, where Adonis was worshipped.

BISTONES: a people in Thrace.

BOSPORUS: the channel of Constantinople; in general, any Greek strait. Literally "Ox-ford."

BOREAS: the North Wind.

BRAURONIA: a name of Artemis from her cult and temple in the deme or district of Brauron in Attica.

CALCHAS: the prophet who accompanied the Greek army at Troy.

CALLICHORUS: a sacred spring near Eleusis.

CAPANEUS: one of the Seven against Thebes, whom Zeus struck with lightning because he defied the god.

CASTALIA: a spring on Mt. Parnassus sacred to Apollo and the Muses.

CAUCASUS: the rough mountains between the Black and the Caspian seas.

CECROPIAN: referring to Cecrops, first king of Attica and founder of Athens.

CENTAURS: mythical creatures, half-man, half-horse.

CHALCIS: chief town of Euboea on the Euripus strait; there is also a town in Aetolia by this name.

CHALYBES: a people who lived on the south shore of the Black Sea; they were noted for their work in iron.

CHRYSE: a goddess whose altar Philoctetes was pointing out at Chryse in the Troad when he was stung by a serpent; also an islet near Lemnos.

CITHAERON: a mountain in Boeotia.

CLEISTHENES: an Athenian leader around 510 B.C. who took power when the sons of Pisistratus were banished.

CLYTAEMESTRA: the proper spelling in Greek for the person known generally as Clytemnestra, wife of Agamemnon of Argos.

COCYTUS: the river of moaning in Hades; also a river in Epirus.

CORYBANTS: priests of Rhea Cybele, the earth goddess of Phrygia in Asia Minor.

CORYCIAN: referring to nymphs in Corycia, a city in Cilicia.

CURETES: the Cretan demi-gods who took care of the infant Zeus.

CYBELE (RHEA): the earth-mother goddess of Phrygia in Asia Minor.

CYLLENE: the highest mountain in the Peloponnesus near Arcadia, sacred to Hermes who was said to have been born there.

CYNALOPEX: the nickname of a pander in Aristophanes' *Lysistrata*: a mongrel between dog and fox.

CYPRIS: a name for Aphrodite, goddess of love, from one of her favorite islands, Cyprus.

DANAE: daughter of Acrisius, king of Argos, visited by Zeus in her tower-prison in the form of a shower of gold; she became the mother of Perseus.

DANUBE: a large river in eastern Europe.

DAULIA: or Daulis; a town in Phocis, the home of Tereus, Philomela, and Procne.

DELPHI: the seat of Apollo's famous oracle on the south slope of Mt. Parnassus in Phocis.

DEO: another name for Demeter, the goddess of crops and fruits.

DIOMEDES: son of Tydeus, succeeded Adrastus as king of Argos. He was one of the Epigoni (sons of the Seven against Thebes) and fought in the Trojan War.

DIONYSUS: the Greek god of wine.

DIRCE: or Dirke; wife of Lycus, king of Thebes. She was killed by Amphion and Zethus because she mistreated Antiope, their mother.

DODONA: an oracle of Zeus in Epirus; he gave his responses by the rustling of oak leaves.

EDONIAN: referring to the Edoni, a people in Thrace, of whom Lycurgus, son of Dryas, was king.

EILITHYIA: the Greek goddess who aided women in childbirth.

ELEUSINIAN: referring to the shrine of Demeter and to the great festival held at Eleusis, a small village near Athens.

EPAPHOS: son of Zeus and Io, who was born on the Nile river where his mother ended her wanderings.

ERECHTHEUS: son of Hephaestus and an early king of Athens.

ERINYES: the Furies who pursued evil-doers.

ETEOCLES: son of Oedipus of Thebes, brother of Polynices, Antigone, and Ismene.

ETEOCLUS: son of Iphis; he came from Argos to Thebes with the famous Seven.

EURIPUS: the narrow strait between Boeotia and the island of Euboea.

EUROTAS: a river in Sparta; hence a reference to anything Spartan.

EURYDICE: the wife of Creon of Thebes, who succeeded to power after Oedipus.

EURYSTHEUS: king of Tiryns at whose bidding Hercules performed his twelve labors.

EVIUS: an epithet of Bacchus, god of wine.

GORGONS: three women, daughters of Phorcys (Phorkis) and Ceto, who had serpents for hair, bronze claws, and huge teeth; Medusa was their mortal sister.

GORGOPIS: in the myth of Athamas and Ino of Boeotia, another name for Ino. Phrixus and Helle are part of the same group of legends.

HADES: the lower world of the Greeks.

HECATE: a moon goddess with many attributes and forms; she was worshipped at crossroads.

HELENUS: son of Priam and a well-known Trojan prophet.

HELICON: a mountain range in Boeotia sacred to Apollo and the Muses.

HERA: wife of Zeus and queen of the Olympian gods and goddesses.

HERACLES: or Hercules; the famous hero who performed the labors laid on him by Eurystheus.

HERMAE: pillars surmounted by the head of Hermes and equipped with male members which were found lopped off by vandals just before the Sicilian expedition sailed from Athens in 415 B.C.

HERMES: the Greek messenger god, son of Zeus and Maia, born in a cave on

Mt. Cyllene in Arcadia. He presided over commerce and invention as well as sports.

HIPPIAS: a son of Peisistratus, tyrant of Athens; he was banished in 510 B.C.

HIPPOMEDON: an Argive chieftain, one of the Seven against Thebes.

HYBRISTES: a river in Asia, so-called for its turbulence (*hybris*, insolent violence).

IACCHOS: another name for Bacchus or Dionysus.

IDA: a mountain near Troy, the first of the messenger-beacons in Aeschylus' *Agamemnon*.

INACHOS: the father of Io; he was the son of Oceanus and Tethys and the first king of Argos.

IOLCUS: the home of Pelias and Jason as well as Alcestis, wife of Admetus, in Magnesia in Thessaly.

ISMENUS: a small river in Boeotia into which the brook named for Dirce flowed.

ITALIA: Italy.

KANOBOS: Canopus in lower Egypt just east of Alexandria.

KERCHNEIA: a lake in Argolis.

KISTHENE: a place near the sea in Asia Minor opposite Lesbos where Aeschylus locates the Gorgons.

KOLCHIS: a country in Asia between the Black Sea and the Caucasus.

KORE: a name for Persephone, daughter of Demeter; it means the "maiden."

KRONOS: or Cronus; the father of Zeus.

LABDAKOS: or Labdacus; father of Laius, king of Thebes, and grandfather of Oedipus.

LAIUS: king of Thebes and father of Oedipus.

LAPITHAE: a mythical people in the mountains of Thessaly ruled by Pirithous, a half-brother of the Centaurs who fought for control of the land with the Lapithae.

LARISSA: a town and a plain on the Peneus river in Thessaly.

LEIPSYDRION: a waterless district near Mt. Parnes in Attica.

LEMNOS: an island in the Aegean northwest of Lesbos.

LERNA: a region in Argolis near Argos with a marsh and a small river of the same name; here Hercules killed the Lernaean Hydra.

LOXIAS: another name for the god Apollo.

LYCIA: a region on the southwest coast of Asia Minor.

MACISTUS: a mountain in southern Euboea, one of the beacon-stations of the *Agamemnon*.

MAEOTIS: an inland sea on the borders of Europe and Asia north of the Black Sea: the Sea of Azov.

MAIA: the mother of Hermes by Zeus; she was the eldest of the Pleiades, the daughters of Atlas and Pleione.

MEDIA: a region of Asia Minor south of the Caspian Sea.

MEGAREUS: son of Eurydice and Creon of Thebes who offered himself as a sacrifice to Ares for deliverance of Thebes from the Seven who attacked it. Euripides calls him Menoeceus.

MELEAGER: son of king Oeneus of Calydon, he was one of the Argonauts and killed the Calydonian boar.

MENELAUS: brother of Agamemnon of Argos, he ruled at Sparta.

MENOECEUS: father of Creon and Jocasta of Thebes.

MEROPE: queen of Corinth, wife of king Polybus, the foster-mother of Oedipus of Thebes.

MESSAPION: a mountain in Boeotia, one of the beacon-stations in the *Agamemnon*.

MOLOSSIAN: referring to a powerful people in Epirus, noted for their fine dogs.

MYCENAE: a city in Argolis nine miles from Tiryns; Agamemnon's capital.

NESTOR: an old Greek from Pylos in western Peloponnesus; he fought at Troy.

NIOBE: daughter of Tantalus and wife of Amphion, king of Thebes. Because she took excessive pride in her children, Apollo and Artemis killed them and Niobe herself was turned to stone by Zeus.

NYSA: the name of several mountains sacred to Dionysus; he was said to have been raised near or upon one of them.

OLYMPIA: a place full of temples in northwestern Greece, the seat of the Olympic games.

OLYMPUS: the mountain range between Macedonia and Thessaly whose highest peak is covered with snow; the home of the Greek gods.

ORSILOCHUS: a Trojan who was killed by Teucer in *Iliad* 8.274.

ORTHRYS: the two-headed hound, offspring of Echidne, who begot the Sphinx, the Hydra, the Chimaera, and the Nemean lion.

PALLAS: Athena, goddess of wisdom.

PAN: a silvan deity of Arcadia.

PANDION: a king of Athens, son of Erechtheus, and the father of Procne and Philomela.

PAPHOS: one of two towns of the name on the west coast of Cyprus, where Aphrodite landed after her birth from the sea waves.

PARIS: son of Priam of Troy, the judge in the beauty contest between Aphrodite, Athena, and Hera, in which he received Helen as a prize from Aphrodite.

PARNASSUS: a mountain range stretching southeast through Doris and Phocis with its highest part a few miles to the north of Delphi.

PARTHENOPAEUS: the son of Meleager and Atalanta, one of the Seven against Thebes.

PATROCLUS: son of Menoetius of Opus and of Sthenele, the best friend of Achilles at Troy; he was killed by Hector, son of Priam.

PELASGIA: a general term for Greece, from its most ancient inhabitants, the Pelasgi.

PELIAS: father of Alcestis and king of Iolcus; he was killed by his daughters at the suggestion of Medea.

PELOPS: the patronymic ruler of southern Greece, the Peloponnesus.

PEPARETHUS: a small island in the Cyclades group in the Aegean Sea.

PERSEPHONE: the daughter of Demeter, goddess of crops, who was stolen away to Hades by Pluto and whose return to earth in the spring symbolizes the revival of nature each year.

PHASIS: a river in Colchis near the Black Sea on its east coast.

PHERES: father of Admetus of Thessaly, king of Pherae.

PHINEUS: king of Salmydessos, husband of Cleopatra, who was daughter of Boreas and Oreithyia. When Phineus rejected Cleopatra, his new wife Idothea blinded the sons of Cleopatra and shut them in a vaulted tomb.

PHOCIS: a region in northern Greece where Delphi is located.

PHOEBUS: a name for the god Apollo.

PHORKIS: a sea god, son of Pontus and Ge (sea and earth) and father of the Gorgons and the Fates; his wife was Ceto.

PHRYGIA: a region in west-central Asia Minor.

PIERIA: a district on the southeast coast of Macedonia, the seat of worship of the Pierides, or Muses.

PITTHEUS: king of Troezen, son of Pelops, father of Aithra, and grandfather of Theseus of Athens.

PLEIADS: or Pleiades; the daughters of Atlas the Titan, comrades of Artemis. When pursued by the hunter Orion in Boeotia they prayed for rescue and were transformed into doves which the gods placed in the heavens as a constellation.

POLYBUS: king of Corinth, foster-father of Oedipus of Thebes.

POLYDORUS: father of Labdacus of Thebes, grandfather of Laius.

POLYNICES: son of Oedipus, brother of Eteocles, Antigone, and Ismene; he married Aegeia, daughter of Adrastus, king of Argos, and was killed at Thebes.

POSEIDON: the god of the sea.

PRIAM: king of Troy.

PYTHIAN: referring to Apollo at his shrine in Delphi; an epithet from the fact that he killed Pytho, the serpent of the caves of Mt. Parnassus.

PYTHO: a name for Delphi.

RHEA: or Cybele, the earth-mother of Asia Minor.

SALMYDESSOS: a town in Thrace on the Black Sea Coast.

SARDIS: the seat of the Lydian monarchy in Asia Minor.

SARONIC: a gulf between Attica and Argolis.

SCAMANDER: the small river of the Troad famous in the *Iliad*.

SCYROS: an island in the Aegean Sea east of Euboea where Thetis concealed her son Achilles to keep him from the Trojan war.

SCYTHIA: a wild region in southern Russia between the Carpathian mountains and the Don river.

SEMELE: mother of Dionysus by Zeus, and daughter of Cadmus of Thebes.

SIDON: a city in Phoenicia.

SIPYLOS: a mountain on the borders of Lycia and Phrygia where Niobe was changed to stone.

SISYPHUS: a son of Aeolus and a king of Corinth whose wickedness was punished in Hades by his struggle to roll a rock uphill.

SPARTA: a region in south-central Greece; it is also called Lacedaemon or Lacedaemonia.

STROPHIUS: king of Phocis.

STRYMON: a large river which formed the boundary between Thrace and Macedonia.

TANTALUS: son of Zeus and the nymph Pluto, father of Pelops and Niobe; he was punished in Hades by thirst which he was unable to quench.

TEREUS: king of Thrace, husband of Procne, in the myth about Philomela.

TEUCROS: son of Telamon and Hesione, was the best bowman among the Greeks at Troy.

THEBES: an important city in Boeotia, where Oedipus was king.

THEMIS: daughter of Ouranos and Ge (sky and earth), she married Zeus. She is the personification of law, custom and the general order of things.

THEMISKYRA: a town in Pontus on the Thermodon river.

THERSITES: son of Agrius, an ugly, talkative commoner in the Greek army at Troy.

THESPROTIAN: referring to Thesprotis, a region in Epirus.

THERMODON: a river in Pontus in Asia Minor where the Amazons lived.

TMOLUS: a mountain in Lydia in Asia Minor.

TYDEUS: son of Oeneus and Periboea and father of Diomedes; see *Iliad* 14.113-120 for his genealogy.

TYNDAREUS: father of Helen, who became wife of Menelaus of Sparta.

ZACYNTHUS: an island in the Ionian Sea near the coast of Elis in Greece.

ZEPHYR: the west wind.

ZEUS: the father of the gods and their ruler, the personification of the heavens.

BIBLIOGRAPHY

Aristotle, *Poetics*, edited by A. Gudeman; Berlin, Weidmann, 1934. Translated by Lane Cooper, *Aristotle On the Art of Poetry*; rev. ed., Cornell University Press.

Arrowsmith, William, "The Cyclops of Euripides," *The Hudson Review* 5 (1952).

Bieber, M., *The History of the Greek and Roman Theater*, Princeton University Press, 1939.

Bowra, C. M., *Sophoclean Tragedy*; Oxford University Press, 1944.

Burckhardt, Jacob, *Griechische Kulturgeschichte*, ed. R. Marx; II, 266–317; Leipzig, A. Kröner.

Campbell, A. Y., *The Agamemnon of Aeschylus*; see my review in *Classical Philology* 33 (1938), 417–419.

Dixon, M. MacNeile, *Tragedy*; 3d ed., London, E. Arnold, 1929.

Fergusson, Francis, *The Idea of a Theater*; Princeton University Press, 1949.

Fitts, Dudley, and Robert Fitzgerald, translations of *Oedipus at Colonus*; *Alcestis*; *Antigone*; see my reviews in *Classical Philology* 38 (1943), 155; 33 (1938), 347. D. Fitts, ed., *Greek Plays in Modern Translation*; see my review in *The Western Review* 12 (1948), 244–246. Fitts-Fitzgerald, translation of *Oedipus Rex*; see my review in *The Classical Weekly* 43 (1950).

Flickinger, R. C., *The Greek Theater and Its Drama*; 4th ed., University of Chicago Press, 1936.

Gayley, C., *Classic Myths in English Literature*; Ginn, 1939.

Geffcken, J., *Die griechische Tragoedie*; 3d ed., Leipzig, 1925.

Goheen, Robert F., *The Imagery of Sophocles' Antigone*; Princeton University Press, 1951.

Graves, Robert, *The Greek Myths*; Penguin Books, 1955.

Greene, W. C., *Moira: Fate, Good, and Evil in Greek Thought*; Harvard University Press, 1944.

Haigh, A. E., *The Attic Theater*; 3d ed. by A. W. Pickard-Cambridge, 1907.

————, *The Tragic Drama of the Greeks*; 1896 (reprinted 1925).

Harsh, P. W., *A Handbook of Classical Drama*; Stanford University Press, 1944.

Harvey, Sir Paul, *Oxford Companion to Classical Literature*; 1937.

Havelock, E. A., *The Crucifixion of Intellectual Man*; Beacon Press, 1950.

Highet, Gilbert, *The Classical Tradition*; Oxford University Press, 1949.

418 · Bibliography

Howald, E., *Die griechische Tragoedie*; Munich, 1930.

Jaeger, W., *Paideia*; English translation by Gilbert Highet: chapters on Aeschylus, Sophocles, Euripides; Oxford University Press, 1939.

Kitto, H. D. F., *Greek Tragedy, A Literary Study*; London, Methuen, 1939; Anchor Books A 38, paper-bound.

Kranz, Stasimon, *Untersuchungen zu Form und Gehalt der griechischen Tragoedie*; Berlin, Weidmann, 1933.

Lesky, A., *Die griechische Tragoedie*; Leipzig, A. Kröner, 1938.

Little, Alan M. G., *Myth and Society in Attic Drama*; Columbia University Press, 1942; see my review in *Journal of American Folk Lore* 56 (1943), 309–310.

Murray, G., *A History of Ancient Greek Literature*, chapters 9, 10, 11, 12; New York, D. Appleton, 1897.

Nestle, W., *Die Struktur des Eingangs in der attischen Tragoedie*; Stuttgart, 1930.

Nicoll, Allardyce, *The Development of the Theater*; 1929.

Nietzsche, F., *The Birth of Tragedy*; 1872.

Norwood, Gilbert, *Greek Tragedy*; 2d. ed., London, Methuen, 1928.

Parker, W. R., *Milton's Debt to Greek Tragedy in Samson Agonistes*; Johns Hopkins Press, 1937; see my review in *Classical Philology* 34 (1939), 178–179.

Pickard-Cambridge, A. W., *Dithyramb, Tragedy, and Comedy*; Oxford University Press, 1927.

———, *The Theater of Dionysus*; new ed., Oxford University Press, 1948.

Pohlenz, M., *Die griechische Tragoedie*; Leipzig, 1930.

Rose, H. J., *A Handbook of Greek Literature*; London, Methuen, 1934.

Schadewalt, W., *Monolog und Selbstgespraeche; Untersuchungen zur Formgeschichte der griechischer Tragoedie*; Berlin, 1926.

Schmid, Wilhelm, *Geschichte der griechischen Literatur*; Muller Handbuch VII, 1, 2; Munich, Oskar Beck, 1934, pp. 1–523; Schmid-Stählin, VII, 1, 1, 1929, pp. 629–659.

Sheppard, J. T., *Greek Tragedy*; Cambridge University Press, 1911.

———, *Aeschylus and Sophocles*; New York, Longmans, Green, 1927.

Shipley, J. T., editor, *Dictionary of World Literature*; New York, Philosophical Library, 1943; see my articles on Greek theater, Roman theater, eccyclema, cyclic chorus, cothurnus, coryphaeus, satyr play, proscenium, anagnorisis, and choregus.

Thomson, George, edition of Aeschylus, *Oresteia*; Cambridge University Press, 1938, 2 vols.; see my review in *The Classical Journal* 36 (1941), 366–368.

———, *Aeschylus and Athens*; London, 1941.

——, *Studies in Ancient Greek Society*; London, Lawrence and Wishart, 1949.

——, "The Social Origins of Greek Tragedy," *The Modern Quarterly* 1 (1938), 233–264.

Thomson, J. A. K., *Irony*; Harvard University Press, 1927.

Webster, T. B. L., *Introduction to Sophocles*; Oxford University Press, 1936.

Whitman, C. H., *Sophocles: a Study of Heroic Humanism*; Harvard University Press, 1951.

Wilamowitz-Moellendorf, Ulrich von, *Einleitung in die griechischen Tragoedie*, 3d reprint from 1st ed. (1889) of Euripides' *Heracles*, Chapters 1–4 (1921), 43–103, "Was ist eine attische Tragoedie?"

Wilhelm, A., *Urkunden dramatischer Auffuehrungen in Athen*; Vienna, 1906.

Wright, W. C., *A Short History of Greek Literature*, chapters 12, 13, 14; New York, American Book Co., 1907.

Ziegler, Kurt, article "Tragoedie" in Pauly-Wissowa, *Realenzyklopaedie*, II Reihe, Band VII (1936), columns 1899–2075.